Essential Paediatrics in Primary Care

W0230578

Essential Paediatrics in Primary Care covers the breadth of paediatric practice, written with the frontline experience of the challenges and dilemmas faced in diagnosing and treating children in primary care in mind. The practical text continues to offer clear, evidence-based guidance about managing children in primary care, including when referral to hospital is appropriate, and has been fully revised and updated in this second edition. The concise, list-based format facilitates a confident and knowledgeable diagnosis to be reached in the short time available in general practice.

This book is invaluable for general practitioners and GP trainees wanting to keep abreast of recent progress in paediatric care and in preparation for Membership of the Royal College of General Practitioners (MRCGP) and similar qualifying specialist examinations and is an ideal aide-mémoire for nurse practitioners and health visitors and a useful guide for medical students and junior doctors considering a career in general practice.

Essential Paediatrics in Primary Care

Second Edition

A SAHIB EL-RADHI
MRCPCH, DCH, PhD
Consultant Paediatrician and Honorary Senior Lecturer
BMI Chelsfield Park Hospital
Orpington, UK

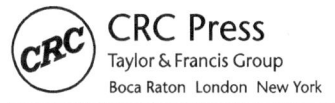

CRC Press
Taylor & Francis Group
Boca Raton London New York

CRC Press is an imprint of the
Taylor & Francis Group, an **informa** business

Second edition published 2026
by CRC Press
2385 NW Executive Center Drive, Suite 320, Boca Raton, FL 33431

and by CRC Press
4 Park Square, Milton Park, Abingdon, Oxon, OX14 4RN

CRC Press is an imprint of Taylor & Francis Group, LLC

© 2026 A Sahib El-Radhi

First edition published in 2013

ISBN: 978-1-032-64287-1 (hbk)
ISBN: 978-1-032-60906-5 (pbk)
ISBN: 978-1-032-64288-8 (ebk)

DOI: 10.1201/9781032642888

Typeset in Minion Pro
by Apex CoVantage, LLC

Contents

Foreword

In the 12 years or so that has passed since the publication of the first edition of this book, we might perhaps ask whether the generalist care of children in the UK has changed very much. This group of patients remains a large proportion of the day-to-day work of primary care teams, and probably a greater element of GPs work as members of those teams.

Workload pressures on primary care teams have increased without doubt, and the size of these teams has increased in themselves. The latter is no doubt a good thing as part of expert generalist care, though the advantages that might accrue to child health care have yet to be clearly evaluated. Clearly unchanged are the key descriptors of primary care that apply to children as all other patients: first access, continuity, family context and all the rest.

This is all against the backdrop of enormous high level structural change in how the NHS in England is organised, most of which has had minimal advantage to child health, if any. Such change is less evident in Scotland, Wales and Northern Ireland. We should also remind ourselves that the preservation of generalist child health care is an important and valuable function within UK general practice, and something not seen necessarily in other countries.

The core content of learning about paediatric generalist care, or what can be described as essential in the words of the title of this book, does change over time, and this is reflected in the new edition. The accessible style remains; readers can go straight to a subject of their choice and find key information and guidance at a glance. The text is still in 18 content areas which are easy to navigate. What has been tweaked is some of the details – for example in allergy, transgender and autism/ADHD – where care is emergent and usually challenging for specialists and generalists alike. Red flag issues remain highlighted, illustrating the key primary care role in the identification of serious or acute children's disease, where improvement can always be made.

Content matches for the most part the curricular objectives for the Royal College of General Practitioners examinations and assessments which will be a relief for GP Registrars, though also of benefit to established GPs using this text for their continuing professional development.

In the end, the responsibility of primary care teams, as well as specialist paediatricians, is to help children realise their potential by the various means at their disposal: prevention, diagnosis and treatment *inter alia*, and the information contained in this revised account will certainly help them to do that.

John Spicer FHEA MBBS MA FRCGP
GP, Croydon
Tutor in Clinical Ethics and Law
Queen Mary and City
St George's, University of London
UK

Preface

Since the publication of the first edition of this book in 2013, remarkable progress has been made in paediatric health. The scientific progress achieved in the past 11 years, on the one hand, and the lack of books specific to paediatrics in general practice, on the other, provided the impetus to write this new edition.

The second edition of *Essential Paediatrics in Primary Care* constitutes a major revision of the paediatric practice based on a complete review of the previous edition, in addition to the progress on paediatric health issues made in recent years. The book aims to provide primary health practitioners (PCPs) and other healthcare professionals with relevant and up-to-date information.

The book is written primarily for PCP and GP trainees. However, the hope is that nurse practitioners, health visitors, medical students and other health professionals who deal with health issues of children will also find the book useful.

The book is written by a long-experienced paediatrician, who worked for many years in several European and Middle Eastern countries.

There is a huge and increasing amount of information available on the internet, which has meant that parents and carers of children are nowadays better informed. However, this information is of variable quality and often difficult to use when a case presents at a GP practice. As for the professional side, although guidelines, meta-analysis and the outcomes of many randomized controlled trials (RCTs) have also been available and easily accessible online during the past two to three decades, PCPs are usually very busy, and often have little time to utilize this information. In addition, the information is often not concise, practice-based or easy to execute in practice. Rigorous efforts have been made to collect evidence-based information which is only relevant to the GP practice. The hope is that this new edition will provide a stimulus and a guide that can influence the practice of PCP colleagues.

The book is structured in 18 clinical chapters covering almost all areas of paediatrics seen in general practice, presenting the evidence base where relevant and, where this is lacking, reaching a consensus view of the paediatric practice based on recent scientific publications and the author's own experience. Less detail is given on areas of clinical practice generally undertaken in secondary or tertiary centres. Many areas of paediatric practice in primary care are suffering from inadequate information. This book tries to address this significant knowledge gap by providing practical information on these areas.

It is not possible to cover all health problems with the same degree of detail in this book. In a continuing effort, this edition addresses the full spectrum of problems related to the health and welfare of children and youths that are faced by practitioners and other health professionals. The aim, as in the previous edition, is to be concise and reader-friendly with a short book. The information presented in this book has been carefully checked and selected to aid decisions on how to deal with a sick child.

The book can be read cover to cover but is probably best used for rapid reference. I hope that the book will be beneficial to primary care colleagues and that by applying the sound and accurate scientific information provided, children who are attending primary care will also benefit.

Acknowledgements

The author is grateful to his family for their encouragement and understanding while this book was being prepared. I wish to thank Sami El-Radhi (son of Sahib) and Gassan Ahmad (nephew of Sahib) for providing the excellent drawings in this book. I express appreciation and thanks to the Childhood Eye Cancer Trust (www.chect.org.uk) which very kindly supplied four images on eye cancer (Figures 1.3, 7.2, 13.3, 13.4). The Trust is helping to fight eye cancers, particularly retinoblastoma. I also wish to thank Meningitis UK (www.meningitisuk.org) for providing the images showing a meningococcal rash (Figures 4.4, 4.5). This national charity's aim is to raise awareness and fund research to eradicate all forms of meningitis and associated diseases, particularly through vaccination. I also thank the British Thoracic Society for kindly granting permission to reproduce the summaries of asthma management as shown in Figure 9.2. Finally, I acknowledge the kind permission of Richard Ashton and Barbara Leppard to reproduce the following images from *Differential Diagnosis in Dermatology*, Third Edition (Radcliffe Publishing, 2005): Figures 1.5, 4.2, 4.3, 4.7, 4.8, 6.1, 17.1–17.11, 17.13 and 17.14.

CHAPTER 1

Newborn

NEONATAL HEALTH PROMOTION (See Table 1.1)

TABLE 1.1 Health promotion offered to children up to 4 months of age

When	Intervention
Antenatal	Provide advice and support on:
	• Perinatal mental health and psychological wellbeing for parents. The mental health should be enhanced through information, education and communication activities. Various novel interventions (e.g., internet and mobile-based interventions) have proven effective for mental health promotion.
	• Strategies that focus on increasing breastfeeding rate, providing vaccination.
	• General health and wellbeing, including engaging in physical activity; healthy eating; cessation of smoking, consuming alcohol or misusing illegal substances.
	• Maternal vaccination up to date with inactivated influenza and pertussis.
	• Prevention of obesity (body mass index [BMI] >30 kg/m^2) as the main driver for metabolic dysfunction in pregnancy, e.g., gestational diabetes and type 2 diabetes.
	• Healthy weight gain during pregnancy of 11.5–16 kg for women of normal weight and BMI 18.5–24.9.
	• Daily intake of 400 micrograms of folic acid until 12 weeks pregnancy.*
Baby after birth Day 5 of life	• Immediate and continuous kangaroo mother care of skin-to-skin.
	• General examination with particular emphasis on eyes, heart and hips.
	• Vitamin K administration.
	• Advice on ways to prevent sudden infant death syndrome (SIDS), including safe sleep arrangement.
	• Neonatal hearing screening.
	• Sharing information to ensure a smooth transition from the midwifery to health visiting service.
	• Neonatal blood spot screening (heel prick) See Box 1.1.
Mother postnatal	• Mental health problems, particularly depression and anxiety, in this period is very common, affecting up to 20% of women and causing morbidities and mortality. About 8% of fathers also experience some mental problems.
6–8 weeks	• Second baby check at GP surgery. It is useful for both parents to be present.
8 weeks	• Vaccination. See Table 1.2.

* A dose of 5 mg is recommended if the pregnant woman has a high risk of neural tube defects (NTDs), e.g., family history of NTD, being diabetic, or taking antiepileptic or retroviral drugs.

DOI: 10.1201/9781032642888-1

TABLE 1.2 Routine recommended immunization schedule

During pregnancy	Pertussis, inactivated seasonal flu vaccine, tetanus, up to date hepatitis B if at risk of acquiring hepatitis B in pregnancy (Live vaccines, e.g., BCG, oral polio, are not recommended)	
8 weeks	DTaP/IPV/Hib/HepB	Thigh
	MenB	
	Rotavirus (oral drops)	
12 weeks	DTaP/IPV/Hib/HepB	Thigh
	PCV	
	Rotavirus (oral drops)	
16 weeks	DTaP/IPV/Hib, HepB	Thigh
	MenB	
1 year (on or after child's first birthday)	Hib and MenC	Upper arm/thigh
	PCV	
	MMR	
3 years 4 months old (or soon after)	DTaP/IPV	Upper arm
12–13 years (boys and girls)	HPV 2 doses 6–24 months apart	Upper arm
14 years	TD/IPV	Upper arm
Children eligible each year	Attenuated Influenza virus vaccine	Both nostrils

DTaP = diphtheria, tetanus and pertussis; IPV = polio virus; Hib = Haemophilus influenza type B; PCV = pneumo-coccal conjugate vaccine; MenB = meningococcal group B; MenC = meningococcal group C; MMR = measles, mumps, rubella; HPV = human papillomavirus; TD = tetanus and diphtheria.

BOX 1.1 Newborn screening

Neonatal screening tests
- For each screening programme, there must be a clear pathway of referral to secondary and, if necessary, tertiary specialists.
- Physical examination, within 72 hours and again at 6–8 hours, to include screening for congenital dislocation of the hips (CDH), should be performed as soon as possible after birth and a further examination at 6–8 weeks (see next section).
- Physical examination, including screening for CDH, should be performed as soon as possible after birth and a further examination at 6–8 weeks (see next section).
- Growth monitoring, including length if indicated. Nine-centile charts should be used.
- Hearing screening. Currently selective or high-risk screening, rather than universal screening, is used. The distraction test at 6–8 months can only produce good results if training and monitoring are of a high standard.
- Universal newborn eye screening (UNES), using red reflex testing, is the standard of care for early identification of congenital cataract.

- Newborn blood spot—Performed on day 5 to screen for rare but serious paediatric diseases, including:
  - ❯ Sickle cell anaemia (SCA)
  - ❯ Cystic fibrosis (CF)
  - ❯ Congenital hypothyroidism
  - ❯ Severe combined immunodeficiency (SCID)
  - ❯ Metabolic diseases (phenylketonuria, maple syrup urine disease, isovaleric acidaemia, glutaric aciduria, homocystinuria)

NEONATAL EXAMINATION (THE BABY CHECK)

Paediatricians or midwives routinely perform neonatal examination 24–72 hours after birth. This period will allow time for the neonate to adapt physiologically from fetal to neonatal life. GPs routinely perform neonatal examination at 6–8 weeks. The examination has the aim to:

➤ Detect congenital abnormalities which may be present in 3–5% of infants. These should be explained to parents and recorded.
➤ Establish a baseline for subsequent examinations.
➤ Ensure there are no signs of infection or metabolic disease.
➤ Perform measurements of weight and head circumference (HC) and plot them on a centile chart. A newborn's weight may decrease 10% below birthweight in the first week but should regain or exceed birthweight by 14 days of life. They should grow at approximately 25–30 gram/day during the first 3 months.

Neonatal examination should include the following areas:

➤ Reviewing **family history**, including maternal diseases (e.g., gestational diabetes), pregnancy issues, sexually transmitted diseases, medications (Box 1.2) and intake of alcohol, tobacco smoke and illegal drugs.

BOX 1.2 The main drugs that may have adverse effects, including teratogenicity, on the unborn baby

- *Addictive substances*: Neonatal abstinence syndrome leading to sedation and respiratory depression. *Cocaine*: Eye and skeletal defects.
- *Alcohol*: Alcohol fetal syndrome.
- *Anaesthetics and sedatives* (e.g., halothane): Alteration of DNA synthesis in vitro.
- *Anticoagulants* (e.g., warfarin): Embryopathy with growth restriction, skeletal and CNS abnormalities.
- *Anticonvulsants* (e.g., phenytoin): Fetal hydantoin syndrome.

- *Analgesics* (e.g., aspirin): Skeletal and hearing defects, cleft lip and palate and hypospadias.
- *Antibiotics* (e.g., aminoglycosides): Eighth cranial nerve toxicity; tetracyclines: Dental discoloration, enamel hypoplasia.
- *Cytotoxic drugs* (e.g., methotrexate): Craniofacial anomalies.
- *Oestrogens*: Masculinization of the female fetus. *Androgens*: Hirsutism and virilization.
- *Psychotherapeutics* (e.g., lithium): Defect of the heart valve (Epstein's anomaly).
- *Tobacco smoking*: A harmful effect on fetal development and cognitive impairment. Both carbon monoxide and nicotine restrict the utero-placental blood flow, causing hypoxia to fetal tissue.

➤ **General examination.** Much information can be gained by simple observation without disturbing the child. Is the general appearance normal? Are they well nourished? Are there any dysmorphic features?

➤ **Skin**
  - ➤ Colour: This is usually red to pink, but varies greatly, depending on the baby's age, race, temperature and whether the baby is unsettled.
  - ➤ Peripheral cyanosis (or acrocyanosis) is a common physiological finding in the first few days of life caused by peripheral circulatory instability. The cyanosis is limited to the extremities.
  - ➤ Mottling (cutis marmorata) is usually a temporary condition, often due to cold. It occurs when the blood flow to tiny vessels under the skin is disrupted resulting in a fine, bluish-red, lace-like pattern.
  - ➤ Capillary haemangioma (see 'Birthmarks' later)

➤ **Skull (Figure 1.1)**
  - ➤ Palpation of the suture lines and the size and tension of the anterior fontanelle. Great variation in the size of the fontanelle exists. In general, a small fontanelle enlarges during the first few months of life, while a large one gradually becomes smaller. A large fontanelle should not cause any concerns as long as the HC is normal and it is not tense or bulging. A persistently large fontanelle may be associated with macrocephaly, hypothyroidism or hydrocephalus. A persistently small fontanelle may suggest microcephaly, cranial synostosis or chromosomal abnormalities.
  - ➤ Measuring the HC around the largest occipital-frontal diameter across the forehead is a significant health indicator and represents brain growth in utero, normally 33–37 cm. If the HC measures above or below the normal for age, the parents' HC should be measured. Macrocephaly is the most common cause of a larger-than-average head, usually inherited from the father.

➤ **Face**
  - ➤ Are there any dysmorphic features?
  - ➤ Petechiae. These are common and do not blanch with pressure.
  - ➤ Both nares should be patent.
  - ➤ Milia on the nose are a common finding.
  - ➤ Snuffles are inspiratory noises which are common and should disappear by the age of 3–6 months.

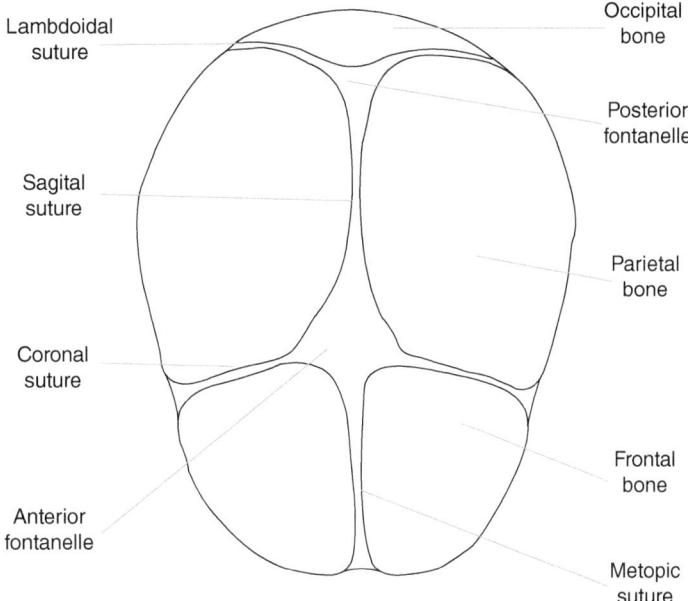

FIGURE 1.1 Skull showing the patent sutures and the two fontanelles.

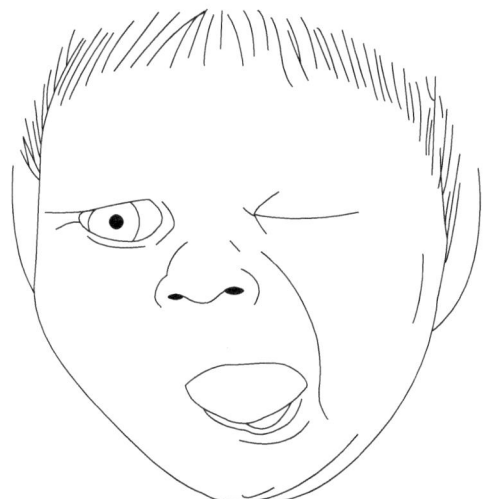

FIGURE 1.2 Right-sided facial nerve palsy. When the infant cries, there is movement only on the non-paralyzed side of the face, the eye cannot be closed and the nasolabial fold is absent.

➢ Mouth for possible precocious dentition (incidence 1:2000) and for complete or submucosal cleft palate (likely if the arch is excessively high or the uvula is bifid).

➢ A unilateral facial palsy (7th nerve palsy) may not become apparent unless the child is crying. The weakness causes flattening and drooping of the affected nasolabial fold, which, in turn, causes an asymmetrical face (Figure 1.2).

➤ **Eye**
  ➢ Establishing that both eyes are of normal size and not microphthalmic.
  ➢ Red reflex with ophthalmoscope. Its presence suggests the absence of cataract or intraocular pathology. White pupillary reflex may suggest cataracts, chorioretinitis, tumour or retinopathy of prematurity (ROP). The presence of such a reflex or a cornea larger than 1 cm in diameter requires urgent ophthalmological referral.

RED FLAGS

- Although it is possible to separate the eyelids with the fingers, this is not recommended as this approach hurts, makes babies cry and they close their eyes even more tightly.
- Small subconjunctival scleral haemorrhage, seen frequently in newborn infants, is transient and harmless, caused by increased intravascular pressure during delivery. Parents can be reassured if it is found.

➤ **Ear**
  ➢ External structural malformation?
  ➢ Unilateral or bilateral pre-auricular skin tags. If pedunculated, they can be ligated tightly at the base by an ENT surgeon or paediatrician.
  ➢ Note that the newborn eardrums are difficult to visualize because the ear canals are often blocked with vernix and amniotic debris during the first few days of life.

➤ **Chest**
  ➢ Breast hypertrophy is common in both sexes and is caused by intrauterine hormonal stimulation. Breasts should never be manipulated, as this may cause infection and abscess. It will usually spontaneously regress.
  ➢ Supernumerary breasts and nipples are common, located along the 'milk line' from the axilla to the pubic symphysis, mostly just below and medial to the normal breast. They may appear as a tiny, pigmented macula. No treatment is required.
  ➢ The newborn respiration is normally irregular with pauses that should not exceed 10 seconds. The respiratory rate is 30–40 breaths/minute when resting.
  ➢ In heart auscultation, an absence of a heart murmur does not exclude congenital heart defects. The heart rate is normally between 120 and 160 beats/minute (see the section 'Congenital Heart Disease').

RED FLAGS

- A respiratory rate >60/minute over 1 hour of observation may suggest cardiopulmonary or metabolic disease.
- Grunting during expiration may signify potentially serious cardiopulmonary disease.

➤ **Abdomen**
  ➤ Before touching the child, the hands should be washed and warm. Palpate lightly first and then more deeply, using two fingers while watching the baby's face for any grimacing or wincing. Palpation must be gentle and painless.
  ➤ Any distension? Any masses?
  ➤ Umbilical hernia, which is common, particularly in children from Africa.
    ➤ Abdominal muscles can be weak, allowing a separation between the two rectus muscles (diastasis recti).
    ➤ The liver edge is usually palpable 1–2 cm below the right costal margin.
    ➤ Palpation of a femoral pulse along the inguinal ligament should elicit the pulsation.

RED FLAG
- Any inguinal hernia (IH) should be referred as soon as possible to a paediatric surgeon. In contrast to IH, umbilical hernia is usually benign and does not require a referral.

➤ **Genitalia**

In males:
  ➤ The glans penis is normally covered by foreskin. Both testes should be completely descended. About 6% of males have one or both testes undescended. If the scrotum is underdeveloped, it suggests an undescended testis. Testes are to be palpated with warm hands. If they cannot be felt, they may be retractile or undescended. Retractile testis can usually be milked down from the inguinal area into the scrotum.
  ➤ Penile length in the term newborn: *24.5–32 mm*. A micropenis has a stretched length shorter than 2.5 standard deviations (SD) below the mean, or about *<22.3 mm*.
  ➤ The orifice of the urethra should be identified and any hypospadias excluded.
  ➤ IH occurs in 1–4% in full-term babies and in up to 30% of low birthweight. *A referral to paediatric surgery prior to hospital discharge is recommended.*

In females:
  ➤ A large labia majora covers and occludes the labia minora and vaginal introitus.
  ➤ Vaginal discharge is frequent and appears on the second or third day of life, sometimes with bleeding (neonatal uterine bleeding), which occurs in about 5% of newborns, and is caused by withdrawal of the maternal hormone. It usually resolves spontaneously.

PRACTICE POINTS
- The foreskin is physiologically adhered to the glans and should not be retracted.
- Palpation of the testes with cold hands may stimulate the cremasteric reflex, causing them to retract to the top of the scrotum and even into the inguinal canals. A misdiagnosis of undescended testis should not be made.

- If testes are not descended at the 6- to 8-week examination, a review is arranged at 1 year of age. If still undescended, the child should be referred to a paediatric surgeon.
- Enlargement of the clitoris is common but must be differentiated from congenital adrenal hyperplasia (CAH). In CAH, the enlargement is marked, resembling a penis, with varying degrees of labial fusion. As the urethra opens below this clitoris, a mistaken diagnosis of hypospadias and cryptorchidism may be made.
  - Transillumination is useful to distinguish a hydrocele from a hernia.

➤ **Extremities**
  ➤ Most newborns have mild bowing of the legs. This often becomes more pronounced when they are toddlers.
  ➤ Often there is a transient positional deformity of the feet caused by the intra-uterine position. If the anomaly can be corrected completely by hand pressure, it is not pathological. A fixed structural deformity such as clubfoot should be referred for further evaluation.
  ➤ The fingers and toes should be checked for number and evidence of in-curving (clinodactyly). Palmar creases should be noted: Single and unilateral palmar crease is a common finding. Clinodactyly and bilateral palmar creases may be associated with chromosomal abnormalities.
  ➤ Partial syndactyly (webbed toes) between the second and third toes is a common minor congenital anomaly, which does not require any surgical repair.
➤ **Back**: Many babies have a pilonidal dimple at the lower end of the back and the top of the cleft. The dimple usually has no significance and will disappear.
  Referral is indicated:
  ➤ If the size is >5 mm and situated >25 mm from the anus.
  ➤ In rare instances when the bottom to the dimple is invisible despite stretching. A referral should be initiated to ensure that the tract is not connected with the spinal cord.
  ➤ If tufts of hair are present over the lumbosacral spine, these suggest an underlying abnormality, e.g., spina bifida occulta, sinus tract or tumour.
➤ **Hip examination**: Check the hip for congenital dislocation (Box 1.3, Figure 1.3).

BOX 1.3 Neonatal hip examination

- Ortolani manoeuvre: The hip is abducted and upward pressure is applied by the finger on the greater trochanter. A dislocated hip will clunk back into the acetabulum.
- Barlow manoeuvre for dislocation: The femoral head is gently pushed out of the acetabulum with a clunk.

- Babies with risk factors (breech presentation, family history of hip dislocation or foot deformity) require ultrasound examination within the first 6 weeks.
- Limited hip abduction is a serious sign and suggests that the hip is dislocated.
- Clicks due to ligaments and asymmetrical skin creases of the thighs are found in many normal babies and are not significant.

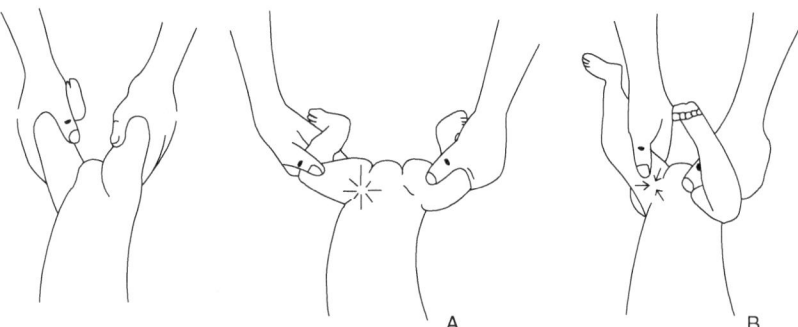

FIGURE 1.3 Hip dislocation tests.

A: The Barlow test is the most important test, aimed at dislocating an unstable hip from the acetabulum. This is performed by applying the index and middle finger along the greater trochanter with the thumb on the inner thigh. Then gently adduct the hip and apply pressure posteriorly. The manoeuvre is positive if a 'clunk' or 'jerk' is felt.

B: The Ortolani test aims at reducing a recently dislocated hip. With the fingers in the same position as noted earlier, gently abduct the hip while lifting the leg anteriorly.

NEUROLOGICAL EXAMINATION

The neurological examination should focus on the following:

➤ Are there any dysmorphic features?
➤ The level of alertness, irritability and spontaneous movements. Reduced movements can suggest weakness.
➤ The quality of the baby's cry: Normal, weak, high-pitched?
➤ Posture and movement of the four extremities. Do they move equally and maintain a normal posture of flexion?
➤ The anterior fontanelle usually closes by 18 months.
➤ HC: Measure three times and take the largest diameter.
➤ Head control. In ventral suspension, the head is down below the level of the body at 0–4 weeks and in the same plane as the body at age 6–8 weeks Muscle tone: Is it normal, increased or decreased? It is assessed by repeatedly flexing and extending the baby's arms and legs.
➤ Primitive reflexes such as:
  ➢ Moro reflex elicited by holding the baby facing the examiner and then allowing the baby's head gently to drop back. The child symmetrically abducts and extends the arms and flexes the thumbs.

➤ Grasp reflex elicited by placing the finger in the palm of each hand.
➤ Asymmetric tonic neck reflex elicited by turning the baby's head to one side and noting the arm's gradual extension on the same side of the turned head and flexion of the opposite arm.
➤ Vision (6–8 weeks): Check that the baby can fixate on and follow a moving object.
➤ Hearing: Check the hearing screening results.

EVIDENCE-BASED INFANT FEEDING

Breastfeeding

➤ Breastfeeding has been described as the single most effective child survival intervention that can reduce the global burden of undernutrition.
➤ Many organizations, including the World Health Organization (WHO), recommend exclusive breastfeeding for the first 6 months of life, with further continuation until the age of 2 years and beyond.
➤ Breastfeeding increases the number of beneficial bacteria, such as *Bifidobacteria*, *Lactobacillus*, and *Clostridium*, in the infant's gut. The composition of gut microbiota can influence the neuronal development, immune system and homeostasis in infants. On the other hand, disorder in the maternal microbiota has been linked with premature rupture of membranes, premature delivery, intrauterine growth restriction and stillbirth.
➤ Oxytocin, a hormone produced in the hypothalamus, is released into the circulation during breastfeeding, promoting milk ejection and inducing powerful antistress effects in addition to decreasing blood pressure and cortisol levels. It also stimulates digestive and metabolic processes. Breast milk can be seen as a potential probiotic.
➤ There are other benefits to breastfed infants, including lower risk of obesity, infections, eczema, leukaemia and sudden unexpected death in infants (SUDI). Benefits to mothers include greater postpartum weight loss and lower rate of diseases, e.g., type 2 diabetes, hypertension, hyperlipidaemia and ovarian and breast cancer.
➤ Promotion of this natural feeding should be initiated prenatally by GPs, obstetricians, midwives and obstetric nurses. Women make decisions about breastfeeding early in pregnancy, sometimes even before they become pregnant.
➤ Healthcare providers must provide support and encouragement for lactation, including provision of educational literature available on the benefits of breastfeeding. Family members and the wider community can play a major supportive role. The global Baby Friendly Hospital Initiative (BFHI, or Baby Friendly Initiative) offers ten steps to successful lactation.
➤ Tongue tie (ankyloglossia) and breastfeeding: There has been a huge increase in the number of infants diagnosed and treated for ankyloglossia. It is possible that the recommended frenotomy may decrease maternal pain during lactation, but there is currently no clear evidence that a lingual procedure leads to a longer duration of breastfeeding.

Formula Feeding

Although breastfeeding is considered superior to formula feeding, many infants receive and thrive well on formula from birth, although this is often not the case if they live in poor countries. In 2018, the WHO revised the BFHI to ensure all mothers were supported to make a fully informed decision about formula feeding.

Studies have shown:

➤ Formula-fed infants are at higher risk for rapid or excessive weight gain compared with breastfed infants, leading later to obesity and metabolic dysfunction. This is caused by a variety of factors, including nutrient composition and the way the formula is prepared and provided to infants.
➤ Infants fed on formula have a decreased number of *Bifidobacteria* compared to those who are breastfed. Microbiota in early life is reported to be essential for brain development and immune system.
➤ A high percentage of mothers using formula for their babies experience negative emotions because of such a decision.
➤ Necrotizing enterocolitis (NEC) is a common and devastating gastrointestinal emergency in premature neonates, causing a mortality rate of 15–30%. Apart from prematurity, a major risk factor for NEC is formula feeding.

COMMON NEONATAL PROBLEMS

Birthmarks

➤ **Milia** are multiple pearly white or pale yellow papules or cysts which are scattered on the face, especially on the nose. They disappear within a few weeks of life. No treatment is required.
➤ **Salmon patch** is by far the most common vascular lesion in neonates and is a midline or symmetrical pink macule over one or both eyelids.
➤ **Blue spots (formerly known as Mongolian spots)** are present at birth in >80% of black and Asian children and in 5–10% of white infants. They may be solitary over the sacral area but can be multiple over the legs and shoulders. Blue spots should not be confused with bruises.
➤ **Erythema toxicum neonatorum** is seen in about half of healthy newborns and is often mistaken for staphylococcal pustules. The well-appearing child and the asymptomatic rash exclude any infection.
➤ **Café-au-lait spots**. Single or a couple of lesions of café-au-lait spots 1–3 cm in length occur in about 20% of all healthy children. Café-au-lait spots are the whole marks of neurofibromatosis and are diagnosed by six or more spots over 0.5 cm in diameter in prepubertal individuals and 1.5 cm in diameter (patch) in postpubertal individuals.
➤ **Infantile haemangiomas** (previously called strawberry nevi) are found in about 10% of all children. They are usually not present at birth, appear in the first few weeks of life, enlarge during early infancy, start regressing after the age of 1 year and disappear around the age of 4–6 years. Lesions greater than 5 cm in diameter may be associated with Kasabach–Merritt syndrome, which is characterized by vascular lesions (haemangioma), thrombocytopenia and chronic consumption coagulopathy as platelets are consumed and destroyed within the haemangioma. A platelet count should be checked in large lesion (see 'Dermatology').

Referral for specialized treatment for haemangioma is indicated if there is:

➤ Localization in a high-risk area: Near the eyes, throat or nose
➤ A risk of airway obstruction
➤ Rapid growth
➤ Recurrent bleeding, infection or ulceration

Umbilical problems include omphalitis, which is a superficial cellulitis of the umbilicus and/or surrounding tissues. It can progress rapidly to systemic infection with high mortality. Immediate referral to hospital is required for parenteral antibiotics. Umbilical hernia is a common finding occurring in 10–20% of infants in Western populations and in about 50% of African children. It is caused by a delay of the umbilical ring closure. The vast majority of cases resolve spontaneously. Parents should be reassured that complications are rare and closure is expected by the age of 4 years. Umbilical granuloma is a solid pedunculated mass which presents with infection and discharge and sometimes bleeding. The area should be clean and dry with application of silver nitrate.

Birth Trauma

➤ **Moulding** of the head is frequent, particularly if the head has been engaged for a long time.
➤ **Cranial caput succedaneum** consists of subcutaneous and extra-periosteal oedema of the soft tissues of the scalp with no limitation to the sutures.
➤ **Cephalohaematoma** is a subperiosteal haemorrhage which is always confined by the cranial suture. Most cephalohaematomas disappear within 2 weeks to 2 months. They require no treatment.
➤ **Intracranial haemorrhage (ICH)** is common in premature infants, particularly in those with birthweights less than 1500 g, with an incidence of 20–40%. ICH may lead to post-haemorrhagic hydrocephalus. Checking the skull sutures and measuring HC are essential each time the baby is seen in clinic.
➤ **Fracture of the clavicle** is a common injury in babies delivered with shoulder dystocia. The infant may be asymptomatic or display pseudo-paralysis on the affected side. Palpable bony crepitations and irregularity at the site of the fracture are the physical findings.
➤ **Brachial palsy**. Injury to the fifth and sixth cervical spinal nerves (Erb's palsy) causes adduction and an internally rotated arm with extension of the elbow and flexion of the wrist. Injury to the seventh and eighth cervical nerves and first thoracic spinal nerve (Klumpke's palsy) is rare and leads to weakness of the hand and absence of the grasp.

INFECTIONS

Congenital and Perinatal Infections

Infections may occur during pregnancy (congenital infections), labour and childbirth (perinatal infections) or through breastfeeding (postnatal infections). Newborns experience the highest rate of infection during the first 28 days of life (neonatal infections). These infections are caused by:

➤ Group B streptococci (GBS) are a leading contributor to adverse maternal and neonatal outcomes, causing thousands of deaths of mothers and babies. Invasive GBS infections cause sepsis, meningitis and pneumonia in the first week of life (early onset) or between 7 and 89 days of life (late onset). Classically, the congenital infections are grouped by the acronym TORCH (T = toxoplasma, O = other, R = rubella, C = cytomegalovirus, H = herpes simplex virus).
➤ Toxoplasmosis.
➤ Cytomegalovirus.
➤ Syphilis.
➤ Rubella.
➤ HIV.
➤ Parvovirus.
➤ Herpes simplex virus (HSV).
➤ Varicella-zoster virus.
➤ Hepatitis.
➤ Sepsis and meningitis.
➤ Among the viruses, most frequently responsible for congenital infections are cytomegalovirus (CMV), herpes simplex, varicella-zoster, hepatitis B and C, parvovirus, HIV and rubella.
➤ Neonatal SARS-CoV-2 infection. There is currently no clear evidence showing vertical transmission. Most infants of infected mothers are asymptomatic, with some showing a low degree of fever, signs of an upper respiratory tract infection and, rarely, pneumonia.

Symptoms and signs of congenital and perinatal infections are shown in Box 1.4.

BOX 1.4 Symptoms and signs of congenital and perinatal infections

- Subtle, non-specific, pale, unwell-looking
- Skin: Petechiae
- General symptoms: Poor feeding, vomiting, abdominal distension, lethargy, temperature instability, IUGR*
- Eyes: Chorioretinitis
- Ears: Defects with hearing loss
- Dental defects
- Heart: Patent ductus arteriosus, pulmonary artery stenosis
- Pulmonary: Respiratory distress with tachypnoea, congenital pneumonia
- Hepatosplenomegaly
- Neurological: Microcephaly, seizures

* IUGR = intrauterine growth restriction.

Common Postnatal Infections

Eye Infection (Ophthalmia Neonatorum)

This is a common finding, and most eye discharges are benign. Ophthalmia neonatorum is a form of conjunctivitis occurring within the first month of life. The main differential diagnosis includes:

➤ **Viral conjunctivitis** (e.g., HSV and adenoviruses). The onset is acute, unilateral or bilateral with serosanguinous discharge. The condition is usually benign and self-limiting except HSV, which typically occurs 1–2 weeks after birth in association with skin vesicles and may cause keratitis, cataracts and retinopathy.

➤ **Chlamydia** is the most common cause of ophthalmia neonatorum in the UK. The infection usually occurs 5–14 days after birth with a minimal or severe purulent discharge and swelling of the eyelids.

➤ **Gonococcal infection** presents in the first few days of life with a rapidly progressive, profuse, purulent discharge with lid oedema and corneal involvement. The infection is mainly transmitted from the mother's birth canal during delivery. Urgent treatment with systemic antibiotics is needed.

➤ These infections need to be differentiated from the far more common **obstruction of the nasolacrimal duct**, which affects up to 20% of neonates. The obstruction resolves spontaneously in over 95% of cases over the next few months. Some children need frequent reviews, lacrimal sac massage and topical antibiotics. The diagnosis is made by:

    ➤ The history of initial watery discharge, which is sticky and crusty.

    ➤ Refluxing discharge when pressure is applied over the lacrimal sac.

    ➤ The eye is not red and the child is otherwise well.

Red Flags/Consider Referral to Eye Specialist If:

- The discharge is thick and/or purulent and/or rapid, suggestive of bacterial infection (chlamydia, gonorrhoea, staphylococcal).
- If HSV conjunctivitis is suspected, topical steroids should not be applied.
- Both eyes are infected without prior history of a watery eye.
- Gonorrhoeal/chlamydia eye infections are caused by sexually transmitted diseases (STDs).
- The eye infection is causing the child to be unwell or distressed.
- Gonorrhoea/chlamydia are maternal sexually transmitted diseases (STDs). Mothers may be asymptomatic.
- The child is unwell or distressed.
- The inflammation affects the bulbar conjunctive (over the sclera).
- Persistent signs of nasolacrimal blockage for months.
- If Signs of nasolacrimal blockage do not resolve by 1 year of age; *referral for consideration of probing is required.*

RESPIRATORY DISEASES

➤ **Respiratory distress syndrome (RDS).** The primary cause is inadequate surfactant leading to diffuse alveolar atelectasis, oedema and cell injury. Risk factors for developing RDS are mainly prematurity and, to a lesser extent, maternal diabetes and maternal infections. Clinical signs include tachypnoea >60 breaths/minute, subcostal retractions, grunting, nasal flaring and cyanosis.

➤ **Meconium aspiration**. The passage of meconium-stained amniotic fluid (MSAF) occurs in up to 20% of all pregnancies because of intrauterine hypoxia, amniotic infection or pregnancies beyond 42 weeks' gestation. Meconium aspiration syndrome (MAS) is a respiratory distress in neonates (mainly term or post-term babies) born after aspiration of MSAF. Only a small percentage (up to 12%) born with MSAF develop MAS.

➤ **Transient tachypnoea of the newborn (TTN)**. This is a mild and self-limited respiratory distress characterized by (in contrast to RDS):

➣ Tachypnoea, usually without subcostal recession.
➣ Babies with TTN are usually born at term.
➣ More common in babies born by caesarean section.

PRACTICE POINTS

- *Referral of babies with RDS is required.*
- If symptoms and signs of TTN are mild, the baby may be kept at home under observation, provided the condition is stable and improving, the baby is feeding well and there are no parental concerns.

METABOLIC DISEASES

Many metabolic disorders are currently screened at birth (see Table 1.3), including phenylketonuria and congenital aciduria and galactosemia. Most metabolic disorders occur because of missing digestive enzymes that are needed to break down food. Before the screening programme, babies with metabolic disorders presented with lethargy, poor feeding, vomiting and seizures. Other metabolic disorders include:

➤ **Hypoglycaemia** is defined as a blood glucose level <1.7 mmol/L. A level <2.3 mmol/L should be a cause for further evaluation. Prematurity, intrauterine growth restriction, asphyxia and infection are the main causes. The main symptoms include lethargy, jitteriness, apnoea, seizures and poor feeding. Many infants are asymptomatic.

➤ **Hypocalcaemia** is defined as a calcium level <7mg/dL (<1.9 mmol/L). Causes of early hypocalcaemia (during the first 3 days) include prematurity, diabetic mothers and birth asphyxia. Late-onset hypocalcaemia usually presents at the end of the first week of life and is caused by hypoparathyroidism, magnesium or vitamin D deficiency, among others. Symptoms are similar to those of hypoglycaemia.

CONGENITAL HEART DISEASE

The birth prevalence of congenital heart disease (CHD) is around 1%. It is the most serious and most commonly occurring birth defect accounting for about 50% of all major birth defects. The aetiology can be identified in 20–30% of cases and is divided between genetic (10–15%) and environmental causes (85–90%) such as maternal diseases (obesity, diabetes, hypertension, smoking during pregnancy and prenatal exposures to drugs). The most common presentations of CHD are:

➤ Murmur detected incidentally at a routine baby check.
➤ Respiratory distress which mostly manifests as tachypnoea.
➤ Poor feeding leading to an underweight baby.
➤ Cyanosis appearing on the lips and face during feeding.

Diagnostic clues to detect CHD in young infants are listed in Box 1.5.

BOX 1.5 Diagnostic clues to CHD

- Normal findings in a neonate do not guarantee that serious CHD does not exist. On the other hand, the presence of an innocent murmur is common, occurring in at least 50% of children. A common problem in heart auscultation is the difficulty in distinguishing innocent from pathological murmurs (see Chapter 10 Cardiology).
- It is best practice to check the femoral and dorsalis pedis pulses as part of a clinical examination. However, they are often not easily detectable and may occasionally be palpable even in the presence of coarctation.
- In a baby who tires rapidly and sweats during feeding, CHD must be excluded.
- In an infant with respiratory distress, a ventral septal defect (VSD) could be the cause. There may be no murmur at birth, and it can appear by the age of 6 weeks.
- All children with Down's syndrome should undergo an echocardiogram. About 40% have CHD, and the signs are not always clinically detectable.
- A certain percentage of CHD (5–15%) remains undiagnosed in the perinatal period despite antennal ultrasound scans.
- Initial screening for CHD consists of a combination of cardiac auscultation, chest x-ray, pulse oximetry and echocardiography. Pulse oximetry to measure arterial oxygen saturation is an effective screening test to detect CHD.
- Artificial intelligence (AI) has made a major impact in cardiology ranging from prenatal detection of CHD, assisting in analysis of murmur and optimizing the management of patients with CHD.

Early detection of CHD is important because:

➤ Missed or delayed diagnosis of CHD can cause distress to the parents, even if the delay does not cause any harm to the baby.
➤ Preventing the occurrence of certain complications including cardiac failure and arrhythmia, pulmonary hypertension, thromboembolic events and infective endocarditis.

NEONATAL JAUNDICE

Jaundice is common in term and preterm infants during the first few days of life. Jaundice appearing on day 1 of life suggests a haemolysis. Almost every infant will have a total serum bilirubin level that is above the normal maximum adult level of 1 mg/dL = 17.1 millimoles. This physiological jaundice appears on days 2–3 of life. Jaundice appearing after 3 or 4 days of life suggests an infection, e.g., UTI or sepsis. Jaundice after the first week of life can suggest breast milk jaundice, biliary atresia, infection or metabolic disorders, e.g., galactosemia or hypothyroidism (Box 1.6). After the neonatal period, viral hepatitis remains the most common cause of jaundice worldwide. Jaundice should be differentiated from xanthochromia (carotenaemia), caused by carotene deposits in the skin.

Physiology

➤ Physiologic jaundice occurs in most neonates (60–80%) during the first few days of life. It is not a disease and is not present in the first 24 hours, and it is always an indirect hyperbilirubinemia.

➤ The jaundice is caused by increased turnover of erythrocytes and transient inability to conjugate and clear bilirubin.

➤ Breast milk jaundice (BMJ) is nothing else than physiologic jaundice, which may persist for weeks. Mothers should be encouraged to continue breastfeeding, and interrupting breastfeeding to treat BMJ is discouraged. The incidence of BMJ is 2–4% of exclusively breastfed babies during 2–3 weeks of life.

➤ There is no evidence that a well full-term baby without haemolysis will have any ill effects from a bilirubin <400 μmol. The indirect bilirubin is fat soluble and may enter through the blood–brain barrier, causing kernicterus if bilirubin rises more than 425–510 millimole (25–30 mg/dL).

➤ Direct-reacting bilirubin is water soluble, not fat soluble, and therefore does not damage the brain tissue or cause kernicterus. It is, however, associated with serious diseases, such as congenital hepatitis and biliary atresia.

BOX 1.6 Main causes of neonatal jaundice

● *Indirect hyperbilirubinemia*
  ❯ Physiological
  ❯ Haemolytic (e.g., ABO incompatibility)
  ❯ Breast milk
  ❯ Gilbert syndrome
● *Direct hyperbilirubinemia*
  ❯ Congenital hepatitis (e.g., CMV)
  ❯ Infection (sepsis)
  ❯ Intrauterine infection (e.g., toxoplasmosis, syphilis)
  ❯ Biliary atresia
  ❯ Metabolic (e.g., galactosemia)

Investigations

All babies with significant and/or prolonged jaundice may need tests to exclude pathological jaundice (Box 1.7). Guidelines when to refer cases with jaundice are shown in
Box 1.8. First-line investigations are listed in Box 1.7.

BOX 1.7 Baseline tests to establish the cause of hyperbilirubinemia

- Urine
  - Dipsticks to exclude UTI.
- FBC
  - Haemoglobin low in haemolysis; leukocytosis in infection; reticulocytosis in haemolysis.
- LFTs
  - Indirect hyperbilirubinemia suggests physiological or breast milk jaundice. Direct hyperbilirubinemia indicates hepatocellular disease, e.g., hepatitis (usually with a high transaminase level); alkaline phosphatase is raised in bile obstruction.
- PT, PTT
  - For coagulation defects.
- Coombs test
  - Positive to diagnose ABO and Rh incompatibility.
- BG and Rh status
  - To diagnose Rh and ABO incompatibility of the mother and infant.

BG = blood group; FBC = full blood count; LFTs = liver function tests; PT = prothrombin time; PTT = partial thromboplastin time.

BOX 1.8 Guidelines for referring babies with neonatal jaundice

- Clinical jaundice appearing prior to 36 hours of age.
- >300 µmol/L of total bilirubin in a breastfed term infant and >270 µmol/L in a formula-fed term infant.
- Serum bilirubin level increasing by >85 µmol/L per day.
- Direct (conjugated) bilirubin >17.1 µmol/L (= 1 mg/dL).
- Persistent jaundice after 8 days in a term infant; 14 days in premature infants.
- Any hyperbilirubinemia in an unwell or distressed child.
- Any hyperbilirubinemia with anaemia.

PRACTICE POINTS

- Transcutaneous bilirubinometry is a handheld, non-invasive device to measure serum bilirubin that has been shown to be superior to clinical assessment and reduces the need for phlebotomy. It is a useful device to have in clinical practice.
- Indirect hyperbilirubinemia with otherwise normal LFTs is suggestive of Gilbert's syndrome.
- Note that jaundice progresses from the face to the trunk and then to the legs. Therefore, the skin of the face will appear more jaundiced than that of the feet.
- An infant with yellow skin but normal white sclera usually has carotenaemia.

ANAEMIA

Erythropoiesis declines rapidly with the rise of arterial oxygen saturation (from a fetal level of 50–60% to 95% at birth) and remains low for 6–10 weeks. This causes a decline of Hb to 9–11 g/dL in full-term infants and 7–9 g/dL in premature infants. The low Hb is the best stimulus for erythropoiesis and should not be suppressed by blood transfusion unless the child is symptomatic. Anaemia is defined as an Hb level of less than 11 g/dL. The main causes of anaemia in neonates are shown in Box 1.9. Baseline tests are shown in Box 1.10.

BOX 1.9 Main causes of neonatal anaemia

- Blood loss (twin-to-twin transfusion, fetomaternal bleeding, placenta praevia, massive cephalohaematoma)
- Haemolytic anaemia
  - › ABO, Rh or minor blood group incompatibility (e.g., c, E, Kell, Duffy)
  - › Maternal disease (e.g., lupus, autoimmune haemolytic disease
  - › Red blood cell membrane defects (e.g., spherocytosis)
  - › Metabolic defects (e.g., G-6-P-D deficiency)
  - › Haemoglobinopathies
- Infection
- Physiological anaemia
- Iron deficiency anaemia (IDA)
- Red cell aplasia (Diamond–Blackfan syndrome)

BOX 1.10 Baseline tests for suspected anaemia

- FBC: Hb <11 g/dL indicates anaemia, low MCV (<70 fL) and MCH (<26 pg) suggest microcytic, hypochromic anaemia. (Remember that capillary blood samples are 2.7% ± 3.7% higher than venous haematocrits. Warming the foot reduces the difference to around 2%.)
- Reticulocyte count (elevated in haemolysis and chronic blood loss).
- Serum ferritin low in IDA, normal or high in haemolytic anaemia.
- Coombs test.
- LFTs: Hyperbilirubinaemia suggests an acute or chronic haemolysis.
- Reticulocyte count high in haemolytic anaemia and in response to iron treatment.

PRACTICE POINTS

- Anaemia of prematurity is common, is usually normocytic and normochromic and does not respond to iron therapy.
- The time of umbilical cord clamping remains controversial (Box 1.11).
- Mild anaemia is usually asymptomatic; pallor and other clinical symptoms first occur when the Hb falls below 7–8 g/dL.

- By far the most common cause of anaemia is nutritional IDA, which can be easily diagnosed by low Hb, MCV, MCH and ferritin levels. IDA is rare in neonates.
- Premature infants are often comfortable with an Hb of 6.5–7.5 mg/dL. The level itself is not an indication for transfusion unless the infant is symptomatic (e.g., tachypnoeic) or has an infection.
- An iron supplement (2 mg/kg per day as fortified formula or therapeutic iron) should be given to all premature infants for the first year of life. This prophylaxis should start after the baby is 8 weeks old to prevent late anaemia of prematurity.
- Resist the temptation of the parents to add tonics, vitamins or trace metals to iron therapy. These have no scientific value.
- Treatment with oral iron should be given to all children with Hb <11 g/dL for 4–6 weeks. Hb needs to be checked to ensure resolution of the anaemia.

BOX 1.11 Early versus late clamping of the cord

- Early cord clamping (within the first minute after birth) was advocated on the grounds that it can prevent polycythaemia (haematocrit >60%) and decrease the risk of postpartum haemorrhage.
- Delaying clamping of the cord for at least 2–3 minutes does not appear to increase the risk of postpartum haemorrhage and leads to improved iron status, particularly in infants where access to good nutrition is poor, although this increases the risk of jaundice.

(Cochrane search: Pregnancy and Childbirth Groups Trials Register, December 2007)

RED FLAGS

- Ignoring the need to investigate anaemia (even mild) is a mistake; its presence may indicate a serious underlying disorder.
- Iron preparations are an important cause of accidental overdose. Ensure that parents are keeping the medicine away from children. Parents should also be told about common side effects of iron therapy.

BLEEDING (PURPURA)

Core Messages

Purpura indicates extravasation of blood into the skin or mucosal membranes. It is due to vasculopathy, thrombocytopathy, coagulopathy or a combination of these mechanisms. It may represent a benign condition or a serious underlying disorder. Depending on their size, purpuric lesions are either petechiae (pinpoint haemorrhages <1 cm) or ecchymoses (>1 cm in diameter).

TABLE 1.3 Rapid diagnosis of common bleeding disorders using platelets, PT and PTT

	Diagnosis	Platelets	PT	PTT
Well baby	Immune thrombocytopenia	↓	N	N
	Vitamin K deficiency	N	↑	↑
	Hereditary coagulopathy (e.g., haemophilia)	N	N	↑
	Von Willebrand disease N↓	N	N*	
Unwell-appearing	Disseminated intravascular coagulopathy (DIC)	↓	↑	↑
	Infection	↓	N	N
	Liver disease	N	↑	↑

PT = prothrombin time; PTT = partial thromboplastin time.
* This inherited disease is diagnosed by the absence of von Willebrand factor (vWF) concentration.

➤ In contrast to exanthem and telangiectasia, purpura does not blanch in response to pressure. Petechiae, small superficial ecchymoses or mucosal bleeding suggest thrombocytopenia.
➤ In neonates, petechiae are commonly observed on the presenting part during delivery, particularly if the delivery was traumatic. The birth history, the location of the lesions and the absence and the absence of bleeding from other sites help in differentiating from coagulopathy and vasculitis. Baby girls may have some vaginal bleeding noted from 2 to 10 days of life.
➤ The crucial factor in diagnosing and managing an infant with bleeding is determining whether the infant is well or unwell and *requires immediate referral* (Table 1.3).
➤ A well baby is likely to have vitamin K deficiency, hereditary coagulopathy or immune thrombocytopenia, whereas a sick child is likely to have an infection (Table 1.3).

PRACTICE POINTS

- Thrombocytopenia complicates up to 10% of all pregnancies. In a neonate with petechiae, management starts by taking the mother's previous medical history for presence of immune thrombocytopenic purpura (ITP), systemic lupus erythematosus (SLE), drugs and infections during pregnancy. History is more important than extensive tests.
- The crucial factor in diagnosing and managing an infant with bleeding is determining whether they are unwell.

Vitamin K deficiency bleeding (VKDB) (previously called haemorrhagic disease of the newborn) occurs in 1 in 200–400 neonates who did not receive vitamin K prophylaxis.

➤ This is an acquired coagulopathy due to inactivation of vitamin K–dependent coagulation factors (II, VII, IX, X).
➤ Vitamin K 0.5 or 1.0 mgt IM is currently administered to all neonates during the first 24 hours of life. An oral preparation of vitamin K is available in certain instances, e.g., parents' refusal of the vitamin K injection. This is as effective as IM, provided that one dose is given on day 1, day 7 and day 30 of life.

RED FLAGS

- Of all diseases with purpura, those caused by sepsis, such as meningococcal septicaemia, are the most serious and need urgent management at the emergency department. Although invasive meningococcal disease has become uncommon due to vaccination, it still poses a threat to health of children, particularly to those with immunocompromised status, and children still die from this disease every year.
- At birth, most coagulation factors are decreased, and APTT and PT are physiologically prolonged. As petechiae and ecchymoses are common and harmless manifestations of birth trauma, therefore this harmless purpura should not be taken seriously and treated.
- Whenever there are unexplained bruises, non-accidental injury (NAI) should always be suspected. Lesions are suspicious when they are found in areas of the body not normally subjected to injury (trunk, buttocks and cheeks). Additional clues for NAI should be sought: Inflicted cigarette burns, retinal haemorrhages, intraoral injury and skeletal examination. Radiological skeletal survey may be indicated.

APPENDIX

Definitions of Terms

- Embryo   <9 weeks' gestation.
- Fetus   9 weeks' gestation to delivery.
- Miscarriage   Spontaneous loss of pregnancy <24 weeks' gestation.
- Stillbirth   Birth of baby >24 weeks' gestation with no signs of life.

  It is either an intrauterine death (IUD) or intrapartum during labour.
- Abortion   The termination of pregnancy by the removal or expulsion of a fetus or embryo from the uterus, either spontaneous or induced.
- Multiple pregnancy:
  - Monozygotic   A single ovum fertilized by a single sperm which splits (identical twins) into two embryos. About a quarter of twins are identical.
  - Dizygotic   Ovulation of two ova fertilized by two sperm (non-identical twins).
- Term   37–42 weeks
- Preterm   <37 weeks
- Postterm   >42 weeks
- Low birthweight   ≤2500 g
- Small for gestation (also known as intrauterine growth restriction [IUGR]): A birthweight <10th centile for the gestational age. Babies may be:
  - Asymmetrical   Weight on the lower centile than HC.
  - Symmetrical   Weight and HC on the same centile.
- Large for gestation   Birthweight >90th centile for gestational age.
- Perinatal mortality rate: Number of stillbirth + deaths within 7 days per 1000 deliveries.

CHAPTER 2

Growth, Development and Disability

CORE MESSAGES

➤ Growth refers to the increase in body size (weight, height and head circumference) over time (Table 2.1). Linear growth is rapid in utero and in infancy, continues at a steady rate in childhood (3–10 years), accelerates in adolescence (11–18 years) and then slows again and ceases by adulthood.

➤ Growth hormone (GH) has a minor role in fetal growth, but insulin-like growth factor-1 and -II (IGF-1 and II) are essential for fetal and postnatal growth. Cord serum concentrations of both growth factors correlate positively with birthweight.

➤ For decades, short and tall stature had been centred on the GH–IGF-1 axis, as both have been known to stimulate growth by acting on the growth plate, which is located near the ends of bones. Current knowledge indicates that normal growth depends on genes and on multiple other hormones (thyroid, androgens, oestrogen). On the other hand, glucocorticoids in excess and proinflammatory cytokines (tumour necrosis factor-alpha, interleukin [IL]-6) negatively regulate linear growth.

➤ Emotional deprivation and malnutrition early in life have a profound effect on linear growth. This is induced by a decreased circulating IGF-1.

Children need enough calories to grow and develop. The daily calorie requirements for children at different ages are shown in Table 2.2. This is about 80–120 kcal/kg during the first year of life, with subsequent decrease in calories per kg body weight except during puberty, when rapid growth requires increased caloric consumption. Energy expenditure is utilized as follows:

➤ About 12% of energy expenditure is used for daily growth.
➤ 25% is used for physical activity.
➤ 13% for thermic effect and faecal loss.
➤ The remaining 50% is used for basal metabolism.

The principal source of fluid is milk during the early years of life (Table 2.3).

GROWTH MONITORING

Although there is disagreement about the ages when these measurements are made and how often, routine measurement of weight, height and head circumference is

DOI: 10.1201/9781032642888-2

TABLE 2.1 Approximate growth increase during the first few years of life

	Weight	Length (cm)	HC
At birth (term baby)	2.7–4.6 kg	47–55	33–37 cm
0–3 months	25–30 g/day	3.5/month	2 cm/month
3–6 months	20–25 g/day	2.0/month	1 cm/month
6–12 months	12–15 g/day	1.2–1.5/month	0.5 cm/month
1–3 years	8 g/day	0.8–1.0/month	0.25 cm/month
4–6 years	6 g/day	4–5 cm/year	1 cm/year

TABLE 2.2 Calorie requirements at different ages

Age (Years)	Calories per Day	
	Boys	Girls
1–3	1230	1165
4–6	1715	1545
7–10	1970	1740
11–14	2220	1845
15–18	2755	2110
Adults	2550	1940

TABLE 2.3 Daily fluid intake requirements at different ages

Age	mL/kg/Day
0–6 months	150
7–12 months	120
1 year	120–135
2 years	115–125
4 years	100–110
10 years	70–85
14 years	50–60
18 years	40–50

widely accepted among professionals to monitor growth. Benefits of growth monitoring include:

➤ Assessing the overall nutritional status.
➤ Detecting impaired growth, which may be associated with child neglect or abuse.
➤ Detecting overweight children at an early stage.
➤ Detecting other growth disorders as an important diagnostic clue:
   ➢ Rapid growth, e.g., precocious puberty.
   ➢ Constitutional growth delay.
   ➢ Endocrine and chromosomal disorders, e.g., Turner's syndrome and growth hormone deficiency.

➤ Chronic diseases, e.g., coeliac or Crohn's disease.

➤ Syndromes, e.g., Noonan's syndrome or bone dysplasia.

Measurement of Weight

➤ Weight is a useful index to reflect the child's nutritional status.

➤ Infants should be weighed naked or with a nappy at most, subtracting the weight of the nappy afterward. Older children should be weighed with underwear on.

➤ During the first year of life, a child's weight and height may cross at least one centile line. After the age of 1 year, growth measurements in most healthy children tend to stay within the same centile until the onset of puberty unless a growth disorder intervenes.

Measurement of Height

➤ Any child older than 2 years should be measured for height in a standing position. In children younger than 2 years of age, recumbent length is significantly greater than standing height. The length measurement of full-term babies is normally 47–55 cm.

➤ Although it is doubtful about whether there is value in routinely measuring length in neonates or during the first year or two, a baseline length measurement at 6–8 weeks of age should be carried out if the infant was small for dates, failed to thrive or had dysmorphic features. The main benefit of this is to identify very short infants (length <0.4 centile) who may have skeletal or endocrine abnormalities.

➤ Early identification of short stature associated with hormonal deficiencies is important because early treatment improves outcomes for adult height.

➤ The Tanner Whitehouse six-centile growth charts are outdated because of children growing taller (known as 'secular trend'). Instead, the nine-centile growth charts should be used showing the 0.4 and the 99.6 centiles. Only 1 child in 250 lies above or below these centile lines. A child below the 0.4 centile has a significant probability of having an organic cause for short stature (nine-centile charts are available via the link: www.rcpch.ac.uk/growthcharts).

➤ Children who appear unusually short should be checked for sitting height as well. Children with achondroplasia have a normal sitting height but a markedly reduced standing height.

Measurement of Head Circumference

➤ Head circumference (HC) should be recorded carefully following birth and at 6–8 weeks of age.

➤ A large head, known as benign familial macrocephaly (BFM), is by far the most common cause of a large HC in a healthy child, often exceeding two standard deviations or more above the mean. The presence of a large head in one of the parents, usually the father, can help establish the diagnosis.

➤ Children with pathological causes of large HC, which include hydrocephalus, subdural effusion and haematoma, are usually symptomatic with features of increased intracranial pressure (ICP) such as irritability, tense fontanelle, suture separation of the skull, prominent scalp veins and a downward gaze.

➤ If HC measures slightly above or below the normal for age in the absence of symptoms or signs of ICP, two HC measurements over a 4-week period are sufficient. There is no justification for more repeated measurements because these may cause parental anxiety and are of little benefit. GPs must either decide that an enlarged HC is normal or refer the child to paediatrics.

➤ A small HC may also suggest a familial and benign small head with or without developmental delay. Other causes of small HC include premature fusion of the sutures, which is clinically diagnosed by a palpable elevated bony ridge along the length of the fused suture and an abnormal head shape depending on which sutures have closed prematurely (see Chapter 1).

GROWTH DISORDERS

Small for Gestational Age and Fetal Growth Restriction

➤ Small for gestational age (SGA) refers to infants (10–20% of births) who are born below the tenth centile for gestational age or is defined as more than two standard deviations. Early onset (<32 weeks' gestation) is a more severe form caused by chronic fetal hypoxia. It affects the weight, length and HC. Late onset (>32 weeks' gestation) is a milder and more common form of SGA (80% of cases). It affects weight only. These children usually show a rapid catch-up growth during the first year of life.

➤ Low birthweight (LBW) is defined as a birthweight of <2500 g and includes both preterm neonates with an appropriate weight for their gestational age and neonates with a small LBW for the gestational age (SGA). Infants born below the 10th centile for gestational age are also termed SGA.

➤ At least 90% of SGA infants show spontaneous catch-up growth during the first 6 months of age and usually completed within the first two years of age.

➤ Causes for LBW and SGA are often due to maternal diseases include undernutrition, maternal hypertension, diabetes and chronic infections.

➤ Fetal growth restriction (FGR, or intrauterine growth restriction) refers to inappropriate weight gain and abdominal circumference during a certain period of gestation based on two ultrasound measurements. The cause for FGR is often placental dysfunction.

FAILURE TO THRIVE

➤ The UNICEF 2013 report indicates that globally, about one in four children under the age of 5 years suffers from undernutrition, representing the most common cause of failure to thrive (FTT).

➤ Although there is no agreement about a definition of FTT, a child under the age of 5 years whose weight is <0.4th centile on the nine-centile chart or a weight loss that has crossed two centiles is considered to have FTT. WHO growth charts use cutoff values of + 2SD, which approximately correspond to the 2nd and 98th centile. All definitions indicate a caloric intake insufficient to maintain growth. Box 2.1 lists the main causes of FTT.

BOX 2.1 Main causes of FTT

Inadequate Caloric Intake	Inadequate Absorption	Increased Output
• SGA/FGR	• Coeliac disease	• Congenital heart disease
• Breastfeeding problems	• Inflammatory bowel disease	• Hyperthyroidism
• Severe gastroesophageal reflux	• Cystic fibrosis	• Infection
• Psychosocial factors (neglect, abuse)	• Parasitic infection	• Malignancy
• Eating disorder	• Malabsorption	
	• Pancreatic insufficiency	

➤ Children with FTT often have poor scores in cognitive, neurological and psycho-motor development, as well as problems with immunodeficiency and increased rate of infections.

➤ FTT is divided into two main categories: Non-organic (NOFTT) and organic (OFTT) causes. Gastrointestinal diseases, such as malabsorption, coeliac and IBD are the most common causes of OFTT. In children, in contrast to adults, psycho-social causes are far more common than organic causes (only 5–10% of cases). If the history and physical examination do not suggest a specific underlying organic disease in a child with FTT, psychosocial causes are likely, and further investigations are usually unnecessary.

Investigations

➤ Urine for microscopy and culture.

➤ Full blood count (FBC): Looking for anaemia, which is common in malnutrition and chronic infections.

➤ Inflammatory markers (C-reactive protein [CRP] or erythrocyte sedimentation rate [ESR]): High in infectious diseases and malignancy.

➤ Thyroid function test to exclude hyperthyroidism.

➤ Coeliac and pancreatic screening tests in blood.

➤ Liver function tests (LFTs), including bone profile: calcium, phosphate and alkaline phosphatase.

➤ Faecal calprotectin: Its concentrations correlate with the level of mucosal inflammation.

PRACTICE POINTS

- Primary care doctors, who work closely with the community, are in an optimal position to detect FTT in children when they attend the examination. Discussion regarding diet and lifestyle, observation of behaviour in clinic and anthropometric measurements should be documented.
- Investigations should be performed in relation to signs and symptoms of the disease. Inpatient monitoring is not advisable except in extreme circumstances or if OFTT is suspected. Guidelines for referral are shown in Box 2.2.
- In premature infants: When plotting growth parameters, the weeks of prematurity should be subtracted from the postnatal age. For example, if a child is seen at a chronological age of 15 months but was born 3 months early, the corrected age is 12 months. This correction should be done until the age of 2 years.
- SGA babies (weight less than tenth centile for gestational age) whose poor growth dated from the first trimester are symmetrically affected with low weight, height and HC. They often remain underweight for a few years and should not be categorized as FTT. Those with SGA from the third trimester are only underweight, but their height and HC are not affected. They are more likely to catch up with growth. In general, a delay in growth of length and HC occur only in severe cases of FTT.
- Neglect, either nutritional or emotional, is the most common cause of underweight infants and may account for >50% of cases with FTT.
- Children at high risk of abuse are often those with excessive crying during infancy, physical disability, chronic illness or behavioural or learning difficulties.
- Neglected children returning to their parents with no medical or social intervention may face serious reinjury (in about 25%) or death (in about 5%).
- Weight loss in adolescent girls is likely to be due to an eating disorder. The diagnosis can be difficult in the early stages. Asking about self-image and attitude (e.g., by using self-administered four simple questions) towards eating and weight can screen for 'eating disorder risk' in secondary schools.

BOX 2.2 Guidelines on when to refer a child with FTT

- Persistent parental anxiety
- Poor parent–child interaction
- Safeguarding issues
- Features that suggest an underlying illness with the need to exclude organic causes of FTT
- Malnutrition, severe growth faltering, or dehydration

TABLE 2.4 Weight definitions of healthy and overweight children

Classification	BMI (kg/m²)
Healthy weight	18.5–24.9
Overweight	25–29.9
Obesity I	30–34.9
Obesity II	35–39.9
Obesity III	40 or more

EXCESSIVE WEIGHT GAIN (OBESITY)

➤ Childhood obesity has changed from a sign of health and wealth to a disease that is one of the most serious challenges of the 21st century. The number of obese children has tripled over the past 20 years. The definition in children >2 years is provided in Table 2.4. In children up to 24 months, the diagnosis of obesity is based on the weight-to-height ratio on growth charts.

➤ Childhood obesity is linked to adult obesity (60% of prepubertal obese children become obese adults) and risk of increased mortality, cardiovascular disease, hypertension, type 2 diabetes, back pain, osteoarthritis, hyperlipidaemia, non-alcoholic fatty liver disease (NAFLD), cholelithiasis, some cancers and sleep apnoea. It reduces the life expectancy by an average of 9 years. In addition, obesity is associated with a high incidence of psychosocial problems including depression, anxiety, dysfunctional social relationships and low self-esteem.

➤ Obese children often do not eat more than their peers. Genetic factors and reduced energy output (long hours sitting in the front of TV and computer) are more important causal factors. In order to change behaviour and improve the wellbeing of children, parents need to be included in the diet and lifestyle changes.

  ➤ The gut microbiota affects energy homeostasis through immune, hormonal and neural systems and has a potential causal role in obesity.

  ➤ Obesity directly affects the immune system, which contributes to long-term obesity-associated comorbidity such as T2D.

BOX 2.3 Main causes of obesity

- Simple obesity caused by genetic and environmental factors
- Infant of diabetic mother (IDM)
- Polycystic ovary syndrome (PCOS)
- Endocrine (e.g., Cushing's, hypothyroidism, e.g., Turner and Prader–Willi syndrome)
- Drugs (e.g., steroids, pizotifen, anticonvulsants)
- Insulinoma
- Beckwith–Wiedemann syndrome
- Cerebral gigantism (Sotos syndrome)
- Laurence–Moon–Biedl syndrome (polydactyly, learning disability, retinitis pigmentosa)

BOX 2.4 Recommended investigations

● Urine:	● For microalbuminuria for children >6 years with chronic obesity
● T_4/TSH:	● Will confirm or exclude hypothyroidism.
● U&E:	● Deranged in Cushing's syndrome
● Fasting glucose:	● Normal 5.6 mmol/l or < 126 mg
● HbA1C:	● Normal: 5.7–6.4% or 39–47 mmol
● Lipids:	● Including total cholesterol, HDL, LDL and triglycerides
● Ca:	● For suspected cases of hypoparathyroidism
● S. cortisol:	● Cushing's syndrome
● Bone age:	● Normal in simple obesity, delayed in endocrine causes
● LFTs:	● To assess the liver transaminases
● Ultrasound:	● For the liver to explore the presence of NAFLD and to confirm ovarian cysts in PCOS
● CT MRI:	● For suspected cases of Cushing's disease

PRACTICE POINTS

- Obesity due to a syndrome or endocrine cause is rare. Table 2.5 shows the differential diagnosis between simple and endocrine/syndrome causes of obesity.
- A common reason for seeking medical help for child's obesity is parental concern whether the 'child's glands are causing the obesity'. Obesity usually has no 'gland' as an underlying cause.
- Body mass index (BMI) gives no indication of body fat distribution, whereas waist circumference (midway between the tenth rib and top of the iliac crest) is a marker for central body fat accumulation and is more accurate than BMI. Estimated values of waist circumference in boys and girls are provided in Table 2.6.
- Obesity is the main risk factor for hypertension. Blood pressure (BP) should be recorded in any child with obesity at each visit to the surgery. It is elevated in up to 30% of older children with long-standing simple obesity. It is also elevated in Cushing's syndrome and Turner's syndrome. Table 2.7 shows the grades of BP in children.
- Much time is wasted in the clinic by only focusing on advice about food. The child with obesity is aware of this often upset by frequently hearing that they are eating too much dietary restriction is notoriously unsuccessful in treating the condition. Box 2.5 shows evidence-based treatment of obesity.
- The main cause of childhood obesity is not overeating but genetic (usually confirmed by a detailed family history) and decreased energy output. The latter can be estimated indirectly by the total hours spent in the front of the television and computer per day.

- Prediabetes exists in about 5% of obese children. Abnormal fasting glucose and HbA1C levels with elevated levels of low-density lipoprotein (LDL) and low levels of high-density lipoprotein (HDL) are risk factors for cardiovascular disease and stroke.
- The finding of supernumerary digits with obesity raises the likelihood of Laurence–Moon–Biedl syndrome (obesity, polydactyly, retinitis pigmentosa and progressive nephropathy). An uncommon but important physical sign: When the hand is fisted, it may show short fourth and fifth knuckles – a sign seen in pseudohypoparathyroidism and in girls with Turner's syndrome.
- There has been a high prevalence of non-alcoholic fatty liver disease (NAFLD). It is assessed by checking the liver transaminases and through liver ultrasound scan.

TABLE 2.5 Differential diagnosis between simple and endocrine obesity

	Simple Obesity	Endocrine Obesity
History	Long duration	Shorter duration
Family history (obesity)	Often positive	Usually not
Height	Average or above	Short
Physical examination	Otherwise normal	Usually abnormal
Fat distribution	Diffuse	More localized (e.g., truncal)
Bone age	Normal or advanced	Delayed
Sexual development	Appropriate for age	Delayed
Striae	Pink, appear at puberty	Often violaceous, appear early

TABLE 2.6 Estimated values in centimetres of waist circumference in both sexes

Age	Boys			Girls		
	10th	50th	90th Centile	10th	50th	90th Centile
2	43.2	47.1	50.8	43.8	47.1	52.2
5	48.4	53.2	61.0	48.5	53.0	61.4
10	57.0	63.3	78.0	56.3	62.8	76.6
15	65.6	73.5	95.0	64.2	72.6	91.9

TABLE 2.7 Normal systolic (SBP) and diastolic (DBP) blood pressure grades

Blood Pressure	Values	Centiles for Gender and Age
Normal BP	SBP and DBP	<90th
Borderline normal BP	SBP and/or DBP	90–95th
Hypertension	SBP and/or DBP	>95–99th
Significant BP	SBP and/or DBP	>99th

RED FLAGS

- Early-onset obesity occurring in a child should be considered a syndrome if it is associated with:
  - Short stature
  - Delayed psychomotor development
  - Cognitive impairment
  - Cryptorchidism or hypogonadism
  - Dysmorphism
  - Ocular or auditory abnormalities
- Polycystic ovary syndrome (PCOS) should be considered in all female adolescents, particularly in association with:
  - Signs of hyperandrogenism (acne, hirsutism)
  - Ovary dysfunction with oligo-amenorrhea

Management of Obesity

At present, three treatment options are available: lifestyle intervention (nutrition combined with physical activity), medications and bariatric interventions.

BOX 2.5 Treatment strategy (NICE guidelines)

Activity

- Encourage enjoyable activities (walking, swimming, aerobics, gardening) as part of everyday life
- Minimize sedentary activity, e.g., watching TV or computer and video games
- Build activity in the working day, e.g., take the stairs instead of the lift, take a walk at lunch time
- Encourage being active, e.g., dancing and skipping
- Be more active, e.g., walking and cycling to school and shops
- Children should be encouraged to increase their physical activity even if they do not lose weight because of other benefits such as reducing the risk of type 2 diabetes and cardiovascular events
- Children should be encouraged to do at least 60 minutes of moderate exercise each day either in one session or several, each 1 minute or more

Diet

- Starchy food (potatoes, rice, pasta, bread)
- Plenty of fibre-rich foods (oats, beans, peas)
- Eat at least five portions of fruit and vegetables each day
- Low-fat diet and avoiding increasing fat and/or calorie intake
- Eat as little as possible fried food, drinks and confectionaries high in added sugar and food and drinks high in fat (fast food)
- Eat breakfast
- Encourage eating high-fibre bread, whole grain cereal, whole-meal pasta, brown rice
- Help children maintain or work towards weight reduction
- Children should eat regular meals in a pleasant, sociable environment without distraction such as TV watching
- Parents should eat the same food as their children whenever possible
- Get children involved at meal times; they are likely to eat what they made themselves

Drug and Surgical Treatment

➤ Drug treatment is generally not used for children younger than 12 years except in severe cases with comorbidities, e.g., sleep apnoea or raised intracranial pressure.
➤ For children aged 12 years or older, treatment with Orlistat is indicated:
  ➢ If physical comorbidities such as sleep apnoea or orthopaedic issues or severe psychological problems are present.
  ➢ For a trial of 6–12 months with regular review to assess effectiveness, side effects and adherence.
➤ Orlistat (the only approved anti-obesity drug) should be prescribed for children only by a multidisciplinary team with expertise in:
  ➢ Drug monitoring.
  ➢ Psychological support.
  ➢ Behaviour intervention such as increased activity.
  ➢ Nutrition and diet advice.
➤ In the past few years, more drugs have become available to treat obesity including topiramate, phentermine, semaglutide and liraglutide.
➤ Surgical intervention (bariatric surgery) may be considered in exceptional circumstances and undertaken by a multidisciplinary team.
  ➢ Received intensive management in a specialized obesity service.
  ➢ Been found to be generally fit for surgery and anaesthesia.
  ➢ Willing to commit to the need for long-term follow-up.
  ➢ BMI ≥35 kg/m^2 with at least one severe comorbidity such as sleep apnoea, hypertension or NAFLD.
  ➢ BMI >40 kg/m^2 with less serious comorbidity.

NORMAL DEVELOPMENT

Core Messages

➤ Development refers to the way a child grows, changes and develops skills physically, emotionally, cognitively and socially between birth and adolescence.
➤ The perinatal period and the first 3 years of age are the most sensitive times for adequate development. Most brain development is completed during these two periods. Nutrients promote healthy brain development.
➤ Nutrient deficiencies, even before conception and during pregnancy, can result in low birthweight, neural tube disorders and lifelong developmental delays or disabilities.
➤ Early life adversities, such as child neglect and nutrient deficiencies, which are commonly associated with poverty, can have long-term adverse effects on brain development and cognition. On the other hand, positive parent–child relationships with love and affection and a healthy diet are essential to a child's brain development.

Developmental Surveillance Programme (Healthy Child Programme)

➤ Approximately 12–15% of children during the first few years of life experience developmental delay or disabilities ranging from delay in achieving certain developmental milestones to functional impairment in hearing or vision, as well as learning, emotional and behavioural disorders.

➤ In recent years, emphasis has shifted from detecting developmental problems to preventing them. The Child Health Programme aims at preventing diseases, detecting physical and developmental abnormalities and promoting optimum health development with an early intervention. The key components include:
  ➣ Eliciting parental concerns.
  ➣ Obtaining a developmental history.
  ➣ Performing a physical examination.
  ➣ Observing the child and parents.
  ➣ Identifying any risk, which includes detection of disabling conditions such as cerebral palsy, visual and hearing impairment and autism spectrum disorder (ASD).
  ➣ Maintaining records.
  ➣ Discussing the findings with the parents.

The 2- to 2.5-Year Review

➤ The review involves performing health and development assessment, which is usually carried out by health visitors at home or at an appropriate child clinic.

➤ The programme aims at early detection of:
  ➣ Any parental concerns including behavioural problems (e.g., temper tantrum), sleep issues and toilet training.
  ➣ Any developmental delay? Delay in speech and communication in the presence of normal physical development may raise suspicion of ASD.
  ➣ Any ill health?
  ➣ Any growth impairment?
  ➣ Ensuring an up-to-date immunization schedule
  ➣ Promoting a healthy lifestyle and preventing obesity by emphasizing healthy eating habits and encouraging physical activity.
  ➣ Injury prevention involves raising awareness and preventing accidents (such as locked cupboards for medicine).

➤ The Department of Health 2009 guidance on the 2-year review advises that if there are concerns, a formal assessment using validated tools should be used. Recommended tools include:
  ➣ World Health Organization (WHO) growth charts.
  ➣ Age and stages questionnaires (ASQs).
  ➣ Parents' Evaluation of Developmental Status (PEDS).
  ➣ Social and communication questionnaires (SCQs) for early detection of ASD.

➤ Starting in April 2015, National Health Service (NHS) England mandated the use of a standard questionnaire and specified the ASQ-3. In addition, starting in October 2016, the ASQ:SE-2 (S = social; E = emotional development) should be used.

➤ Development is assessed from the answers given by the parents on the ASQ-3.

➤ Ideally, the parents are offered validated questionnaires to elicit parental concerns in advance of the appointment, to be discussed at the check-in. Appropriate questionnaires to use are the PEDS or the ASQ, as both help professionals elicit and interpret parents' concerns about their children's development and behaviour.

Performing a Developmental Assessment

➤ If the developmental surveillance identifies any concerns, clinicians may follow-up with a detailed developmental assessment (Table 2.8).

TABLE 2.8 Summary of detailed developmental milestones

Age in Months	Gross Motor	Fine Motor	Personal/Social	Language and Communication
0–1	Knees under the abdomen. In ventral suspension: Head below the body level.	Hands fisted	Regards human face with interest	Responds to sounds (bell) if active or crying, startles if quiet
2	Prone: Lift head to 45°, knees no longer under the abdomen. In ventral suspension: Head held erect.	Hands open most of the time	Smiles in response	Coos, vocalizes with vowel sounds (ah, uh)
3	Lift head to 45° for sustained period. In ventral suspension, head up above the level of body.	Hands open, holds placed object actively	Anticipates feeding, smiles spontaneously	Chuckles
4	Bears weight briefly on extended legs, rolls front to back	Reach and grasp begin, puts toys to mouth	Excited when toys presented, smiles and vocalizes at self in mirror	Laughs loud, increased vocalization
6	When pulled to sit, no head lag, assists by lifting head, sits leaning forward on arms	Transfer objects from one hand to another, reaches for toy with one-hand approach	Takes solids well, bites and chews, pats at mirror image	Increasing babble, expresses with sounds
9	Sits indefinitely, pulls to stand	Explores pellet with index finger	Imitates waving, straightens arm through sleeve	Non-specific 'Mama' and 'Dada'
12	Stands independently well, walks a few steps.	Helps turn book pages, imitates scribbling	Throws toys away in play	One word besides 'mama' and 'dada'
15	Gets to standing without support, walks well	Tower of 2 or 3 cubes	Starts to handle spoon and cup	4 or 5 words

(Continued)

TABLE 2.8 Summary of detailed developmental milestones (Continued)

Age in Months	Gross Motor	Fine Motor	Personal/Social	Language and Communication
18	Walks carrying objects, runs stiffly	Tower of 3–4 cubes, turns 2–3 book pages	Feeds self with spoon, handles regular cup	Follows simple commands, points to 1–4 body parts
21	Runs well, walks up and down stairs holding rail, kicks a large ball	Tower of 5–6 cubes, completes 3-piece form board	Uses fork, helps with simple households tasks	20–50 words, combines 2 words
24	Jumps with both feet from floor	Tower of 6–7 cubes, threads shoelace through holes, imitates line drawing, ability to thread beads	Feeds self with little spilling, ability to use cutlery, ability to put on coat without help	At least 50 words, 3-word sentences, follows instruction, e.g., close the door, ability to name items/animals
30	Stands briefly on one foot, alternates feet going upstairs	Tower of 8–10 cubes, turns single book pages	Accomplishes toileting, puts on shoes	Names many familiar objects, names many body parts
36	Pedals tricycle, alternates feet going upstairs	Tower of at least 10 cubes, holds crayon in fingers, tries to cut with scissors	Toilet training, dresses with supervision	Recites nursery rhyme, gives first and last name

➤ It is traditional to ask about developmental milestones, particularly in children with suspected developmental delay (DD). Primary care providers (PCPs) may identify any DD during routine checks or when the parents, nursery or school raise concerns.

➤ Although caregivers can provide helpful data about the pattern of development, focus should be on current levels of development rather than past ones. Observing the quality of the skills is essential rather than documenting the age at which the milestone was achieved.

➤ There is no need to memorize detailed lists of milestones. Clinicians may keep a copy of screening testing (Box 2.6). The goal of development assessment is to answer the following questions: Is the child's development in the 'normal range' and comparable to that of their peers? Are the key areas of development (gross motor, fine motor, language and personal/social) developing at the same rate?

BOX 2.6 Rapid screening list for a developmental assessment

- *Antenatal history:* Underlying medical conditions, use of medication and use of drugs, alcohol, tobacco, any infections.
- *Birth and neonatal:* Gestational age, anthropometric data, Apgar score, Result of thyroid-stimulating hormone (TSH) and the universal hearing test.
- *Physical examination:* Growth, dysmorphism, neurocutaneous stigmata, muscle tone, gait, tendon reflexes, cranial nerves, spine, hips, and behavioural observations.
- *Developmental milestone:* Current level across the gross and fine motor, personal and communication.
- *Hearing and vision:* Parental concerns, any family history of problems.

Primitive Reflexes

These reflexes do not usually persist (except the parachute reflex), and their persistence is a sign of abnormal development (Table 2.9).

TABLE 2.9 Some primitive reflexes with the age of disappearance

Reflex	Usual occurrence and disappearance
• Rooting	• From birth until 4 months of age
• Placing	• From birth until about 6 weeks of age
• Moro	• From birth until about 3 months of age
• Palmar grasp	• From birth until 3 months of age
• Atonic neck	• From 2 months until 6 months of age
• Parachute	• From 9 months of age and persists

DEVELOPMENTAL DELAY

Globally, DD affects 1–3% of children under the age of 5 years. It is defined as a delay in two or more developmental key areas of gross/fine motor, speech, language, cognition, social/personal or other activities of daily living. It is subdivided as follows:

➤ Mild DD is functional age <33% below chronological age.
➤ Moderate is functional age 34–66% below chronological age.
➤ Severe is functional age <66% chronological age.

PCPs play a significant role in early identification of DD. It is essential that they have the knowledge and skills to identify DD and provide an appropriate management plan. Identification of a child with DD is usually achieved through:

➤ History: e.g., 'High-risk babies', including prematurity, small-for-date.
➤ The routine 8-week examination.
➤ Parental or professional concerns including health visitors.

What Causes DD?

➤ Genetic causes such as chromosomal deletion.
➤ Perinatal causes such as prematurity, intrauterine growth restriction, birth injury.
➤ Cerebral such as microcephaly.
➤ Toxins, e.g., alcohol and smoking during pregnancy.
➤ Maternal infection (e.g., cytomegalovirus).
➤ Psychosocial causes including neglect.

What Can Be Done in Practice?

➤ Full history (including the neonatal period and any hypoglycaemia) and examination (including developmental examination).

➤ In case the history and/or examination are suspicious of DD:
  ➤ Hearing and vision assessment.
  ➤ Growth parameters including head circumference (HC) measurement.
  ➤ Consider requesting some investigations shown in Box 2.7.

BOX 2.7 Initial investigation for a child with DD

- *Genetic testing*: Chromosomal microarray,* fragile X genetic testing
- *Biochemical/metabolic*: FBC, U & E, CK, TFT, lead, ferritin, biotinides, amino acids, ammonia, urine for organic acids

* Chromosome microarray (array-based comparative genomic hybridization [aCGH].
CK = creatinine kinase; FBC = full blood count; U&E = urea & electrolytes.

  ➤ Parents should be encouraged to do stimulation activities (e.g., massage, playing, reading and singing) and monitor their child regularly using the health booklet.
➤ Currently, chromosomal microarray is the most efficient diagnostic test for global DD, yielding about 15–20% positivity. The standard karyotyping is currently rarely requested. Fragile X syndrome typically causes moderate DD.
➤ *If DD is suspected and/or there is persistent parental concern, a referral should be considered to a developmental paediatrician.*

RED FLAGS

- Any child who is not walking by the age of 18 months should have a CPK blood test to exclude Duchene muscular dystrophy (DMD). About 50% of children with DMD walk later than at 18 months.
- It is essential to distinguish the child who has always been delayed in development from the one who began with normal development and subsequently slowed or regressed developmentally. The latter may indicate neurodegenerative diseases, autism or certain types of seizures.
- Although feeding difficulty (crying, pushing food away and gagging during feeding) often occurs in healthy children, persistent and marked feeding problems may suggest the presence of DD.
- A child with normal motor developmental milestones and good non-verbal problem-solving ability but a delay in social/language development is suspicious for a hearing problem or ASD.

DISABILITY

Disability indicates any restriction or lack of ability to perform an activity which is considered normal for the child's age. Estimates from the WHO put the global prevalence of disability at 15% or one in seven people in the world. Approximately 1.2 million people in the UK have mild or moderate learning disability, and around 200,000 have severe learning disability. Disability includes:

➤ Motor disability such as cerebral palsy or DMD.
➤ Delayed speech and language acquisition.
➤ Cognitive or intellectual disability is a condition of arrested or incomplete development of the body or mind that limits a person's ability to partake in typical activity and social interaction.
1. **Learning disability (LD)**. The WHO defines LD 'as a state of arrest or incomplete development of mind'. LD is characterized by three core features: Reduced ability to understand new or complex information, reduced ability to cope independently in social functioning and onset before adulthood having a lasting effect on development. The severity of LD depends on the person's intelligence (Box 2.8).

BOX 2.8 Severity grades of learning disability

- Mild IQ 50–69
  - 85% with intellectual disability (ID) have this mild severity and likely are recognized to have ID before 5–6 years of age. They have difficulty in comprehension, arithmetic and writing skills. These children are at increased risk for being manipulated by others.
- Moderate IQ 35–49
  - Around 10% of children with LD have moderate-severe LD, with some degree of independence in self-care and significant limitation in reading, writing, math and other skills. They are likely recognized by 3–5 years of age.
- Severe IQ 20–34
  - Severe LD that likely needs continuous support, very limited communication and language of just a few words. They are usually recognized in infancy.
- Profound IQ <20
  - Severe limitation of self-care, severe limitation in language and communication, usually recognized at birth or soon after.

LDs have multiple causes including genetic, syndromic (such as Fragile X syndrome and Down's syndrome) and psychosocial deprivation. Environmental factors include toxic exposure, brain injury and infections. Premature babies and children of families with low income are at higher risk of developing LD compared to full terms babies and to those families with high income. About 60% of cases have no known aetiology.

2. **Specific learning disability (SLD)** is a neurodevelopmental disorder characterized by challenges and difficulties in one or more areas of reading, writing and mathematical skills and is typically diagnosed in early school age. The prevalence of SLD ranges from 5% to 15% among school children (Table 2.10).
   SLD is diagnosed if there is difficulty in at least one of the following areas:
   ➢ Reading (e.g., inaccurate, slow), accounting for 80% of cases
   ➢ Understanding the meaning of what is read
   ➢ Spelling

TABLE 2.10 Summary of some specific learning difficulties

Specific Disability	Brief Description of the Difficulties
● Dyslexia	● This is a neurodevelopmental disorder characterized by reading difficulty, associated impaired learning, perception and phonological process. It co-occurs with psychiatric and other developmental disorders, especially ADHD, speech and language problems. Aetiology is multifactorial and heritability in up to 70%. It affects 5–20% of school-age children.
● Dyscalculia	● Refers to a persistent difficulty performing arithmetic calculation, i.e., having a poor understanding of number sense and their magnitude and relationships between numbers.
● Dyspraxia	● This is characterized by pronounced difficulty in performing purposeful movements and coordination. Approximately 2–6% of children have dyspraxia, and 80% of autistic children have dyspraxia in early childhood.
● Dysphasia	● Defined as a language impairment that affects previously acquired linguistic ability.
● Dysgraphia	● This is a specific learning disability causing impaired legible and automatic letter production. Children spend up to 60% of their time at school writing, which requires about 10 years of practice to reach a level of almost complete automatization. Despite education, 5–10% do not reach a sufficient level of automatization in handwriting.

➤ Writing (e.g., grammar, punctuation)
➤ Understanding number concepts (e.g., calculation)
➤ Mathematical reasoning (e.g., solving math problems)
➤ The diagnosis of SLD requires the persistence of difficulty for at least 6 months, starting during school-age, and is not due to other conditions such as intellectual disorder

PRACTICE POINTS

● Identifying patients with LD by primary care clinicians is central to initiatives for improvement of health of the UK population.
● GPs receive additional financial incentives for maintaining registers of patients with learning disability as part of the Quality and Outcomes Framework (QOF) and offer them annual checks.
● Patients with LD are at risk of having comorbidities throughout their life. If LD is not recognized and managed, patients are likely to exhibit physical and mental ill-health, loneliness. social isolation, unemployment and repeated self-harm. Those children with SLD are at risk of low academic achievement, poor mental health, psychological distress and dropping out of school.
● It is estimated that an average UK GP practice, which provides care for about 2000 patients, will have 6 patients with severe LD and 44 with mild-moderate LD.

CHAPTER 3

Behavioural Disorders

TEMPER TANTRUMS

Core Messages

➤ Temper tantrums are normally dysregulated reactions to frustration. They are present in up to 80% of toddlers and tend to decline with age.
➤ They include excessive screaming, kicking, hitting and breath holding. Their frequency and intensity vary considerably.
➤ Most tantrums can be regarded as a normal part of development, and most parents can expect some tantrums from the age of 18 months up to the age of 4 years. Some attacks can start as early as 6 months. They usually last between 2 and 15 minutes.
➤ Between 18 months and 3 years of age, children are usually very egocentric, want to be independent and self-sufficient and dislike being dominated by their parents. If an adult stands in their way and they cannot reach their goals, they can become frustrated, and a temper tantrum is triggered. By the age of 3 years, temper tantrums often become less frequent and less intense as children learn how to use language and better communicate their wants and needs.

Management Tips

➤ Raising children and managing their behaviour will vary between families. Also parents will have different parenting approaches, and we should be respectful of their decisions. However, if they do ask for help and advice on managing tantrums, there are some techniques that might help.
➤ Parents should not ask children to do something when they must do that anyway, e.g., do not ask 'When would you like to eat or sleep' but rather say 'It is now lunchtime or bedtime'. It is good to have a regular routine – this will give children a feeling of safety, as they will know what is coming next: For example, bath time and then bedtime.
➤ Praising good behaviour will consistently be more effective than criticizing. Punishing and arguing with children is not advised and should be avoided.
➤ Parents should take time each day to share activities and games with their children and let them feel that their parents are enjoying this shared activity.

DOI: 10.1201/9781032642888-3

➤ Parents should allow their children to feel important and grow in self-confidence by giving them little tasks suitable for their developmental ability.

➤ Parents should remain calm and hang on to a sense of humour and not punish the child. Parents must manage their own behaviour before expecting their child to manage their own. Yelling back or spanking will only make the situation worse.

➤ Parents should try not give in to a child during a tantrum; that attitude will only increase their frequency.

➤ Tantrums may be ignored if they are attention seeking and the child is in a safe place.

➤ After the child has calmed down from a tantrum, parents can teach them skills to help avoid tantrums in the future, e.g., how to try to express their feelings without hitting or screaming, how to learn better ways to get what they want, and how to interact successfully with their peers.

➤ Parents increasingly use electronic devices to try to regulate their children's difficult emotions, including tantrums. This is potentially problematic, given that toddlerhood is a critical time for learning basic emotion regulation. Parents should avoid using these devices as a primary way of regulating their children's behaviour.

➤ Parents management training (PMT) is a successful treatment for severe disruptive behavioural disorder in children, either in a group or on an individual basis. The objective is to teach parents effective control strategies.

➤ If, despite the use of these interventions, temper tantrums are worsening in terms of frequency, intensity and duration, *a referral to secondary care should be considered, particularly if*:
  ➢ There is evidence of self-harming or violence against others.
  ➢ There are signs of withdrawal or frustration.
  ➢ There is suspicion of neglect or abuse.

RED FLAGS

- When a child presents with temper tantrums, primary care physicians should check the child for possible coexistent conditions which may cause or contribute, such as hearing or visual impairment, language delay and learning difficulties.
- Beware of the following conditions, which may be associated with tantrums:
  - Epileptic syndromes, such as benign Rolandic epilepsy and complex partial seizures, which may present with emotional/behavioural outbursts of anger. A detailed description of the epileptic seizures and EEG will lead to the correct diagnosis.
  - Severe temper tantrums are sometimes an early symptom of autism, occurring particularly when the child is interrupted from performing their routines or 'rituals'.
  - Prader–Willi syndrome, characterized by mental disability and an eating disorder, is associated with emotional problems, including tantrums and compulsive behaviour.

BREATH-HOLDING SPELLS: CYANOTIC AND PALLID

Core Messages

➤ Breath-holding spells (BHS) are benign, non-epileptic, paroxysmal conditions which affect about 5% of children and is characterized by an episodic apnoea, often leading to changes in postural tone and consciousness, and may end in a seizure. Peak age is 6–18 months. The attacks are unusual in children <6 months and after the age of 5 years. Family history is positive in 25% of cases. The hereditary nature as autosomal dominant has been established.

➤ Although BHS aetiology is still unclear, autonomic system deregulation and increased vagal tone leading to cardiac arrest and cerebral anoxia play an essential role.

➤ About one-third of affected children have two to five attacks a day; another third will have one attack per month, and the remaining third may either have more frequent or less frequent than the first two.

➤ Spells are usually triggered by anger, frustration or pain. The child will recover within 1–2 minutes. A postictal phase (as occurs in seizures) and incontinence do not occur. The child is well between these spells.

➤ Spells follow a typical course: Pain → crying (not in the pallid attacks) → apnoea (lasting about 10 seconds) → cyanosis or pallor → loss of consciousness → possible seizure, which is usually very brief.

➤ Combination attacks (both cyanotic and pale types) occur in 20% of the total cases.

➤ It is important to differentiate between the cyanotic and pallid form because the pallid form may be associated with rhythm abnormalities (Box 3.1) and between BHS and epilepsy (Box 3.2).

BOX 3.1 Differentiating between cyanotic and pallid forms of BHS

- Cyanotic spells are far more common than the pallid form.
- Cyanotic spells are triggered by anger or frustration; the pallid spells are usually triggered by a painful event.
- Crying is the rule in the cyanotic type and very brief or absent in the pallid form.
- Following loss of consciousness, cyanotic spells may be associated with clonic jerks and bradycardia. Pallid spells may be associated with tonic seizure; bradycardia and/or cardiac asystole occur. The tonic and clonic episodes sometimes need to be differentiated from epilepsy (Box 3.2).

BOX 3.2 Differential diagnosis between BHS and a seizure

- Excluding febrile seizures, epileptic seizures are uncommon and ten times less common (0.5%) than breath holding (5%).
- Epilepsy occurs at any age; the age of breath holding is as noted earlier.
- Cyanosis in breath holding occurs first before the onset of a subsequent seizure, while cyanosis occurs after the onset of an epileptic seizure.
- BHS are nearly always stereotyped (as noted earlier); epileptic seizures are unpredictable in the way they occur.

- Recovery is fast in breath holding (1–2 minutes) while the recovery is longer with a seizure.
- There is no postictal phase in breath holding in contrast to seizures.
- The EEG is normal in breath holding and likely abnormal in epilepsy.

Management Tips

➤ The first step of management is to establish the diagnosis by taking a detailed history, which alone can confirm the diagnosis.

➤ BHS are quite distressing to the parents. Explanation and reassurance that the event is benign and that child will grow out of it are the cornerstones of management. There is no permanent neurological damage.

➤ Distracting the child whilst in pain and avoiding situations which lead to breath holding can help. Some parents find splashing cold water on the face helpful in terminating the duration of the spells. These parents may continue doing so, although this might not work for every child.

➤ Cardiopulmonary resuscitation (CPR) is usually unnecessary and unhelpful. When the child is unconscious or fitting, they should be placed on their side in the recovery position.

➤ ECG, Hb and ferritin are usually the only investigations indicated in the pallid form (see 'Red Flags'), and Hb in the cyanotic spells. EEG may be requested if the diagnosis is unclear and the history suggests epilepsy.

➤ Iron has been found to be effective in the cyanotic attacks and the presence of iron deficiency anaemia or iron deficiency alone. Iron therapy can also result in improvement of BHS even in the absence of iron deficiency. Iron has an impact on autonomic nervous dysregulation, as it is a cofactor for many enzymes and neurotransmitters. In severe and frequent cases of BHS, antiepileptic drugs, e.g., piracetam, may reduce the spells.

RED FLAGS

- While some professionals consider BHS an 'attention-seeking behaviour', these spells are not intentional and not voluntary, and the child is unable to control them.
- An ECG is an essential investigation in the pallid spells to exclude prolonged QT syndrome, which is a serious but treatable form of cardiac arrhythmia.

HEAD BANGING AND ROCKING

➤ Sleep-related rhythmic movements manifest as body rocking, head banging or rolling of the head. They are common stereotyped repetitive behaviours, usually seen in healthy children around naptime and bedtime. The typical age of occurrence is 6–9 months, and they often disappear around 18 months of age. They may persist after the age of 2 years in about 3% of children.

➤ The condition typically occurs with the child lying face down, banging the head into a pillow or mattress. In the upright position, the head is banged against the wall or bedside.

➤ When the movements are frequent, occurring outside bedtime and naptime, and/or significantly interfere with normal sleep/daytime function or result in injury, they are considered a rhythmic movement disorder (RMD). Most children with RMD recover in early childhood.

➤ Head banging and rocking may also be caused by attention seeking, for self-stimulation and for self-comfort. Children with developmental delay or neurodisability may also frequently exhibit these head movements.

➤ Management of children is shown in Box 3.3.

BOX 3.3 Management tips for children with head banging and rocking

- Children need to be carefully examined to ensure they are healthy and developing normally. The head should be examined to exclude any injuries.
- Parents can be reassured if the child:
  - ❭ Is healthy and has a normal development.
  - ❭ Is showing this behaviour only at bedtime and naptime.
  - ❭ Has no associated sleep disorder such as sleep apnoea or night terrors and the movements do not interfere with sleep quality, which may result in increased daytime sleepiness.
- Parents can be advised:
  - ❭ To give plenty of attention to the child during the daytime and ignore the head movements at night.
  - ❭ To try soothing routines, e.g., warm bath, before putting the child to sleep.
  - ❭ To not put the child to sleep until they are tired and ready to go to sleep rather than making bedtime a battle of wills.
  - ❭ That padding of the bed is often unnecessary, as there is a small risk of trapping the head.
  - ❭ To remove the child's bed or crib away from the wall or furniture, as this can worsen the noises and cause injuries.
- Although most cases do not require any pharmacological treatment, in rare cases of poor sleep or self-inflicted head injury, benzodiazepines or melatonin may be used.

TEETH GRINDING (BRUXISM)

➤ Bruxism is defined as repetitive jaw muscle activity characterized by teeth grinding. Prevalence ranges from 3.5% to 49% in children.

➤ This unconscious habit usually occurs during sleep. In adults, the habit is often caused by stress. In children, the habit may be caused by:
  - ➢ Improper teeth alignment.
  - ➢ Stress, anger, frustration, or anxiety.
  - ➢ Unknown causes.

➤ Mild and infrequent teeth grinding is usually harmless. Severe grinding may cause damage to the teeth enamel, periodontal tissue and temporomandibular joints; sore jaw; irregularities in the dental arches; dental mobility; and fractures.

➤ Management depends on the cause. Dentists may correct any teeth non-alignment. They may prescribe a plastic mouth guard to be worn at night. If stress is suspected as the cause, parents are advised to help their child relax their body and mind by reading their favourite book and avoiding screens at night. A warm bath before sleep may also help. Frequent and/or severe grinding may require a psychological approach including cognitive behavioural therapy (CBT), stress and relaxation therapy. The use of some drugs, including clonidine or clonazepam, can be of some use in certain cases.

THUMB SUCKING AND NAIL BITING

➤ Thumb sucking is observed in utero as early as 29 weeks' gestation. In infancy, as many as 25–50% are sucking their thumbs. This incidence declines to 15–20% in children aged 5–6 years. It is considered normal until the age of 3–4 years.

➤ Nail biting is found in as many as 45–60% of school-age children to adolescents.

➤ In at least some children, the habit may be considered a form of self-stimulation or self-comfort. Occasionally the habit is caused by stress or tension.

➤ Both habits (thumb sucking and nail biting) may cause some complications including dental problems, deformities of the thumb or nails and paronychia.

➤ Use of averse-tasting substances on the thumb may occasionally help.

➤ The increased use of a pacifier in some societies has resulted in marked reduction in the prevalence of thumb sucking. However, using pacifiers can also have consequences on tooth and speech development.

➤ Malocclusion (upper and lower teeth don't align) can result from pacifier use and thumb sucking. A longer duration of breastfeeding is known to result in a reduction of malocclusion and thumb sucking.

SELF-STIMULATION (MASTURBATION) IN PREPUBERTAL CHILDREN

➤ It is normal for adolescents to masturbate, an act which is almost universal at puberty (90–95% of boys and 50–60% of girls) as a consequence of normal sexual development.

➤ In prepubertal children it can often be regarded as normal behaviour, in particular in infants and toddlers as part of normal development and body exploration. Stimulation of the genitalia is usually done for pleasure and self-comfort.

➤ Typical self-stimulations occur as repetitive and stereotyped episodes of tonic posturing associated with body rocking movements. The child may be seen self-stimulating on an edge of a chair and without actual manual stimulation of the genitalia. During the act, the child is noted to be dazed, flushed and fully preoccupied. The child may grunt and breathe irregularly followed by fatigue and falling asleep. The act is often repeated several times a day.

➤ Although in utero cases of masturbation have been reported, the typical age of onset is a few months old, and it progressively increases until usually ceasing at the end of toddlerhood.

➤ Unlike masturbation in older children and adults, infantile masturbation may involve little or no genital stimulation. This is the main reason why misdiagnosis as seizure or abdominal pain is made.

MANAGEMENT PLAN

- Reassurance that the habit does not pose any health risk or physical injury. Parents have to understand that their child has learned about it and seems to enjoy it. The habit usually ceases by age 3 years.
- Reassurance that the habit does not mean that the child will be promiscuous or sexually deviant.
- A reasonable approach by the parents is to allow the act to be carried out in a private room.
- Self-stimulation only becomes a problem if parents overreact by punishing the child or stopping them by force, bringing too much attention to it or making it appear 'dirty or wicked'. This may trigger emotional harm to the child.
- Some acts may be caused by boredom or inattention. Therefore, the child may be distracted by spending more time with the parents and increasing physical activity.
- Occasionally, this behaviour is associated with abnormality of the genitalia or perineum, such as nappy rash. Therefore, careful examination of this area is important.

Referral Should Be Considered If:

➤ If the child continues doing it in public, particularly if this done deliberately.
➤ If parents suspect that their child has been taught to masturbate by somebody.
➤ If despite adequate steps taken by parents, the frequency of the acts increases.
➤ There is evidence of child abuse.

RED FLAGS
- Misdiagnosis is common when there are no apparent genital manipulations and movements (described as shaking, staring and limb movements) could be misinterpreted as clonic movements of epilepsy.
- Infantile masturbation needs high index of suspicion in terms of safeguarding and risk of sexual abuse. Carefully taking a history, assessing the family and, importantly, viewing video recording of the episode will lead to the correct diagnosis.

TICS

➤ Tics are sudden, rapid, involuntary, non-rhythmic movements and/or vocalizations. This is a common condition affecting up to 20% of school-age children at some point during their childhood. Chronic tics are when they persist >12 months.

➤ The mean age of onset is around 5 years, with an increased frequency of tics occurring between 8 and 12 years. Up to 80% of affected children who developed tics before the age of 10 years experience a significant improvement during adolescence. By 18 years of age, the majority experience mild tics without significant impairment.

➤ Simple motor tics involve one muscle group such as eye blinks, neck twisting or shoulder shrugging. Complex motor tics involve more than one muscle group such as jumping or squatting.

➤ Tourette syndrome (TS) is an inherited neuropsychiatric disease combining chronic (more than 1 year) multiple motor and/or vocal tics. TS affects 0.5–1% of the general population.

MANAGEMENT OF TICS

● Avoid calling attention to the tics, telling the child to stop or control the tics, and avoid allowing the child to become overly excited or stimulated (very exciting video or computer games).

● Provided not have functional impairment from their tics, and that the child does as tics may improve with time, watchful waiting is an acceptable approach.

● There is no cure for tics or TS. Explanation, reassurance and education are the most important parts of management. Habit reversal training, relaxation training and functional intervention are ways to reduce tics.

● Tics of recent onset may improve by providing an immediate reward for successful tic suppression.

● Some patients with frequent and severe tics or with TS may use cannabis as self-medication. This should be avoided in children and adolescents because it is unsafe, because cannabis exposure has potentially harmful effects on cognitive skills and because it is an illegal drug.

Referral should be considered for:
○ Persistent and frequent tics for several months.
○ Tics causing distress to the child or family.
○ Tics interfering with school performance, social or family life.
○ Suspected TS.

> **RED FLAGS**
> - Physical examination, including neurological examination, is essential in patients with tics to exclude underlying neurological diseases. Neuroimaging and EEG should be performed only if clinically indicated and requested by a specialist.
> - In severe cases of tics, including TS, comorbidities are common and should be searched for: Psychiatric disorders, ADHD, obsessive-compulsive disorders, learning and sleep difficulties.
> - There is a tendency for patients with tics to suppress them, especially when attending clinics. In those individuals who do not exhibit any tics during consultation, video recordings can be helpful in addition to a thorough history.

ANOREXIA NERVOSA

Core Messages

The initial assessment should focus on:
Long-term Management

➤ Anorexia nervosa (AN) is a serious mental illness characterized by self-induced starvation, inability to maintain weight and a high incidence of comorbidities and mortality, which is the highest among psychiatric diseases. It mainly affects girls (92%) with an incidence of 0.3–1%. The typical age is 15–25 years. The peak age of disease onset has decreased in recent years.

➤ The aetiology of AN is complex and includes genetic, neurobiological and environmental factors and is higher in a society which places a high value on thinness and body image.

➤ The severity of AN is measured by the degree of weight loss (see later).

➤ In contrast to postpubertal adolescents and adults, prepubertal children affected by AN are at high risk of:
  ➢ Rapid weight loss due to low energy stores.
  ➢ Rapid dehydration, which may affect physical activity and wellbeing.
  ➢ Stunting of growth, including height, when the anorexia persists.

Main Diagnostic Criteria

➤ Disproportionate concern about body weight or shape; unusually low body mass index (BMI) for age; intense fear of gaining weight even as the weight loss continues; rapid weight loss; restrictive eating habits; and obsession with calorie counting, fat content and dieting.

➤ Mental health problems including anxiety, stress, depression and social withdrawal.

➤ Physical signs of malnutrition (dizziness, syncope, hypotension).

➤ Menstrual or other endocrinological abnormalities.

➤ Frequent and strenuous exercise and purging, often using laxatives.

Clinical findings are mostly the results of malnutrition and include:

➤ Weight well below the centile for normal weight:
  ➣ Mild body weight loss: BMI >17.0 kg/m²
  ➣ Moderate body weight loss: BMI 16–16.99 kg/m²
  ➣ Severe body weight loss: BMI <15–15.99 kg/m²
➤ Cardiac arrhythmia or signs of congestive cardiac failure.
➤ Bradycardia, low blood pressure and low body temperature, constipation, hair loss or abnormal body hair growth.
➤ Excoriation on the dorsum of the hand as a result of induced vomiting.
➤ Sleep disturbance.
➤ Full blood count (FBC) often shows anaemia and leukopenia.
➤ Reduced bone mineral density (osteopenia) affecting nearly 90% of female patients.

Practice-Based Management

The vast majority of patients with AN first contact primary care providers, who can arrange the initial assessment and organize long-term management.

THE INITIAL ASSESSMENT SHOULD FOCUS ON:

➤ Checking for dehydration and muscle wasting. Examination of the mouth, looking for possible glossitis and loss of taste (caused by iron or zinc deficiency), bleeding of gums and fissure of the lips (caused by riboflavin vitamin deficiency). Inspection of the teeth: Recurrent induced vomiting can erode tooth enamel leading to pain and dental decay. The patients should be encouraged to see a dentist.
➤ Measurements of weight, height, pulse, blood pressure and body temperature.
➤ Arrangement of first-line investigations including FBC, U&E, liver and thyroid function tests, bone profile, toxicology screen, serum cortisol, pancreatic enzyme levels, blood glucose, ECG and bone mineral density.

LONG-TERM MANAGEMENT:

➤ After an initial assessment: All children and adolescents with features suggestive or suspected of AN should be referred immediately to a community-based, age-appropriate eating disorder service. Other available treatments include family-based treatment (FBT), psychotherapy, CBT and dietary rehabilitation (NICE Guideline [NG69]: Eating disorders: recognition and treatment. Published May 2017, updated 2020).
➤ For AN patients with normal physical and psychiatric status, or those who refuse referrals, primary care physicians (PCPs) are in the best position to help them restore their body weight and improve their clinical status by focusing on FBT. PCPs may continue to monitor patients' physical and mental health, prescribe medications and play a key role to help with their recovery.
➤ FBT has shown a significant improvement in adolescents' BMI. It also educates parents that they are not responsible for AN in their children, offering them strategies for weight gain and developing healthier relationship with their children.

➤ PCPs can arrange nutritional rehabilitation with the help of a dietitian, putting a target weight gain of 0.25–0.5 kg/week. They also can encourage the patients to engage in social activity, spending time with supportive family members or friends, attending enjoyable gatherings and exploring intellectual pursuits or hobbies they enjoy.

➤ Frequently prescribed medications include selective serotonin reuptake inhibitors, SSRIs, benzodiazepines (e.g., clonazepam) and atypical antipsychotics, particularly olanzapine and risperidone, may help patients with their symptoms of delusion and anxiety.

➤ Rates of recovery from AN at 1–2 years follow-up with the best available treatment lie in the range of 13–50% across age groups. Only around 30% are expected to recover after 9 years. Death (around 10%) is usually due to cardiac arrhythmia or electrolyte disturbance.

RED FLAGS

● The diagnosis of AN can be difficult because patients can be in denial of their disease and do not view their behaviour and issues with body image as abnormal.

● While patients with AN may not present with primary features of anorexia, patients often present to their family physicians for secondary complaints such as amenorrhoea or severe fatigue.

● The diagnosis of AN should not be made before considering other diagnoses which present with weight loss. These include inflammatory bowel diseases, malignancy, diabetes, depression, Addison's disease and hyperthyroidism.

● Patients may develop peripheral oedema in the early stages of refeeding. This has to be distinguished from cardiac failure by the absence of other signs of cardiac failure.

● With height reduction, weight loss will be underestimated if assessment is based on BMI alone.

AUTISM

Core Messages

➤ Autism describes individuals with a specific combination of impairments in social communication and repetitive behaviours beginning early in life. The clinical criteria of ASD are shown in Box 3.4.

➤ Diagnosis before the age of 18 months is difficult. However, infants may show early features of ASD, e.g., poor eye contact, failure to respond to name, reduced social interaction and visual attention, temper tantrums and delayed language development.

➤ Together with these core symptoms, co-occurring psychiatric and/or neurological disorders are common, particularly anxiety, ADHD, depression and epilepsy. About

---

BOX 3.4 Diagnostic criteria of autism

- A. *Difficulty in social communication and social interaction*
  Lack of the following:
  › Social reciprocity
  › Non-verbal communication
  › Developing and maintaining relationships
- B. *Restricted, repetitive behaviours and interaction* (two out of four must be present)
  › Stereotyped, repetitive behaviours
  › Insistence on sameness
  › Highly restricted, fixed interests
  › Hypersensitivity or hyposensitivity
- C. *Symptoms must be present in early development but may not manifest until late*
- D. *Symptoms must cause clinically significant impairment in current functioning*
- E. *Not better explained by intellectual disability or developmental delay*

40% of autistic children have diagnostic features of anxiety, compared to 2–24% in the general population.

➤ Autism is a lifelong disorder which has shown an increased prevalence. Approximately 1–2% of children in the UK and in the United States are affected, with rates of diagnosis increasing each year.

➤ Although ASD is defined as a developmental disorder because symptoms appear within the first 2 years of life, it is generally considered a lifelong disorder.

➤ Neuroimaging studies of children with ASD revealed abnormalities in the cerebral cortex, temporal lobes and cerebellum. These changes are not specific and thus non-diagnostic for ASD. There is also evidence of early brain overgrowth most apparent in the early years of life.

➤ Around 50% of autistic children have an IQ within the normal range or above. The other 50% have comorbid intellectual disability, which would put them in the IQ <70 range.

➤ Several studies have shown that autism is associated with enlarged cerebral volume (macroencephaly). As head circumference (HC) is an index of total brain volume, HC should be measured and documented every time a child with autism attends a paediatric clinic or GP surgery.

Early Diagnosis of Autism

A child usually below the age of 3 years is suspected of having autism if there is:

➤ Delay, regression of language (e.g., less than 10 words by the age of 2 years) or frequent repetition of words or phrases.

➤ Reduced or absent social skills including smiling and/or social responsiveness such as cuddles by parents, sharing of enjoyable games with other children.

➤ Absent or delayed response to name being called (despite normal hearing).

➤ Repetitive stereotyped behaviour such as body rocking, spinning or opening and closing door.
➤ Frequent and severe screaming and tantrums.

Practice-Based Management

➤ An accurate diagnosis of autism is not expected in a primary care setting. It requires an assessment involving a multidisciplinary team consisting of several health professionals. If the diagnosis is inaccurate, children with ASD will fail to receive tailored early interventions to improve their development. Conversely, a wrong diagnosis for a child who has no ASD will have a detrimental effect on their future.

Preschool children (less than 3 years) with suspected autism usually require:

➤ Physical and neurological examination, including developmental assessment, looking for any skin stigmata related to neurocutaneous syndromes such as neurofibromatosis.
➤ Hearing and vision testing.
➤ Reviewing the child after a period of "watchful waiting" is appropriate.
➤ *A referral to a local multidisciplinary team, a neurodevelopmental paediatrician or a child and adolescent psychiatrist if:*
  ➣ A child shows significant limitations or impairments to activities of daily living caused by features suggestive of autism (see 'Early Diagnosis of Autism').
  ➣ The family has significant concerns about their child's development or functioning.

For Confirmed Cases

➤ Following specialist assessment, the child may be allocated a key worker from the local autism team to coordinate services and support the child and family for:
  ➣ Enhancing social and communication skills such as engagement groups, peer support and CBT.
  ➣ Liaison with the local multidisciplinary autism team.
  ➣ Modifying any environmental factors that might trigger behaviour changes to routine or noise levels.
  ➣ Arranging speech and language therapy.
  ➣ Arranging engagement with support groups, online support groups, CBT.
➤ For school-age children: A number of programmes and approaches are available including social skill training programmes. Increasingly, interventions are delivered within the school such as peer-to-peer interactions, with an emphasis on social skills.
➤ Sleep disturbance and circadian sleep alteration are frequent in children with ASD. A low blood concentration of melatonin has been detected during the night and may be responsible for sleep disturbance. Treatment with melatonin can improve sleep disturbance in patients with ASD.

RED FLAGS

- Some autistic features are present in a number of neurological disorders in children and should not be mistaken for ASD. These include neurofibromatosis, tuberous sclerosis, visual or hearing problems, intellectual disability, ADHD and mood or anxiety disorders.
- Autism should not be ruled out because of good eye contact, smiling and showing affection to other family members; reports of normal language milestones; and a previous assessment that concluded that there was no autism.

Autism Support Groups

➤ The National Autistic Society. www.autism.org.uk. Email: nas@nas.org.uk. Tel: +44 (0) 20 7833 2299
➤ Autism Advice & Info UK. www.oassis.co.uk/autism-info. email: oassis@cambian-group.com. Tel: 0800 1973907

ATTENTION DEFICIT HYPERACTIVITY DISORDER

Core Messages

➤ ADHD is the most common neurodevelopmental disorder in children and adolescents, with a worldwide prevalence of 5%. Up to 40% of young people continue to experience symptoms into adulthood. Core symptoms with hyperactivity-impulsivity and inattentiveness should be typically present in early childhood, around 2–3 years of life, and continue for at least 6 months (Box 3.5). The disorder is caused by genetic and environmental factors.

BOX 3.5 Diagnostic criteria of ADHD

- The presence of developmentally inappropriate levels of hyperactivity, impulsivity and/or inattentive persistent symptoms for at least 6 months.
- Symptoms occurring in different settings (at home and school).
- Symptoms are causing impairments in the patient's life.
- Some symptoms and impairments occurred in early to mid-childhood.
- No other disorder better explains the symptoms.

➤ Although these symptoms tend to cluster together, some people are predominately hyperactive and impulsive, while others are more inattentive. While hyperactive-impulsive symptoms are associated with aggression and accidental injury, inattention is more associated with academic impairment, low self-esteem and low overall impaired functions in daily life.

➤ People with ADHD are at increased risk of substance misuse and addiction, criminal behaviour, sleep disturbance, educational underachievement, anxiety, depression, gambling, teenage pregnancy and self-harm. Around one-half will have at least one psychiatric comorbidity apart from ADHD, and around one-quarter will have two or more coexisting disorders.

➤ ADHD can lead to considerable cognitive and behavioural impairments affecting social behaviour, schoolwork and family life. In adults, problems include high crime rates and addiction.

➤ Neuroimaging showed small differences in the structure and functioning of the brain between people with and without ADHD. However, these differences are nonspecific and cannot be used to diagnose ADHD.

Practice Management

➤ For children and young people, the current guidelines specify that a diagnosis requires a full assessment completed by a specialist within secondary care and that PCPs should not diagnose or initiate treatment for ADHD. The specialist is also required to differentiate ADHD from other developmental and mental health diseases as well as evaluate for comorbid disorders.

➤ The specialist is defined by the National Institute for Health and Care Excellence (NICE) as a 'psychiatrist, paediatrician or other health care professional with training and expertise in the diagnosis of ADHD'. Currently, in the majority of cases, PCPs will initiate referral to secondary care services or to the Child and Adolescent Mental Health Service (CAMHS).

➤ Although recent reports indicate limited recognition by PCPs of ADHD cases, mainly because of lack of training and education, GP knowledge is better already, and it is hoped in the future that with necessary training, a primary care ADHD specialist will be created to take over assessment and treatment, particularly if patients have been known to the practice for a long period and are without psychiatric or physical disability.

➤ Preschool children with ADHD: Primary treatment consists of parental training on social skills and stress management to decrease the child's ADHD symptoms and improves social skills.

➤ For school-age children, CBT and computer-based cognitive training programmes are available, in addition to social skill training and behavioural modification techniques. CBT is generally reserved for those who do not adequately respond to medication or choose not to take them. Parents should also be offered a group-based parent training/education programme. Daily behavioural report cards reduce teacher-rated ADHD symptoms and improve academic outcomes.

➤ In addition, since 2008, there has been a rapid expansion in the number of specialist clinics in England and Wales for ADHD and autism, but waiting times are still very long, and a lot of parents will decide to go to the private sector.

➤ Healthcare professionals should stress the value of a balanced diet, reducing screen time and ensuring regular exercise. The strict elimination of artificial colouring and additives from the diet are not recommended unless these appear to influence behaviour. *If they do, then a referral to a dietitian is indicated.*

➤ Drug treatment, although effective, should always form part of a comprehensive treatment plan that includes psychological, behavioural and educational advice and interventions. That is the mainstay of treating ADHD, according to national and international guidelines.

➤ As indicated, drug treatment should be initiated by a specialist trained in the diagnosis and management of ADHD, taking into consideration the BNF reference for recommended drugs for ADHD doses, interactions and side-effects.

➤ Despite the estimated high prevalence of ADHD of around 5%, the prescription rates are less than 1%. Recently, concerns have been raised regarding over-diagnosing children and adults with ADHD and over-prescribing the medication, especially in the private sector.

ADHD Support Group

National Attention Deficit Disorder Information and Support Service, ADDISS. www.addiss.co.uk. Email: info@addiss.co.uk. Tel: 020 8952 2800

ANXIETY DISORDERS

➤ Anxiety is a sustained state of elevated apprehension, arousal and vigilance that occurs in the absence of a clear and immediate danger. It is associated with lower cognitive performance, academic underachievement, sleep disturbance, functional impairment and increased risk of other psychiatric disorders (Box 3.6).

BOX 3.6 Major features of anxiety disorders

- Generalized anxiety disorder is characterized by excessive, difficult to control, diffuse anxiety, accompanied by insomnia, difficulty in concentration, irritability, fatigue and muscle tension.
- Separation anxiety disorders producing common statements such as:
  > I am afraid to go anywhere without my parents.
  > I am afraid that my parents will leave and never come back.
  > I am afraid something bad will happen and I'll never see my parents again.
  > I want my parents with me when I go to bed.
  > I get frightened if my parents leave the house without me.
- Social anxiety disorder, also called social phobia, is the overwhelming fear of social situations such as meeting new people or socializing.
- Selective mutism: Language competence in some situations but not in others.
- Generalized anxiety disorders: Fear/worry about everyday events and problems.
- Panic disorders: Repeated and unexpected panic attacks producing physical symptoms such as sweating and palpitations.
- Specific phobias: Persistence of unreasonable fear associated with a specific object or situations that are causing clinically significant distress:
  > Blood, injections, or injury.
  > Agoraphobia: Fear of leaving home, entering shops, crowds and public places and open places.

➤ Among young people, anxiety disorders have the highest prevalence, with as many as one in ten youngsters meeting the criteria for an anxiety disorder by the age of 16.

➤ Children and young people are at risk of developing anxiety disorders and depression if they experience negative life events such as separation from parents, death of a family member and emotional and physical trauma in early life, including abuse. Heritability of anxiety disorders is in the range of 30–60%.

➤ Anxiety subgroups include various forms of phobias (such as agoraphobia), obsessive-compulsive disorder (OCD), social anxiety and post-traumatic stress disorder (PTSD).

➤ OCD is an anxiety disorder characterized by intrusive thoughts that produce apprehension, fear or worry leading to repetitive behaviours. Its incidence in adults is about 2%, and a third to a half of them report the onset of their symptoms in childhood.

➤ The amygdala (the collection of nuclei buried beneath the temporal lobe) shows increased activities with emotional stimuli and has been associated with severe symptoms of childhood anxiety.

Management

➤ Psychotherapy, medication or a combination of them is the current treatment for anxiety.

➤ CBT can effectively treat individuals with anxiety disorders, although specifically focused on social anxiety. It can help the individual recognize anxious feelings and modify them into self-coping.

➤ Selective serotonin reuptake inhibitors (SSRIs) are drugs which have the highest supporting evidence.

➤ Exposure therapy is the current therapy of choice for specific phobias. This involves gradual and increasing the length of times exposed to the feared object or situation by using imaging approaches, phobic stimuli or situations performing the activity, which are more effective in multiple sessions rather than a single one.

DEPRESSION

➤ Depression is defined as a cluster of specific symptoms with associated functional impairment, with a prevalence estimated at 2.8% for children under the age of 13 years and 5.6% for young people aged 13–18 years.

➤ Common presenting symptoms include persistent low mood, diminished ability to feel pleasure and joy, loss of energy, low concentration, disturbed sleep, weight changes, self-injury and suicide. Suicide is the most important consequence of depression, which is the second most common cause of death among people aged between 15 and 29 years.

➤ Aetiological factors are genetic, environmental and neurobiological. Child abuse (sexual, neglect), stressful life events and childhood trauma are major risk factors. Children with a parent suffering from depression are 4–6 times more likely to develop depression.

➤ Recent evidence suggests the presence of dysregulation in the immune and inflammatory systems contributing to depression. Individuals with autoimmune diseases (e.g., rheumatoid arthritis, inflammatory bowel diseases) are more likely to develop comorbid depression. Patients with depression have increased inflammatory markers including interleukin (IL)-1 beta, IL-6, tumour necrosis factor (TNF) alpha and C-reactive protein (CRP). Higher CRP is associated with greater symptom severity. This is likely related to the gut microbiome, which is synthesizing more than 90% of serotonin in the gut.

➤ Assessment of severity of depression in primary care (based on NICE guidelines):
At least one of the following key questions are present on most days, most of the time, for at least 2 weeks:
  ➤ Persistent sadness or low mood
  ➤ Loss of interest and/or pleasure
  ➤ Fatigue or low energy
If any key symptoms are present, the following associated questions should be asked:
  ➤ Poor or increased sleep
  ➤ Poor concentration or indecisiveness
  ➤ Low self-confidence
  ➤ Poor or increased appetite
  ➤ Suicidal thoughts or acts
  ➤ Agitation or slowing of movement
  ➤ Guilt or self-blame

Many GP surgeries use PHQ-9 questionnaires to make a tentative depression diagnosis. The form can be obtained from: https://patient.info/doctor/patient-health-questionnaire-phq-9

Management (Box 3.7)

➤ Healthcare professionals in primary care, schools and other relevant community settings should be trained to detect symptoms of depression to be able to assess children and young people who may be at risk.
➤ Evaluation of children and young people should include psychosocial risk factors: Age, gender, family structure, family history of depression, bullying, any form of abuse (e.g., physical, sexual), comorbidities such as alcohol, any traumatic event and ethnic and cultural factors.
➤ A child or young person should be offered advice on the benefits of regular exercise and encouraged to follow a structured and supervised exercise programme of at least three sessions per week of moderate duration for 45 minutes to 1 hour.

Self-Harm

➤ Self-harm (SH) is defined as non-fatal intentional acts of self-poisoning (prescribed or over-the-counter), used in over 60% of cases, or self-injury (e.g., self-cutting) or less commonly hanging/asphyxiation.

BOX 3.7 Guidelines on the management of depression

- All children and young people with mild depression:
  - ❯ Discuss the choices available of psychological therapies including digital CBT, group CBT or interpersonal psychotherapy (IPT).
  - ❯ If their needs are not met, or for those who do not want intervention, individual CBT or family therapy is offered.
  - ❯ Antidepressants should not be used for the initial treatment.
  - ❯ If these interventions are ineffective within 2–3 months, *referral to CAMHS should be carried out.* Factors that favour watchful waiting include:
  - ❯ No worsening symptoms.
  - ❯ No family history of depression.
  - ❯ Good social support.
  - ❯ Symptoms are intermittent or of less than 2 week's duration.
  - ❯ Patient is not actively suicidal or self-harming.
  - ❯ No disability or mild associated disability.
- All children with moderate-to-severe depression should:
  - ❯ Be assessed by CAMHS.
  - ❯ Receive CBT or family therapy and possibly antidepressant medication as appropriate for them.
- If individual needs are not met:
  - ❯ They should be offered specific psychological therapy (CBT, IPT or short-term family therapy).
  - ❯ Antidepressants should not be offered without psychotherapy. All antidepressant drugs have significant risks when given to children with depression, with the exception of fluoxetine, which is the only antidepressant for which benefits outweigh the risks. Recommended starting dose (child 5–17 years) should be 10 mg daily. This dose can be increased to 20 mg after 1–2 weeks.
  - ❯ Children on antidepressants should be carefully monitored for side effects, and it can take up to 6 weeks for the full effect of treatment to be apparent.
  - ❯ If treatment with fluoxetine is not tolerated, other antidepressants may be considered (e.g., sertraline or citalopram).

(Based on NICE guidelines CG28, published in 2005 and updated in 2019)

➤ SH is a significant and increasing global problem in children and adolescents. It is often repeated in >50%, which is the strongest risk factor for subsequent SH and future suicide.

➤ People with ASD are at high risk of self-injurious behaviours (hand biting, hair pulling, self-cutting), suicidal ideation and suicide.

➤ In a school survey, 13% of young people aged 15 or 16 reported having self-harmed at some time in their lives. In children aged 5–15 years, 1.3% have tried to harm themselves. Risk factors of self-harm are shown in Box 3.8.

BOX 3.8 Risk factors associated with self-harm

- People who are disadvantaged and from a lower socioeconomic background.
- Poor relationship with family members, child–parent conflicts.
- Any form of abuse.
- Previous SH.
- Bullying, cyberbullying.
- Relationship breakdown with friends (also romantic relationships).
- Chronic physical illness, e.g., disability, pain.
- Alcohol, substance abuse.
- Mental illness, e.g., depression, psychosis.
- Stressful events, such as bereavement.

Management Guidelines for Self-Harm in Primary Care

➤ The management of self-harm consists of:
  ➢ Assessment
  ➢ Referral
  ➢ Treatment
➤ All children and young people who have self-harmed should normally be admitted overnight to a paediatric ward and assessed fully the following day by a psychiatric team before discharge. A review in primary care should be offered within 48 hours.
➤ All children and adolescents who have self-harmed should be offered a psychosocial assessment, which should focus on key problems facing the individual. They must also be assessed for the risk of recurrence of SH and risk of suicide.
➤ CBT helps people identify and evaluate ways to deal with emotional experiences and their thinking. Problem-solving therapy (PST) helps individuals with the skills/problem-solving strategies to manage relationships and deal with different emotions. Mentalization-based therapy (MBT) and dialectical behavioural therapy (DBT) have been found effective in reducing the risk of future SH.
➤ NICE guidelines (www.nice.org.uk) provide useful information on initial management of SH and the provision of longer-term support for children and young people aged 8–18 years.
➤ Other supporting organizations include the Royal College of Emergency Medicine and the Royal College of Psychiatrists.

SUBSTANCE ABUSE

➤ The UK has one of the highest rates of recorded illegal drug misuse in the Western world. In particular, the UK has comparatively high rates of heroin and crack cocaine misuse. Cannabis (commonly known as marijuana, weed or pot) is the most likely used drug followed next by cocaine and stimulants such as amphetamine and opioids. Degrees of severity are shown in Table 3.1.
➤ A reported 30–60% substance use disorders (SUDs) are estimated to be hereditary. The risk of developing SUDs correlates with the number of affected first- and second-degree relatives.

TABLE 3.1 Degrees of severity of substance abuse

	Mild	Severe
• Age of starting	• >15 years	• <15 years
• Family history	• No	• Yes
• Type of drug	• Cannabis	• Heroin
• Administration of drug	• Oral, inhalational	• IV
• Circumstance	• Group setting	• Alone
• Frequency	• Occasional, weekend	• Daily
• Premorbid personality	• Happy	• Depressed
• Family support	• Present	• Absent
• School performance	• Good	• Poor
• Recognition of school achievement	• Present	• Absent
• Comorbidities	• No	• Present

➤ ADHD is a potential precursor to SUDs. More than 50% of children with ADHD initiate alcohol intake at an early age and can later engage with other substance misuse.

➤ Risk factors for substance abuse in children and young people include parental use of substances, poor parental monitoring, association with delinquent or substance-using peers, history of being abused, mental health problems, domestic violence, low academic achievement.

➤ About one-third of all cases of hepatitis B, over 90% of hepatitis C and 5.6% of HIV infections in England are associated with injecting drugs.

➤ Substance abuse is defined as a maladaptive pattern of substance use leading to clinically significant impairment or distress as manifested by one of the following (occurring within a 12-month period):

➢ Recurrent substance use resulting in a failure to fulfil major role obligations at work, school or home (e.g., repeated absences or poor work performance).

➢ Recurrent substance use in hazardous situations, e.g., driving a car.

➢ Recurrent substance-related legal problems (e.g., arrest for conduct disorder).

➢ Continued substance use despite persistent or recurrent social or interpersonal problems caused or exacerbated by the effects of the substance abuse (e.g., physical fights). Box 3.9 shows risk factors leading to substance abuse.

BOX 3.9 Some of the risks caused by substance abuse

Behavioural/Social

● Interruption of a child's normal development
● Domestic violence, physical and sexual abuse
● Mental illnesses (depression, anxiety, suicidal attempts)
● Legal problems (arrests, imprisonment)
● Unemployment

Impact on Health

- Substance-related CNS disorders, e.g., psychosis
- Stress-related gastrointestinal disease
- Malnutrition
- Hepatitis B and C, HIV
- Self-harm, death

Education

- Poor school performance
- Expulsion from school
- Isolation, low self-esteem

Management

➤ Children are always innocent; this is why they always need protection to remain happy and healthy. Careful parental monitoring of their children is essential.

➤ Clinicians have the responsibility to perform a health assessment including their physical and mental health issues, their personal, social and educational circumstances, any drug use, what type and how often taken.

➤ Counselling should include recommendation on testing for hepatitis B, C and HIV, immunization (e.g., hepatitis B) as well as insuring appointments with GPs, school nurses or health visitors.

➤ Psychosocial intervention such as CBT. Detoxification for people who are opioid-dependent and who expressed the choice to become abstinent. Methadone (or buprenorphine) is the first-line treatment in opioid detoxification.

➤ NICE guideline "Drug Misuse Prevention" (2017) is comprehensive and for readers who wish more detailed information on this subject.

1. Department of Health. Drug misuse and dependence: UK Guidelines on clinical management. www.nta.nhs.uk/guidelines-clinical-maangement.aspx
2. NICE guideline NG64: Drug misuse prevention: Targeted interventions (NICE 2017). www.nice.org.uk

CONDUCT DISORDERS

➤ A conduct disorder (CD) is a psychiatric disorder defined as a repetitive and persistent pattern of behaviour that violates the basic rights of others or major age-appropriate societal norms or rules. A type of CD is oppositional defiant disorder (ODD). Worldwide prevalence is 3.2% in children and adolescents, with about 70% affecting boys.

➤ CD includes stealing, lying, truancy, delinquency, repeat disobedience and aggressive behaviour toward people and animals, bullying, threatening and destruction of property.
➤ CD can occur in children <10 years of age (childhood onset), aged 10 years and greater (adolescent onset) and ODD, which is characterized by persistently hostile or defiant behaviour outside the normal range but without aggression or antisocial behaviour. The prognosis is particularly poor in childhood-onset disorder because of its likely persistence.
➤ CDs often occur with other disorders such as ADHD and substance use or abuse, depression, learning disability and (rarely) psychosis and autism.
➤ Although CD is moderately hereditary, multiple environmental factors for CDs include marital discord, abusive parents, social isolation, poverty and overcrowding and substance misuse.

Diagnosis is based on the presence of at least three of the following criteria exhibited in the past 12 months, with at least one present in the last 6 months:

➤ Bullies, threatens or intimidates others.
➤ Initiating physical fights.
➤ Use of weapons that can cause serious physical harm to others.
➤ Being physically cruel to people or animals.
➤ Deliberately setting fires.
➤ Stealing while confronting a victim (e.g., mugging or purse snatching).
➤ Rape.
➤ Destroying property.
➤ Breaking into someone else's house.
➤ Often lying to obtain goods or favours.
➤ CDs may cause major problems including:
  ➢ Affecting the child's development.
  ➢ Interference with learning and prospect of employment.
  ➢ Isolation and difficulty making friends.
  ➢ Low self-worth and depression.
  ➢ Disruption of family life, running away from home.
  ➢ Early unprotected sexual activity with the risk of sexually transmitted diseases (STDs) and teenage pregnancies.

Management may include the following steps:

➤ Provision of increased attention and affection to the child with CD from parents who should agree on how to handle their child's behaviour.
➤ Relationship-enhancing strategies such as children and parents spending time and playing together.
➤ Discipline at school and home should be fair and consistent. This will help children to learn to live within the social rules and law.

➤ Children need to be praised and rewarded often, especially if they improve their behaviour.

➤ NICE Guidelines (TA12. www.nice.org.uk) recommend group-based parent-training/education programmes in the management of children with CDs. Individual-based programmes are only recommended where the family's needs are too complex for group-based programmes. These programmes achieve a substantial and sustained change in behaviour.

➤ Methylphenidate, the most frequently prescribed medication for the treatment of ADHD, was found to decrease CD symptoms.

CHAPTER 4

Fever and Common Febrile Infectious Diseases

INTRODUCTION

Fever is a frequent reason for consultation to GP surgeries, estimated to be around 30% of the total visits. When fever is associated with multiple symptoms, it is often considered the dominant symptom, probably because of the prevailing fever phobia among medical professionals and parents. Many decisions concerning investigation and treatment of febrile children are based on the presence of fever alone. One of the most important tasks for primary care clinicians is to differentiate between an ill febrile child who needs prompt attention, such as hospitalization, and a well child who can be sent home. Although antipyretics are usually prescribed and recommended for febrile children, the principal indication for their use is not to reduce body temperature but to make the child comfortable.

Febrile illnesses have their highest incidence in early childhood, less than 5 years of age. The chapter briefly describes the classification and management of fever and some common infectious diseases usually seen in primary care. Some of these diseases are no longer seen because of the protective immunization. It is not intended to describe these common diseases in detail. There are books on childhood infectious diseases on the market for more detailed information.

FEVER

Fever is, by definition, an interleukin-1 (IL-1)–mediated elevation of the thermoregulatory set-point of the hypothalamic centre. In response to an upward displacement of the set-point, an active process occurs in order to reach the new set-point. This is accomplished physiologically by minimizing heat loss with vasoconstriction and by producing heat with shivering.

Clinically, fever is an elevation of body temperature above the normal daily variation (by 1°C [1.8°F] or greater above the mean of the variation). An infant or child is generally considered to have a fever if their body temperature is 38°C or higher. (A slightly lower temperature is accepted as fever if the temperature measurement is taken at the axilla.)

DOI: 10.1201/9781032642888-4

CLASSIFICATION OF FEVER

Fever is classified into three groups (Table 4.1). This classification is clinically useful for further management. For example, an upper respiratory tract infection is the most common cause of fever with localized signs. Urinary tract infection is the most common bacterial cause without localized signs in febrile children.

TABLE 4.1 The principal three classes of fever

Class	Most Common Cause	Usual Duration of Fever
Fever with localized signs	URTI	<1 week
Fever without localizing signs	Viral infection, UTI	<1 week
Fever of unknown origin	Infections, JIA	>1 week

JIA = juvenile idiopathic arthritis; URTI = upper respiratory tract infection; UTI = urinary tract infection.

Fever with Localized Signs (with a Focus)

The most common febrile illnesses encountered in paediatric practice belong to this category. Upper respiratory tract infections (URTIs), including tonsillitis, are the most common causes of infections in childhood and reasons for doctor consultations. Fever is usually of short duration, either because it settles spontaneously (subsequent to a common viral infection) or because a specific treatment (such as an antibiotic) has been administered to treat a bacterial infection, e.g., streptococcal tonsillitis. Diagnosis is usually straightforward and based on the history and physical examination. Investigations are rarely needed.

Fever without Localized Signs (without a Focus)

Fever without a focus (FWF) is defined as an acute febrile illness without an apparent source, which lasts for less than 1 week, and where the history and physical examination fails to find a cause. About 20% of all febrile episodes demonstrate no localized signs on presentation. The most common cause of FWF is a viral infection, mostly occurring during the first few years of life. Such an infection should be considered only after excluding urinary tract infection (second most common cause) and bacteraemia (Box 4.1). Bacteraemia is usually associated with an ill appearance. Bacteraemia indicates the presence of bacteria in the blood, while septicaemia suggests tissue invasion by the bacteria, causing tissue hypoperfusion and organ dysfunction. Neonates, young and ill-looking children and those with immunodeficiency or sickle cell anaemia are more at risk of septicaemia. Primary healthcare clinicians facing a case of FWF must decide who can be safely managed at home and who requires a referral to hospital.

BOX 4.1 Causes of fever without a focus

Common	Uncommon
• Viral infection	• Occult bacteraemia
• UTI	• Drug fever
• Connective tissue/	• Occult abscess
• Autoimmune disease	• Sinusitis
• Post-vaccination	• Brucellosis
	• Malaria

BOX 4.2 Causes of PUO

Infections (60–70%)
- Viral (e.g., Epstein–Barr)
- Sinusitis
- Endocarditis
- Occult abscess
- Endocarditis
- Occult abscess
- Tuberculosis
- Kawasaki's disease
- Brucellosis

Collagen/Vascular (about 20%)
- Juvenile idiopathic arthritis
- Systemic lupus erythematosus
- Kawasaki disease

Malignancy (5%)
- Leukaemia
- Lymphoma
- Neuroblastoma

Miscellaneous (5%)
- Drug fever
- Factitious fever

Undiagnosed (5%)

Pyrexia of Unknown Origin

Pyrexia of unknown origin (PUO) is characterized by fever without a focus to explain the fever, which persists for 1 week or longer and where no cause is found despite a week of basic investigations in hospital. Causes of PUO are listed in Box 4.2.

The patient's history should include a search for animal exposure, ingestion of raw milk or travel abroad; prior use of antibiotics; and exposure to infections or unwell contacts.

Physical examination should include checking for tenderness over the sinuses, bones and muscles and palpation of lymph nodes; eye examination looking in particular for uveitis as an early clue for rheumatoid arthritis; bulbar conjunctivitis for leptospirosis; and choroid tubercles for tuberculosis (TB).

The prognosis of PUO is better in children than in adults, mainly because of the higher incidence of infection and lower incidence of malignancy. Death may occur in just under 5% of patients, primarily due to neoplastic cases.

PRACTICE POINTS

- There is no evidence that fever causes brain damage or that antipyretics prevent febrile seizures. There is also no evidence to suggest that reduction of body temperature reduces morbidity or mortality from a febrile illness. If there is a morbidity or mortality, it comes from the underlying illness and not from the fever.
- Viral infections are the main causes of childhood febrile illnesses in 90–95% of cases and in 40–60% in FWF. It is essential to identify a bacterial cause in the minority of children who may need antibiotics.
- Children with a viral infection often appear well with good eye contact, have reasonable levels of activity and playfulness and are usually eating and drinking satisfactorily. Children <3 months of age and those with immunodeficiency, sickle cell anaemia, asplenia and/or with body temperature >39.5°C should be considered as having bacterial infections until proved otherwise. Empirical antibiotic treatment and referral to hospital should be considered.
- Roseola infantum (caused by human herpesvirus [HHV]-6) is the most common febrile exanthem in children <3 years, occurring in about 30% of children. Onset of fever is abrupt (sometimes triggering a febrile seizure) and characteristically continuous, often with temperatures as high as 40–41°C and without a focus. The temperature usually drops abruptly on the third or fourth day of fever onset, coinciding with the appearance of a rash. Characteristically, the child becomes well and afebrile when the rash erupts.
- While the risk of bacteraemia is negligible with temperatures of 38–39°C, a strong correlation exists between the incidence of bacteraemia and higher temperatures: It is 7% with temperatures of 40–40.5°C, 13% with temperatures of 40.5–41.0°C and 26% with a temperature higher than 41.0°C.

RECURRENT FEBRILE ILLNESSES

➤ Recurrent fevers (RFs) are defined as three or more febrile episodes during a 6-month period, with symptom-free intervals of at least 7 days separating the episodes. Causes are listed in Table 4.2. Infections such as viral URTIs are by far the most common causes of RF in children. These infections occur at irregular intervals and usually resolve within a week.

➤ Recurrent febrile infections are a source of great concern to parents and a common reason to bring children for medical advice. Risk factors for this group are shown in Box 4.3.

➤ It has been estimated that normal young children may have as many as 12–16 infections per year if they attend nursery, 9 infections per year if a sibling attends school, and 6 or 8 per year if the child or a sibling is not at school. Fortunately, these infections decline with age.

TABLE 4.2 Main causes of recurrent fever

Infectious Causes	Non-Infectious Causes
• Viral (URTI, EBV)	• Immune-mediated (CD, SLE)
• Bacterial (UTI, brucella)	• Neoplasms
• Fungal (histoplasmosis)	• Drug fever
• Parasitic (malaria)	• Periodic fever syndromes (see next)
• Relapsing fever (*Borrelia*)	

CD = coeliac disease; EBV = Epstein–Barr virus; SLE = systemic lupus erythematosus; URTI = upper respiratory tract infection.

BOX 4.3 Risk factors predisposing to recurrent fever

- Attending nursery or a sibling attending a nursery or school
- Immunodeficiency, including neutropenia and asplenia, immunoglobulin A (IgA) deficiency, DiGeorge syndrome (thymic hypoplasia)
- Sickle cell anaemia
- Underlying chronic disease such as ciliary immotility
- Neurodisability (e.g., causing aspiration and pneumonitis)
- Left-to-right cardiac shunt
- Genetic causes of periodic fevers

RELAPSING FEVER

➤ Relapsing fever is the term usually applied to RFs caused by numerous species of *Borrelia* and transmitted by lice or ticks. Human body lice transmit *Borrelia recurrentis* (the causative organism of the epidemic louse-borne RF) from infected humans to other humans.

➤ Ticks are the vectors for at least 15 different species of *Borrelia* that acquire it from rodents (rats, mice, squirrels) and cause endemic tick-borne RF. The most well-known tick-borne disease is Lyme disease, caused by *Borrelia burgdorferi* and transmitted to humans by the bite of a tick infected with these bacteria.

➤ Relapsing fever is characterized by rapid onset of high fever, which recurs in paroxysms lasting 3–6 days, followed by an afebrile period of similar duration. In the UK, Lyme disease is still an uncommon infection, but the cases are increasing annually.

PERIODIC FEVER SYNDROMES

➤ Periodic fevers are also relapsing fevers, but tend to have rhythmic recurrences. They are mostly genetic and characterized by organ-specific inflammation causing overlapping symptoms including arthralgia/arthritis, skin rash, abdominal pain, conjunctivitis and occasionally neurological symptoms. Onset of symptoms usually occurs in early childhood and often before the age of 1 year. A summary of periodic fevers is shown in Table 4.3.

➤ Cyclic neutropenia is an autosomal dominant disease, which is easily diagnosed by recognizing the periodicity of symptoms in association with isolated neutropenia every 3 weeks. During the phase of neutropenia, patients often suffer from stomatitis, oral ulcers, fever and lymphadenopathy. When asymptomatic, the neutrophil count is usually normal.

TABLE 4.3 Summary of the main causes of periodic syndromes

Category/ (Inheritance)	Fever Periodicity	Symptom	Diagnosis	Therapy
FMF (AR)	3–6 weeks	Polyserositis, abdominal and chest pain, arthritis	Gene testing	Colchicine, anakinra
CN (AD)	3–4 weeks	Pharyngitis, stomatitis, repeated bacterial infections	Neutrophils < 500	Antibiotic, CSF
TRAPS (AD)	Variable	Muscle cramps, arthralgia	Gene testing	Steroids
HIDS (AR)	4–8 weeks	Abdominal pain, arthralgia, diarrhoea	Gene testing, high IgD	Steroids, statins
PFAPA (familial)	3–4 weeks	Aphthous stomatitis, pharyngitis, lymphadenitis	High inflammatory markers	Steroids, tonsillectomy

AD = autosomal dominant; AR = autosomal recessive; CN = cyclical neutropenia; CSF = colony-stimulating factors; FMF = familial Mediterranean fever; HIDS = hyperimmunoglobulinaemia D and periodic fever; TRAPS = tumour necrosis factor receptor–associated periodic syndrome.

TABLE 4.4 Antipyretic effect of paracetamol doses on fever

Dose	Expected Temperature Reduction (°C)
5 mg/kg	0.3–0.4
10–15 mg/kg	1.2–1.4
20 mg/kg	1.4–1.6

MANAGEMENT OF FEVER

Assessment
History, focusing on:

➤ Onset, duration and the degree of fever recorded at home
➤ Presence of similar symptoms in other family members
➤ Pattern of feeding, degree of activity, playfulness at home
➤ Pre-existing disease
➤ Previous administration of antibiotics

Physical examination, which focuses on:

➤ *Level of activity*: Eye contacts, playfulness, well or ill appearing?
➤ *Skin colour*: Is the colour of the skin, lips and tongue normal? Does the child look pale, or is their skin mottled or ashen? Are lips blue or cracked?
➤ *Respiratory rate*: Are there signs of nasal flaring, tachypnoea? Is the respiratory rate normal for the child? Is there evidence of grunting, intercostal recession or trachial tug?
➤ *Hydration*: Do the child's skin, eyes and mucous membranes appear normal or dry? Is there a reduction in urine output?
➤ *Other*: Does the child have a rash, blanching or a non-blanching?

Investigation, taking into consideration that:

➤ In a child with localized signs of infection, the investigation should be minimal and focusing on a diagnostic test most likely to provide a diagnosis.
➤ In a child without localized signs, urine check for infection is essential.

Measurement of Body Temperature

An ideal thermometer should have the following characteristics:

1. Accuracy, i.e., a reliable thermometer for predicting fever, reflecting core body temperature.
2. Easy and convenient usage by patient and practitioner.
3. Short duration of temperature measurement.
4. Comfort and avoidance of embarrassment.
5. No cross infection.
6. Not influenced by ambient temperature.
7. High safety factor.
8. Low cost and cost-effectiveness.

Common sites for temperature measurements and thermometers are shown in Box 4.4.

BOX 4.4 Measurements of body temperature

● Most hospitals and GP surgeries use the electronic thermometer. The major advantages of these electronic devices are their rapid response and the ease in reading the digital measurement. Each thermometer or site for temperature measurement has numerous advantages and disadvantages:
  ❯ Axilla, although the site has the advantages of being safe, easily accessible and comfortable, it requires supervision, otherwise displacement may occur. Measurement takes longer than at ear tympanic membranes which is not cost-effective, and measurement in this site is inaccurate.

> ❯ Tympanic thermometry appears to provide an accurate assessment of core body temperature in about 2 seconds. In addition, this technique is clean, safe and cost-effective
> ❯ Oral temperature measurement, although accurate reflecting core temperature, it is not recommended in children aged <5 years who have the highest rate of febrile episodes.

TREATMENT OF FEVER

Antipyretics

➤ Antipyretics are mainly used to lower fever and reduce pain. The primary goal of treating febrile children with antipyretics is to improve the overall comfort rather than focusing on lowering body temperature, and thereby reducing the parents' anxiety. Improving the comfort and evaluating for serious illness (usually fever persists without achieving comfort in serious illness) should be the therapeutical goal of fever management.

➤ The choice of antipyretics has been narrowed to paracetamol and ibuprofen following the recommendation against aspirin use. Before that, aspirin had an advantage over paracetamol because of its low cost and its anti-inflammatory effect. Ibuprofen is more expensive and has more side effects than paracetamol. The degrees of fever reduction by paracetamol are shown in Table 4.4. A dose higher than 15 mg/kg/ is not beneficial.

➤ Antipyretics aim to treat symptomatic fever, which may be associated with pain, discomfort, delirium and excessive lethargy. Antipyretics serve here to improve the child's wellbeing and allow the child to take fluid.

➤ In children who are well and playful with minimal symptoms and fever under 39°C, antipyretic medications may not be necessary. This constitutes a substantial proportion of febrile children.

➤ Physical measures such as a cooling fan or tepid sponging are discouraged. These are unnecessary and unpleasant for the child. It is more helpful to keep the room cool and open the windows and not to overdress or overcover the child with blankets.

➤ It is helpful to educate parents and explain to them that fever is there for a reason and can help fight the infection. As long as the child is comfortable and has a fever below 39°C, do not aggressively reduce it. This approach can help to alleviate parental anxiety.

Combining Antipyretics

Many parents expect antipyretics to normalize body temperature and prevent fever recurrence. Antipyretics do no normalize body temperature, and fever continues due to the underlying cause, triggering parental concerns. This can lead to increased antipyretic use, including alternating antipyretics, and increased health service use. Alternating antipyretics is an increasingly common practice among parents. Many health professionals recommend parents use alternate antipyretics, although this practice has many disadvantages listed in Box 4.5.

BOX 4.5 Reasons for not recommending combined antipyretics

- There is a lack of scientific evidence for the safety of this practice.
- The practice may suggest to parents that fever is a grave sign, thus increasing their fever phobia.
- The practice may increase the incorrect dosing, particularly that of ibuprofen.
- There is no evidence that greater antipyretic doses influence the underlying disease or duration of fever.

Indications for Referral

Febrile children should be considered for hospital admission if:

- They are under 3 months of age.
- They appear toxic or ill-looking (irritability, inconsolable crying, lethargy).
- There is a history of PUO or prolonged fever.
- Serious bacterial infection (SBI) is suspected or present.
- They present with bloody diarrhoea, increased abdominal tenderness or drowsiness.
- There are associated skin petechiae.
- An infant has a fever >40°C without a focus.
- The child has their first febrile seizure (FS).
- There is tachypnoea, grunting, rash, headaches or vomiting.
- If there are concerns about parental cooperation and attending a follow-up appointment is not assured.
- They have significant risk factors, such as immunodeficiency or sickle cell anaemia.
- They have abnormal laboratory results such as WBC >20,000 or high C-reactive protein (CRP).
- The patient is a young child with urinalysis suggestive of urinary tract infection (UTI).

VIRAL EXANTHEMS

An exanthem (from Greek, 'a breakout') is defined as a widespread skin eruption usually occurring as a symptom of an acute viral disease (see Table 4.5).

TABLE 4.5 Some clinical characteristics of viral exanthems

Disease	Incubation Time (Days)	Infectious Period (Days)	Characteristics of the Exanthem
Measles	8–12	• 4 before and 4 after the onset of the rash	• The exanthem appears at the peak of symptoms, first behind the ears and then spreads to the face, neck, trunk and extremities. The rash begins to clear on the third day.

(Continued)

TABLE 4.5 Some clinical characteristics of viral exanthems (Continued)

Disease	Incubation Time (Days)	Infectious Period (Days)	Characteristics of the Exanthem
Varicella	10–21	• 2 before the onset of the rash until all vesicles have crusted, or 5–7 days after the start of the rash	• Macules rapidly progressing to papules and to vesicles on the face and scalp (may appear first on the back and trunk), which spread to the trunk and extremities. After 7 days the vesicles begin to crust, and children are no longer infectious.
Rubella	14–21	• 1–2 days before the rash and 3 days after	• The rash usually starts behind the ears before spreading around the head and neck, trunk and legs. The rash fades after 3 days, and usually the child is no longer infectious.
Erythema infectiosum	4–20	• 1–2 days before onset of the rash and probably not infectious after the rash appears	• Starts on the face with a 'slapped cheeks' appearance, resembling scarlet fever. The rash spreads to the trunk and extremities in 1–4 days after onset of the facial rash. It disappears after 2–4 days.
Roseola infantum	5–15 (mean about 10)	• 1–2 days before onset of fever and 1–2 days after the fever subsides	• The rash is pink or red and appears predominately on the neck and trunk, lasting 24–36 hours. Characteristically, the child becomes well and afebrile when the rash erupts.

Measles

Core Messages

➤ Measles is a highly contagious disease, which was one of the leading causes of child mortality and morbidity globally. Mortality rate ranged from 0% to 0.1% in high-income countries to 3% to 30% in low-income countries. Between 2000 and 2019, an estimated 25.5 million deaths were averted due to the remarkable success of vaccination against measles.

➤ Figure 4.1 shows the rapid decline in measles notifications since the introduction of measles vaccination; deaths have declined likewise.

➤ Clinical course:

  ➢ The pre-exanthem stage begins like a common cold, with abrupt fever (from 39° to 40.5°C), sneezing, dry cough and conjunctivitis. About 24 hours prior to the appearance of exanthem, Koplik's spots can be detected in about 80% of cases as tiny, about 1-mm, whitish spots in the buccal mucosa opposite the lower molars, followed by a rash.

  ➢ Pharyngitis, cervical lymphadenopathy and occasionally a mild splenomegaly.

  ➢ The infectivity decreases considerably with the onset of the rash.

  ➢ During the acute and post-measles phases, children are immunosuppressed and susceptible to opportunistic infections, particularly those with malnutrition and vitamin A deficiency, immune deficiency (e.g., HIV infection) and immune suppression (e.g., organ transplant).

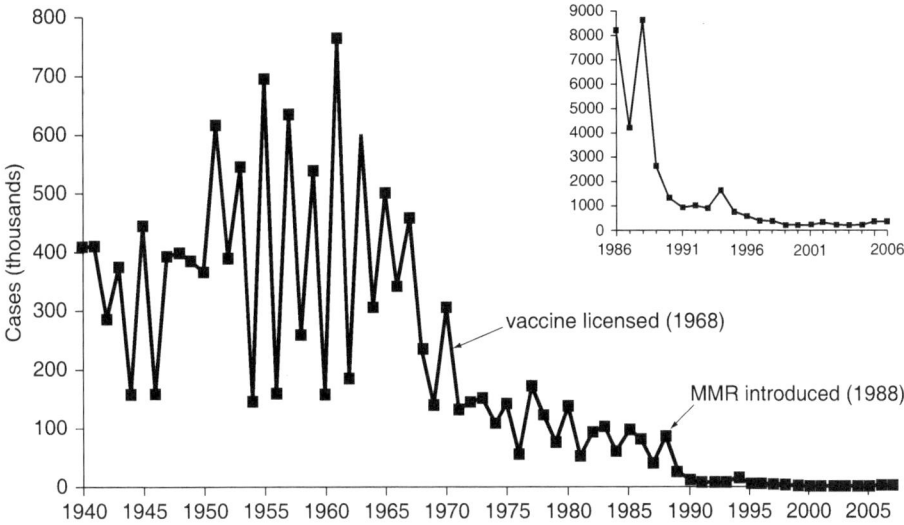

FIGURE 4.1 Measles cases in England and Wales, 1940–2007. There was an increase in the number of confirmed cases of measles in 2009 and a major outbreak in Wales in 2013.

➢ In 1988, the measles-only vaccine was replaced by measles-mumps-rubella (MMR) given at 12–13 months and again at 3–5 years of age (Box 4.6). Contraindications for MMR are shown in Box 4.7.

BOX 4.6 Recent information on MMR vaccine

- MMR are serious diseases that can lead to severe disability and death. Successful herd immunity was achieved for measles in the UK by 2017, reaching the WHO 95% coverage target and resulting in the UK's measles elimination status.
- MMR vaccine effectiveness in preventing measles is 95% after one dose and 96% after two doses.
- MMR outbreaks have occurred in several regions, usually due to suboptimal vaccine coverage. The WHO recommends measles vaccination in infants as early as 6–9 months in areas of measles outbreaks. The vaccine is safe for this age group and produces excellent immune response.
- There is a small increased risk of febrile seizures ranging from 1:1700 to 1:1150 after administered doses of the MMR vaccine.
- In the past few years, immunotherapy has increasingly been used in cancer therapy to improve survival. The MMR vaccine has anticancer activity by activating the host's innate and adaptive antitumour immunity.

BOX 4.7 Contraindications to the MMR vaccine

- Women who are pregnant or trying to conceive (women should be advised to avoid conception within 28 days after vaccination).
- Immunocompromised individuals, including those who are receiving chemotherapy or high doses of steroids, with the exception of HIV-infected patients who have no signs of AIDS.
- People receiving blood products such as immunoglobulin. In this case, MMR administration should be deferred for 3 months.
- Children who are unwell with acute illness. Children with symptoms such as a mild cough or runny nose due to URTI may still receive the MMR vaccine.

Management

➤ Investigations: The diagnosis is mainly clinical, and investigation is usually not required. Full blood count (FBC) often shows leucopoenia and lymphopenia. Measles-specific IgM antibody is diagnostic.
➤ Gamma globulin (0.25 mg/kg) within 5 days of exposure to measles virus prevents the disease and is indicated for certain susceptible individuals including:
  ➤ Immunocompromised patients
  ➤ Pregnant non-immune women
  ➤ Children < 1 year of age
➤ Oral vitamin A (400,000 U) should be given in two doses in 24 hours. It can decrease mortality in children in developing countries and help to avoid eye damage and blindness.
➤ Ribavirin and interferon alpha can be used in severe cases of measles.

Mumps

Core Messages

➤ Mumps is a paramyxovirus infection which begins with swelling and tenderness of one or both parotid glands. About 30–40% of infections are subclinical.
➤ There has been a dramatic reduction in mumps cases since the introduction of MMR vaccination in 1988. Vaccine effectiveness in preventing mumps is 74% after one dose and 86% after two doses.
➤ Following an incubation period of 16–18 days, the parotid swelling peaks in 2–3 days and subsides within 3–7 days. Swelling of the submandibular glands occurs frequently, either accompanying the parotid swelling or alone in about 10% of cases.
➤ The infectious period starts 1 day before the parotid swelling and ends 3 days after the swelling has subsided.
➤ Common complications include the following: Meningoencephalitis occurs in more than 50% of cases, but only 10% of cases are clinically apparent. Orchitis usually occurs within 8 days of the onset of parotitis, mainly in postpubertal boys. The affected testis is tender and swollen. Infertility is rare even with bilateral orchitis. Oophoritis may present as pelvic pain and tenderness, mainly in postpubertal

females. Other less common complications are pancreatitis, arthritis, neural deafness, myocarditis and thyroiditis.

➤ Diagnostic IgM antibodies are detectable within the first few days of infection.

Rubella

Core Messages

➤ The incubation time of rubella is 14–21 days. The infection is usually mild, and children usually present with sore throat, rash (distinctive light-red or pink), lymphadenopathy (prominent in the posterior cervical and suboccipital areas) and low-grade fever (rarely exceeding 38.0–38.5°C) for several days. The infectious period is 1–2 days before the rash appears.

➤ In older children, particularly in females after puberty, the infection is more severe and prolonged. There are usually painful and visibly enlarged lymph nodes, involving postauricular, occipital and posterior cervical nodes, with polyarthralgia or arthritis.

➤ Infection with rubella virus is particularly important to diagnose because of possible fetal-maternal transmission causing congenital rubella syndrome (Box 4.8).

➤ Prevention of maternal rubella used to be through routine vaccination of all girls aged 11–14 years and women of childbearing age. The use of the MMR vaccine has been very successful in preventing congenital and acquired rubella. Outbreaks still occur in developing countries where vaccination is not widespread.

➤ Contraindications to MMR vaccination are shown in Box 4.9.

BOX 4.8 Congenital rubella syndrome

This syndrome may occur if a mother is infected within the first 20 weeks of pregnancy, particularly during the early weeks. It manifests as:

- Eye disease
- Auditory
- Heart
- Hepatic
- Neurological
- Blood

- Cataract, retinopathy, glaucoma
- Sensorineural deafness
- Pulmonary stenosis, patent ductus arteriosus
- Hepatitis
- Microcephaly, neurodisability
- Thrombocytopenic purpura, anaemia

Varicella

Core Messages

➤ Varicella, caused by varicella-zoster virus (VZV), is highly infectious via the respiratory route, causing two distinct clinical syndromes: Varicella resulting from a primary infection and herpes zoster resulting from reactivation of the virus. Figure 4.2 shows a typical skin rash of varicella.

➤ Varicella is usually a benign disease, although complications can occur, including skin and soft tissue staphylococcal infection, respiratory (e.g., pneumonia in about 1%),

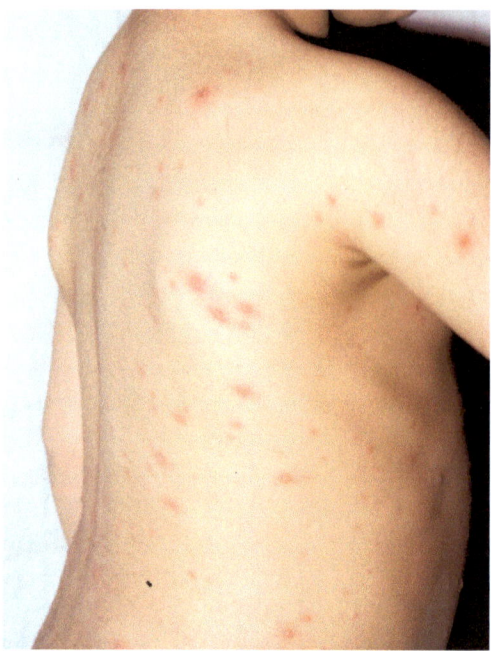

FIGURE 4.2 Typical rash of varicella infection

thrombocytopenic purpura, cerebellar ataxia and encephalitis. The World Health Organization (WHO) estimates that VZV is responsible for 4.2 million severe complications and 4200 related deaths globally.

➤ In patients with impaired cellular immunity and those receiving cytotoxic drugs, varicella is often severe and may be fatal. Severe varicella occurs in children with leukaemia and lymphoma, and the mortality is about 20%. Children with hypogammaglobulinaemia recover normally from varicella.

➤ When maternal varicella develops within 4 days of delivery, neonates develop severe varicella within 5–10 days postpartum (Box 4.9).

BOX 4.9 Congenital varicella infections

● Infection with varicella during pregnancy may produce congenital varicella syndrome (e.g., skin scarring and loss, microcephaly, cataracts, limb malformation). The risk of infection is highest if the infection occurs within the first 20 weeks of pregnancy.

● Delivery within 1 week before or after the onset of maternal varicella infection may cause severe infection within 5–10 days postpartum. The disease is associated with a mortality of around 20% due to disseminated chickenpox, usually with severe pneumonitis. The disease requires varicella-zoster immunoglobulin (VZIG) and aciclovir.

● If there was an interval of >1 week between maternal varicella and parturition, neonates receive sufficient protective transplacental antibody to the virus.

● For these reasons, pregnant women with unknown immunity to VZV should have their VZV IgG status checked.

Management

➤ The majority of patients require no special treatment. Itching can be relieved by simple soothing lotions such as calamine and oral antihistamine. Fever is managed with paracetamol. Aspirin should not be administered because of the risk of Reye's syndrome. Ibuprofen is contraindicated, as it has been linked to developing secondary skin infections.

➤ Patients with severe varicella or with complications should receive aciclovir. This antiviral drug reduces the duration of fever.

➤ Zoster (shingles) can be treated with oral aciclovir within 72 hours of onset of symptoms. This can reduce the duration of viral shedding and postherpetic neuralgia.

➤ VZIG is recommended for those who test seronegative within 10 days (ideally within 7 days) of exposure to VZV. The duration of protection is 3 weeks. VZV vaccination information is shown in Box 4.10.

BOX 4.10 Information on varicella-zoster-virus (VZV) vaccination

● Two varicella vaccines have been licensed in the UK since 2003 for use in susceptible individuals: Varilrix (Glaxo SmithKline) and Varivax (Aventis Pasteur MSD). Both vaccines contain live attenuated VZV.

● Two doses of vaccine are given 4–8 weeks apart and provide 75% protection against varicella and over 90% protection against severe infection. Immunity may wane over time, causing a mild varicella if exposed to VZV.

● At present, varicella vaccine is not offered routinely in the UK, but it may be given to:
  › Close contacts of varicella who are at high risk of complications from varicella or zoster.
  › High-risk children within 3 days of exposure to chickenpox. Varivax (but not Varilrix) is licensed for postexposure prophylaxis.

● Approval for the quadrivalent measles–mumps–rubella–varicella (MMRV) vaccine occurred in 2005 in the United States and in 2006 in Europe. The vaccination is very effective at reducing varicella.

Erythema Infectiosum (Slapped Cheeks)

Core Messages

➤ Erythema infectiosum, or fifth disease, is an acute benign, communicable disease caused by parvovirus B19. It usually affects children aged 5–15 years.

➤ The rash is diagnostic (Figure 4.3), with bright red cheeks, often followed by a lacy rash spreading onto the trunk. There may be mild flulike prodromal symptoms. Complications from parvovirus are uncommon and are shown in Box 4.11.

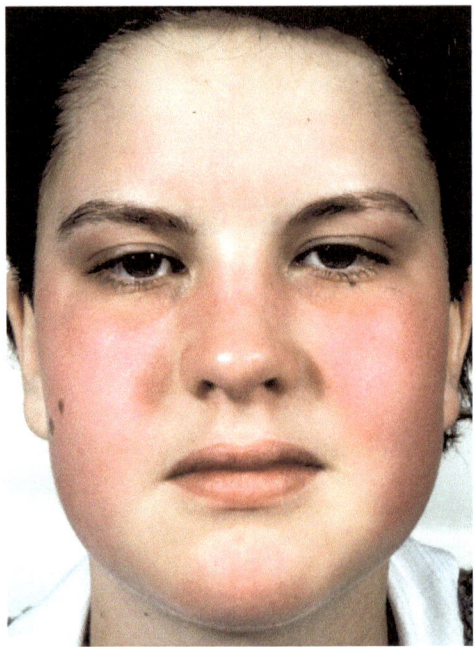

FIGURE 4.3 Example of a child with erythema infectiosum (slapped cheek) or fifth disease.

BOX 4.11 Complications of parvovirus infection in pregnancy

Arthritis	● Often symmetrical, affecting the wrists, hands, knees and ankles. It usually resolves within a few days. In some cases it may persist for 2 months or longer, causing diagnostic difficulty in differentiating it from juvenile idiopathic arthritis. Arthritis is seen mainly in female adults.
Aplastic anaemia	● A transient anaemia affecting particularly those with chronic haemolytic anaemia such as thalassaemia, sickle cell anaemia and spherocytosis.
Fetal hydrops	● Miscarriage and fetal loss in non-immune pregnant women
CNS infection	● Rarely meningitis, encephalitis or neuropathy.

Roseola Infantum (Exanthema Subitum)

Core Messages

➤ Herpes human virus-6 is a ubiquitous DNA virus that has two distinct species: HHV-6A and HHV-6B. Following primary infection, it remains latent within lymphocytes, monocytes and bone marrow cells. Its reactivation is responsible for a variety of diseases in immunocompetent and immunocompromised people (Box 4.12).

➤ Roseola infantum (RI) (sixth disease) is caused by HHV-6, identified in 1988 and, less commonly, by HHV-7. The virus is recognized as a major cause of febrile illness, with viraemia and a high temperature (40.0°C and higher), sometimes with viral rash (Box 4.12).

➤ RI is the most common febrile exanthem in children under the age of 3 years. Approximately 30% of children develop this disease, most commonly aged 6–24 months.

➤ Children with RI may develop a short period of irritability and malaise before the onset of fever, which is abrupt (sometimes triggering a febrile seizure in 10–15% of cases) and characteristically continuous, with temperatures often as high as 40–41°C. Fever usually persists for 3–4 days in about 75% of cases and for 5–6 days in the remaining 25%. The temperature usually drops over a period of a few hours, coinciding with the appearance of the rash.

➤ Clinical findings include mild pharyngitis and suboccipital or posterior cervical lymphadenopathy.

➤ Laboratory findings commonly show leukocytosis of 12,000–20,000 with a slight increase in neutrophils.

➤ HHV-6 is not sensitive to acyclovir but is sensitive to ganciclovir and foscarnet.

BOX 4.12 Manifestations and possible complications of HHV-6

● **In immunocompetent** • Febrile illness, roseola infantum, febrile seizures, ophthalmic diseases (e.g., uveitis), encephalitis, hepatitis, myocarditis, temporal lobe epilepsy, multiple sclerosis, PUO

● **In immunocompromised** • Post-transplant (e.g., haemopoietic or organ) severe encephalitis, pneumonitis, hepatitis

---

BACTERIAL DISEASES

Meningococcal Disease

Meningism

➤ Neck stiffness, or meningism, refers to an abnormal position of the neck or restricted range of movement and is usually associated with pain with passive and active movements.

➤ Meningism is extremely important and requires immediate evaluation because of the possibility of infection (Box 4.13). Non-infectious causes include torticollis (wry neck), sleeping in an awkward position and dystonic drug reaction. In contrast to children with non-infectious meningism, those with an infectious cause usually look ill and have a fever.

BOX 4.13 Some causes of stiff neck (meningism)

Infectious • Meningitis, pneumonia (particularly an upper lobe pneumonia), upper respiratory tract infections with lymphadenitis

Non-infection • Muscular torticollis, congenital abnormality of the cervical spine, dystonia (e.g., caused by drugs), hysteria, Sandifer's syndrome (gastro-oesophageal reflux)

Presentation (Box 4.14)

➤ Meningococcal disease (MCD) has two main clinical presentations: Meningitis and septicaemia, which may occur together. Septicaemia is more common, sudden and unpredictable and progresses more rapidly and more dangerously than meningitis. Septicaemia is associated with high mortality and long-term sequelae among survivors.

➤ Factors that increase the risk of MCD are shown in Box 4.15.

BOX 4.14 Assessment and management of children with suspected MCD

Presentation

- Symptoms/signs of meningitis and septicaemia are nonspecific: Viral-like symptoms with fever, vomiting, lethargy, irritability, headache, myalgia, arthralgia, leg pain, bulging fontanelle.
- More specific symptoms/signs: In the early stages, the rash may be blanching and maculopapular, but it nearly always develops into a non-blanching, petechial rash within 8–9 hours after onset. The child appears ill with tachycardia and tachypnoea, with or without neck stiffness, and prolonged capillary refill time (CRT).

Level of Consciousness Using AVPU

- Alert
- Responding to Voice
- Responding to Pain
- Unresponsive

CRT

- Press for 5 seconds on the big toe, finger or sternum.
- Count the seconds it takes for the skin to return to normal.
- If the CRT >2 seconds, the possibility of MCD should be considered.

Prehospital Treatment with IV or IM Penicillin

- Adults and children aged 10 years or older: 1200 mg
- Children 1–9 years: 600 mg
- Infants: 300 mg

BOX 4.15 Factors that increase the risk of MCD

- Infants <1 year
- Immunodeficiency (HIV, organ transplant)
- Asplenic patients
- People on high doses of steroids
- Complement defects (C5–C9)
- The use of complement inhibitor drugs such as ravulizumab
- Microbiologist dealing with *Neisseria meningitis*
- Chronic diseases (e.g., type 1 diabetes, renal insufficiency)
- People travelling/living in areas where *N. meningitis* is endemic

Prevention

➤ Vaccination is the most effective method for preventing the disease (Table 4.6).

TABLE 4.6 Scheduled meningitis vaccinations

Vaccine	Vaccination Programme	Reported Reactions
MenB	• 1st dose: 8 weeks • 2nd dose: 16 weeks • Booster at 1 year	*Local at injection site*: Pain, swelling, redness
MenC	• 1st dose: 1 year of age (as Hib/MenC)	*Generalized reactions*: Chills, fatigue, malaise, headache, myalgia, nausea, arthralgia diarrhoea
MenACWY	• 14 years	

PRACTICE POINTS

- If meningeal infection is suspected, IM antibiotics should be administered prior to hospital transfer. Benzyl penicillin should be carried in GP emergency bags.
- For suspected meningitis without a rash, NICE recommends urgent transfer without giving antibiotics, mainly to enable administration of dexamethasone within 4 hours of the first dose of antibiotics and because the disease progresses more slowly than septicaemia.
- If urgent transfer to hospital is not possible (e.g., in remote locations or if adverse weather conditions), then antibiotics should be administered in primary care.
- Antibiotics can be administered via IV or IM. Penicillin is withheld if the patient has a clear history of penicillin anaphylaxis. A history of a rash following penicillin is not a contraindication.
- Primary healthcare professionals should identify and treat those close contacts who were exposed to large particle/droplet secretions from the respiratory tract of the patient.
- All children should have a review with a paediatrician 4–6 weeks after hospital discharge.
- Late-onset sensory, neurological, orthopaedic and psychosocial effects of MCD may not become evident until years after the illness. These include:
  - Hearing loss: A hearing assessment should be carried out as soon as possible.
  - Neurodisability including learning, motor and neuro-developmental deficit and epilepsy.
  - Psychological and behavioural problems including post-traumatic stress disorder.

Scarlet Fever

➤ The incidence of scarlet fever in the UK declined from 1940s to the mid-2010s but increased markedly thereafter. There were more than 30,000 reported cases in 2018, the highest number in nearly 50 years.

➤ Scarlet fever is caused by certain strains of haemolytic streptococci in the throat producing an erythrogenic toxin. It can also be caused by streptococcal skin infection. It mostly affects children aged 5–15 years. The incubation time is 2–4 days. The disease is notifiable in the UK. The infections have long been recognized to cause outbreaks in schools and nurseries.

➤ Onset is usually sudden with fever (temperature usually ranges from 39° to 40.5°C), sore throat (tonsillitis often with petechiae on the palate), vomiting and headaches.

➤ A rash appears typically on the second day of illness and is characterized by an erythematous punctiform eruption that blanches on pressure and spares the area around the mouth (circumoral pallor). It appears typically on the neck and chest, later on the trunk and legs. The rash is more prominent in skin creases, with confluent petechiae. The skin feels rough to the touch.

➤ Initially the tongue has a thick white coating, which develops in a few days into typical strawberry tongue. There might be tonsillitis with exudates with cervical lymphadenopathy.

➤ From 6 to 10 days after the eruption, peeling (desquamation) begins and usually lasts several weeks.

➤ Apart from the rash and the tongue, there is essentially no difference between streptococcal tonsillitis, viral tonsillitis (including Epstein–Barr virus [EBV] infectious mononucleosis) and scarlet fever. Normal throat culture for streptococci and anti-streptolysin O (ASO) titres favour a viral aetiology. Scarlet fever can be differentiated from Kawasaki's disease by an older age at onset, absence of conjunctival involvement and rapid response to penicillin (Box 4.16).

➤ Complications include peritonsillar or retropharyngeal abscess, acute rheumatic fever, glomerulonephritis, meningitis, otitis media osteomyelitis and arthritis.

BOX 4.16 Antibiotic therapy for children with scarlet fever

- Birth to 6 months: Oral clarithromycin for 10 days
- Non-pregnant adults and children aged 6 months to 17 years: Azithromycin for 5 days or clarithromycin for 10 days
- Pregnant or postpartum (within 28 days of childbirth): Erythromycin for 10 days
- Children should not return to school or nursery until 24 hours after starting antibiotic treatment.
- In addition to prompt antibiotic treatment, good hand hygiene and disinfection of households such as toys is recommended.

Tuberculosis

Core Messages

➤ After four decades of steady decline in the incidence of tuberculosis (TB), the annual case rate levelled off in 1985 and has increased since then. In 2019 an estimated 10 million people globally had TB, including a total of 550,000 cases of childhood TB, with around 80,000 deaths. Less than half of the children with TB were diagnosed and treated.

➤ Children usually acquire the infection from adults who have active disease and are expectorating tubercle bacilli. Children themselves are usually non-contagious; therefore every effort should be made to identify the adult source to enable eradication of the source bacilli.

➤ In older children, primary infection is asymptomatic in most cases. Radiologically, a parenchymal lesion is usually not visible, but hilar adenitis is prominent and may cause compression of the adjacent soft bronchus, causing wheezing and nonproductive cough. With increased compression, or following perforation of an infected lymph node into the bronchus, segmental atelectasis may ensue.

➤ Other presentations are erythema nodosum, phlyctenular conjunctivitis, and miliary TB, which presents with no specific symptoms and signs such anorexia, weight loss, night sweats and dyspnoea. Ophthalmoscopy may detect typical choroidal tubercle.

➤ Neonatal TB occurs through vertical transmission of infection from mother to infant via the placenta or amniotic fluid. Neonates present with feeding difficulty, failure to thrive, jaundice, respiratory distress or hepatosplenomegaly. Chest x-ray shows bronchopneumonia.

➤ HIV infection may occur in association with TB, which presents as unresolving pneumonia. The infection carries a high mortality rate despite adequate anti-TB and anti-HIV therapy.

Diagnosis

➤ Confirmed TB requires *Mycobacterium tuberculosis* to be confirmed by culture or nucleic acid amplification test (NAAT), such as Xpert MTB/RIF assay (Box 4.17). This test simultaneously detects *Mycobacterium* and resistance to rifampicin.

➤ Unconfirmed TB: Bacterial confirmation is not obtained despite the presence of symptoms/signs as well as radiological evidence suggestive of TB.

➤ Unlikely TB: This is a case without bacteriological confirmation of TB and with criteria for confirmation not met.

BOX 4.17 The diagnosis of TB

● History of contact with an infectious case
● Signs/Symptoms suggestive of TB:
  ❯ Persistent cough >2 weeks, unremitting cough
  ❯ Weight loss/failure to thrive, including an unexplained weight loss or drop in the growth centile
  ❯ Low-grade fever

> ⟩ Identification of *Mycobacteria* (positive in about 30–40% of cases) from sputum, gastric fluid, pleural fluid, CSF or other tissues, or by polymerase chain reaction (PCR). Acid-fast smear is positive in 10–20% of cases, A molecular test (NAAT) is more sensitive than smear microscopy.
> ⟩ Chest x-ray: 'Unresolved pneumonia', with enlarged mediastinal lymphadenopathy.
> ⟩ Positive tuberculin test (Figure 4.4).

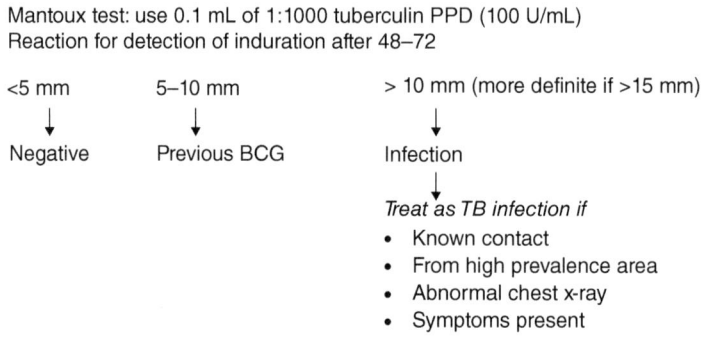

FIGURE 4.4 Diagnosis of tuberculosis by the outcomes of a Mantoux test.

Management

➤ Bacille Calmette–Guérin (BCG) vaccination has been used since 1921 and has been shown to give 70–80% protection against TB but is less effective in adults. The BCG vaccine is no longer given as part of the routine childhood vaccination schedule, but only to those children considered at risk of developing TB (Box 4.18). BCG vaccine administered intravenously has recently been found to provide superior protection from TB compared to intradermal BCG.

➤ Drugs used for treatment of TB are shown in Box 4.19. A 6-month regimen for drug-susceptible TB with isoniazid (INH), rifampicin and pyrazinamide for the first 2 months followed by INH and rifampicin for the remaining 4 months is recommended. If drug resistance is possible, initial treatment should include ethambutol, streptomycin, amikacin or ciprofloxacin until a drug susceptibility result becomes available. Recent evidence supports the use of a 4-month treatment regimen combining these drugs in the initial phase and has shown similar efficacy and safety compared to the current standard regimen of 6 months.

BOX 4.18 Indications for BCG vaccination

BCG vaccination is offered to:

- All infants living in areas of the UK where the annual incidence of TB is ≥40/100,000.
- All infants with a parent or grandparent who was born in a country where the annual incidence of TB is ≥40/100,000.
- Previously unvaccinated children aged 1–5 years with a parent or grandparent who was born in a country where the annual incidence of TB is ≥40/100,000.
- Previously unvaccinated tuberculin-negative children aged from 6 to under 16 years of age with a parent or grandparent who was born in a country where the annual incidence of TB is ≥40/100,000.
- Previously unvaccinated tuberculin-negative individuals under 16 years of age who are contacts of cases of respiratory TB.
- Previously unvaccinated, tuberculin-negative individuals under 16 years of age who were born in or have lived for at least 3 months in a country with an annual TB incidence of ≥40/100,000.

BOX 4.19 Standard treatment of TB for 6 months

- Isoniazid
- Rifampicin
- Pyrazinamide
- Ethambutol

- 10 mg/kg once daily for 6 months (maximal dose 300 mg)
- 15 mg/kg once daily for 6 months (maximal dose 600 mg)
- 35 mg/kg once daily for 6 months
- 20 mg/kg once daily for 2 months

Malaria

Core Messages

➤ Malaria is caused by protozoal infection transmitted by *Anopheles* mosquitoes. The four species of protozoa that commonly infect humans are *Plasmodium vivax*, *Plasmodium ovale* (benign tertian malaria), *Plasmodium falciparum* (malignant tertian malaria) and *Plasmodium malariae* (benign quartan malaria).

➤ The number of malaria cases and deaths is estimated at 200–300 million and around 400,000 people, respectively. About 70% of all malarial deaths occur in children under the age of five years. *P. falciparum*, the most prevalent malaria parasite in Africa and much of Asia, is responsible for cerebral malaria and the overwhelming majority of malarial deaths.

➤ Most cases of malaria imported to the UK are *P. falciparum* (about three-quarters of cases) and *P. vivax*, with 1500–2000 cases each year (total number of cases of all forms).

➤ *Plasmodium* is an intracellular pathogen that directly invades two cell types in humans:

➤ Hepatocytes, where they replicate for 7 days, then rupture into the bloodstream.

➤ Erythrocytes, where they replicate over 48 hours before rupturing out as merozoites capable of invading new erythrocytes.

➤ Typical symptoms include paroxysm of fever, lethargy, headache, cough, anorexia, vomiting, diarrhoea and abdominal pain. Physical examination reveals pallor, splenomegaly (detected in almost 100% of cases) and hepatomegaly. The presenting symptoms of *P. falciparum* infection are an irregular pattern of fever, severe headache, irritability, delirium, coma, hyperpyrexia, convulsion and meningism. Infection is most likely to occur within 3 months of return from malaria-endemic areas, especially if antimalarial prophylaxis has been inadequate or not taken.

➤ A typical tertian paroxysm (*P. vivax* and *P. ovale*) is characterized by fever with rigour, which often triggers febrile seizures. The next stage is marked by high fever, up to a temperature of 41°C. In tertian infection, the paroxysm recurs at 48-hour intervals, while in quartan infection, the paroxysm recurs at 72-hour intervals. The third stage is characterized by a drop in body temperature to normal, with sweating.

➤ Malaria can present as PUO only, without other associated signs such as anaemia or splenomegaly.

Complications include the following:

➤ Malaria has significant effects on the QT interval that are proportional to disease severity. Several antimalarial drugs are associated with QT interval prolongation. Drug-related QT interval prolongation is a potential risk for ventricular arrhythmia.

➤ Nephrotic syndrome may occur with *P. malariae* infection.

➤ Blackwater fever, a state of acute intravascular haemolysis accompanied by haemoglobinuria, may occur as a complication of *P. falciparum*.

➤ Human parvovirus B19 infection may occur, adding to the severity of anaemia. This virus is highly erythrotropic, infecting erythroid progenitor cells.

Diagnosis

➤ Diagnosis is easy when children present with typical paroxysms of fever. Children may, however, present with non-specific symptoms such as sore throat, pallor, myalgia and gastrointestinal and respiratory symptoms.

➤ Definitive diagnosis is made via Giemsa-stained blood smear (thick and thin smears), which are used in addition to the blood slides.

➤ Laboratory findings include anaemia, with Hb concentrations of 50–110 g/L, and leukopenia. Thrombocytopenia, hyponatraemia and hypoglycaemia may also occur.

Management

➤ All countries with endemic *P. falciparum* malaria have updated their treatment policy from monotherapy with drugs such as chloroquine, amodiaquine and sulfadoxine–pyrimethamine to the currently recommended artemisinin-based combination therapy (ACT), which is highly effective, well tolerated (Box 4.20) and unlikely to cause drug resistance. Currently, all episodes of malaria should be treated with at least two antimalarial medications.

➤ Treatment of *P. vivax* or *P. ovale*:
  ➢ Primaquine 0.5 mg/kg/day is recommended.
  ➢ Oral 3-day course of chloroquine, which can be used for benign malaria.

BOX 4.20 First-line treatment for malaria

- Artemether–lumefantrine (AL)
- Artesunate–amodiaquine (AS+AQ)
- Artesunate–mefloquine (ASMQ)
- Dihydroartemisinin–piperaquine (DAP)
- Artesunate–pyronaridine (ASPY)
- Artesunate–sulfadoxine–pyrimethamine (AS+SP)

Prophylaxis of Malaria

➤ Malaria vaccine (2021): RTS,S/ASO1 malaria vaccine should be used for the prevention of *P. falciparum* malaria in children living in regions with moderate-to-high transmission as defined by the WHO.

➤ Malarone Pediatric tablets should be started 1–2 days before entering a malaria-endemic area and continued for 1 week after leaving:
  ➢ 1 tablet daily for 3 days for a body weight of 11–21 kg.
  ➢ 2 tablets once daily for 3 days for a body weight of 21–31 kg.
  ➢ 3 tablets once daily for 3 days for a body weight of 31–40 kg.
  ➢ 4 tablets once daily for 3 days for a body weight over 40 kg.
  ➢ Travelers should be warned about the importance of avoiding mosquito bites, of taking prophylaxis regularly and seeking medical assessment urgently if a child becomes ill within 1 year and especially within 3 months of return from the malaria-endemic area.
  ➢ Proguanil is usually used with chloroquine (only occasionally alone) for the prophylaxis of malaria. The drug(s) should be used 1 week before entering a malaria-endemic area and continued for 4 weeks after leaving.
  ➢ Some drugs used for prophylaxis and treatment of malaria, in particular primaquine, should not be administered before checking for glucose-6-phosphate dehydrogenase (G6PD) deficiency status. This drug can cause severe haemolysis in case of deficiency.

Brucellosis

➤ Brucellosis is primarily a zoonotic infection caused by small, non-motile, gram-negative coccobacilli of the genus *Brucella.*

➤ There are four important species pathogenic to humans: *B. melitensis* (Malta fever, found primarily in goats and sheep), *B. abortus* (abortus fever, in cattle), *B. suis* (swine) and *B. canis* (dogs).

➤ The infection is transmitted to humans through direct contact with infected animals or their products and through consumption of infected milk, milk products or meat. More than half a million cases per year occur worldwide.

➤ Clinically, brucellosis is characterized by the following features:

   ➢ Symptoms and signs include fever, arthritis, arthralgia, backache, anorexia and weight loss, tender hepatosplenomegaly and lymphadenopathy. These symptoms and signs are more severe with *B. melitensis*.

   ➢ Fever occurs in almost every patient (90–100% of cases), often insidiously over the course of several days. Fever may also manifest as periodic fever, with symptoms lasting a few days or weeks followed by symptom-free intervals that last weeks and months, or as PUO.

➤ Complications include spondylitis, osteomyelitis, granulomatous reaction of the eye, meningitis or meningo-encephalitis. *Brucella* endocarditis is rare and may be responsible for the majority of deaths due to the disease.

Laboratory Findings

➤ FBC, looking for anaemia, leukopenia and lymphopenia

➤ Liver function tests: Raised liver enzymes

➤ The diagnosis is established by positive culture of *Brucella* organisms from blood or bone marrow aspirate or positive serological tests (agglutination titre of >1:80).

Management

Antibiotics are the cornerstone of management:

➤ In children >12 years of age, a combination of doxycycline 5 mg/kg/day BID for 3 weeks plus gentamicin 5 mg/kg/day IM for the first 5 days is the recommended therapy.

➤ In children <12 years of age, a combination of trimethoprim–sulfamethoxazole (Septrin) for 3 weeks and a 5-day course of gentamicin IM are the recommended therapy.

➤ Rifampicin has also been used successfully in combination with streptomycin in the treatment of *Brucella* endocarditis.

Lyme Disease

Core Messages

➤ Lyme disease (LD) is a multisystem inflammatory disease caused by the spirochete *Borrelia burgdorferi*. It is transmitted by infected ticks. There are around 3000 cases of new confirmed Lyme disease in the UK each year.

➤ LD is divided into three stages:
  ➣ The first stage occurs 3–30 days after the tick bite and is characterized by an annular skin rash (erythema migrans), which develops at the site of the bite. Associated features include flulike symptoms such as fatigue, myalgia and low-grade fever (occurring in about 50% of cases) and regional lymphadenopathy. Antibiotics at this stage can prevent subsequent stages. The prognosis is excellent with adequate antibiotic therapy.
  ➣ The second stage (early dissemination) follows 2–12 weeks after the tick bite and is characterized by disseminated infection causing:
    ➣ Carditis (most commonly presenting as atrioventricular block or myocarditis)
    ➣ Aseptic meningitis, polyneuritis or encephalopathy
    ➣ Cranial nerve involvement, most commonly presenting as facial nerve palsy
    ➣ Intermittent arthritis
  ➣ The third stage (late dissemination) is characterized by oligoarticular arthritis and acrodermatitis chronica atrophicans, occurring between 6 weeks and 2 years after the tick bite in 50–80% of patients. Arthritis may be the presenting manifestation of LD.

Diagnosis of LD depends on:

➤ Characteristic, clinical features, in particular, the appearance of erythema migrans (80–90%) in addition to exposure to an endemic site.
➤ Specific IgM antibodies against *B. burgdorferi* appearing 3–4 weeks after the infection and peaking after 6–8 weeks. Specific IgG antibodies usually become detectable in the second month after the onset of infection.

Treatment

➤ Adults and children aged ≥12 years:
  ➣ Doxycycline 100 mg twice (or 200 mg once daily) for 21 days
  ➣ Amoxicillin 1000 mg three times daily for 21 days (if doxycycline is not suitable)
  ➣ Azithromycin 500 mg once daily for 17 days (if doxycycline and amoxicillin are not suitable)
➤ For children aged 9–12 years:
  ➣ Doxycycline 5 mg/kg/day twice daily on day one, followed by 2.5 mg in one or two divided doses for a total of 21 days.
  ➣ Amoxicillin 30 mg/kg three times daily for 21 days.
  ➣ Azithromycin 10 mg/kg once daily for 17 days (if doxycycline and amoxicillin are not suitable)
➤ For children aged <9 years:
  ➣ Amoxicillin 30 mg/kg three times daily for 21 days
  ➣ Azithromycin 10 mg/kg once daily for 17 days (if amoxicillin is not suitable)
    Note:
➤ Use of doxycycline and azithromycin for treating LD is off-label but is recommended by national and international guidelines as first-line treatment.

➤ The antibiotic treatment described earlier applies to patients being treated in primary care for LD with erythema migrans and/or non-focal symptoms. Different regimens may be applied by specialists, e.g., for arthritis or meningitis: Antibiotic therapy should continue for 4 weeks and includes third-generation cephalosporins with ceftriaxone 100 mg/kg/day or cefotaxime 50 mg/kg/day.

➤ A Jarisch–Herxheimer reaction may develop in the first 24 hours of treatment with any antibiotic for LD. This is a systemic reaction caused by the release of cytokines when antibiotics kill large numbers of bacteria. Symptoms include fever, chills, myalgia and headache. The reaction is self-limiting and usually resolves within 24–48 hours. It may be mistaken for an allergic reaction.

CHAPTER 5

Allergy

GENERAL

➤ Allergy, a term coined in 1906 by Von Pirquet, is an overreaction of the immune system to a normally harmless substance called an allergen. Definition of terms of allergy and the four distinct types of allergic reactions are shown in Box 5.1. Allergens include aero-allergens (e.g., pollens, faeces of the house dust mite) causing allergic rhinitis and asthma, foods, domestic animals, insects, moulds, drugs and industrial chemicals.

➤ Of the two types of lymphocytes, Th1 and Th2 cells, Th2 produce interleukins 3 and 4 (IL-3, IL-4) to promote IgE synthesis on allergen stimulation. IgE has a physiological function in protecting against parasite infestations, which are associated with a very high level of IgE. The fetus makes IgE from 11 weeks of gestation.

➤ In Western countries, almost 30% of the populations develop one or more allergic diseases, ranging from mild transient eczema, to hay fever, to severe life-threatening asthma or systemic anaphylaxis. Table 5.1 shows an overall prevalence of allergies in these countries.

➤ There has been an increasing prevalence of allergic diseases over the last few decades worldwide, and the global burden of allergic diseases continues to increase. Although allergy is more prevalent in affluent countries, the prevalence of allergic diseases is also increasing globally as populations move from rural to urban environments. Many environmental factors appear to be responsible for this increase, including:
  ➤ Increased exposure to allergens.
  ➤ The modern lifestyle with its insulated homes, high indoor humidity and wall-to-wall fitted carpets that contribute to house dust mite proliferation.
  ➤ Changing dietary habits, with greater consumption of processed food and less natural food.
  ➤ The hygiene theory: Infection suppresses those immunological reactions responsible for allergic responses. With the decline of infections, the prevalence of allergy has increased. In support of this theory is the lower prevalence of atopy among children of large families or those attending daycare nurseries compared with those of small families or those not attending nurseries. Also, children who experienced numerous febrile episodes during the first year of life have a lower incidence of allergy than those with fewer febrile episodes.

DOI: 10.1201/9781032642888-5

BOX 5.1 Definitions of the terms and types of allergic reactions

- Atopy
  - Refers to a genetic predisposition to produce IgE antibodies. The exact mode of inheritance is unknown. Up to 30% of populations are atopic.
- Allergic reaction
  - An immune response to a harmless substance, usually protein (= allergens).
- Sensitization
  - A process by which the immune system produces antibodies. For an allergic reaction to occur, a person needs to have been in contact with allergens previously before sensitization develops.
- Antigen
  - Any substance (e.g., microbes, toxins) that causes the immune system to react.
- Mast cells
  - Types of immune cells located in connective tissue, particularly under the skin, that contain chemicals such as histamine.
- Immune
  - Recognition and reaction to harmful/foreign substances by the immune system response to defend the body.
- Type 1 reaction (anaphylactic)
  - An immediate (within few minutes up to 2 hours) reaction by IgE antibodies, which bind to the receptors of the mast cells and basophils, causing rupture of the membrane and releasing mediators such as histamine, heparin and tryptase, causing the immediate reaction.
- Type II reaction (cytotoxic)
  - Caused by IgG antibodies to the antigens on the cell surface.
- Type III reaction (immunocomplex)
  - Due to either IgE or IgM antibodies which bind with the antigen to form antigen–antibody complexes.
- Type IV reaction (cell-mediated)
  - A delayed reaction whereby lymphocytes and macrophages play a major role.

TABLE 5.1 Prevalence of various allergic diseases in Western countries

Prevalence	Average Cases Reported (%)
Asthma	20–30
Seasonal allergic rhinitis	20
Perennial allergic rhinitis	11–15
Atopic dermatitis	10–15
Food allergy	6–8
Cow's milk allergy	2–3
Egg allergy	2

DIAGNOSIS OF ALLERGY

A detailed allergy-focused history exploring exposure to potential allergens is essential and is often diagnostic. Symptoms are either caused by immunoglobulin E (IgE)–mediated or non-IgE-mediated reactions. Allergy history should include any:

➤ Family history of atopy (asthma, hay fever, food allergy, atopic dermatitis or urticaria).
➤ Seasonal respiratory and/or nasal symptoms which may suggest seasonal allergens such as pollens?
➤ Perennial symptoms (runny and itchy nose and eyes, sneezing etc) occurring throughout the year, particularly at the end of the summer, suggesting allergy to house dust mites?
➤ Symptoms occurring shortly after acquisition of a pet and relief when the child is away from the house, which suggest allergy to animal dander.
➤ Symptoms of asthma occurring in a damp musty basement, suggesting allergy to inhaled fungal spores.
➤ Symptoms produced by dusting or carpet cleaning, suggesting allergy to house dust mites.
➤ Symptoms occurring after moving to a new house or during trips, suggesting environmental causes of allergy.

Physical examination often contributes to the diagnosis, for example:

➤ Mouth-breathing and frequent, habitual wiping of a runny nose with the palm of the hand suggest allergic rhinitis.
➤ The presence of seasonal conjunctivitis with watery eyes and periorbital oedema makes the diagnosis of allergic conjunctivitis most likely.
➤ Examination of the skin may reveal patches of atopic dermatitis, which is often associated with allergic rhinitis and asthma.
➤ Chest examination may reveal tachypnoea, wheezing and subcostal recession.
➤ Normal physical examination is a common finding and does not exclude allergy.

Laboratory Tests

➤ **Total IgE:** Levels of IgE increase with age and vary in different populations. The mean concentration of IgE in atopic individuals is higher than in non-topic people. However, some atopic patients have normal IgE levels. This suggests that low levels of IgE may be more useful in excluding atopic diseases than elevated levels are in confirming their presence. Furthermore, many non-allergic conditions can be associated with high levels of IgE (Box 5.2).
  ➣ Allergen-specific IgE test measuring the levels of different IgE antibodies. It has a high specificity of around 90%, i.e., a positive test indicates sensitization, but has low sensitivity, i.e., a negative test does not exclude mild sensitization.
➤ **Skin prick testing (SPT)** is currently the most used test to identify allergens. Infants and young children show less pronounced reactions compared with older children and adults.

BOX 5.2 Non-allergic diseases with increased IgE levels

Infection
- Systemic candidiasis
- Mononucleosis

Neoplasm
- Non-Hodgkin's lymphoma
- Ascariasis

Pulmonary
- Cystic fibrosis
- Haemosiderosis

Skin Disorder
- Erythema nodosum

Immunodeficiency
- Primary immune deficiency
- Hyperimmunoglobulinaemia

Vascular-Rheumatic
- Kawasaki disease
- Rheumatoid arthritis

Others
- Low level of vitamin D

➤ **Intradermal test (IDT)** is uncommonly used, but it is more sensitive and less specific compared to SPT. It can be used to evaluate both immediate IgE-mediated allergy and delayed-type hypersensitivity.

➤ **Patch test** is the gold standard method in diagnosing contact allergy (e.g., contact dermatitis, atopic dermatitis or urticaria) to confirm a delayed cell-mediated type IV hypersensitivity reaction. It involves the application of diluted allergies to the back of a patient for 48 hours, which are read a day later. The test is less used compared to SPT.

➤ **Directoral challenge** is the gold standard test for diagnosis of allergy, particularly food allergy. It is performed by introducing the suspected allergen (usually food, an extract or aerosol) in gradually increasing amounts under medical supervision to diagnose or rule out allergy. Challenge testing is generally indicated if there is a need for definitive diagnosis or if the history is equivocal and symptoms improve during an elimination diet.

MANAGEMENT

➤ All clinicians, including primary care physicians, need to have basic knowledge and competence to manage mild allergic diseases and recognize when a referral is required. Taking an allergy-focused history is vital.

➤ The key aspects of allergy management include patients' education, awareness of allergen triggers and avoidance, what to do in case of emergency and preventative measures to avoid allergic reactions.

➤ Until recently, UK and US guidelines recommended avoidance of an allergen, such as peanut, in infancy to prevent the development of allergy. Such an avoidance has not been effective, and the prevalence of allergy have continued to increase.

➤ Most recently, attention has focused on allergen immunotherapy (AIT), which is a disease-modifying therapy consisting of a titrated oral administration of the culprit allergen (e.g., peanut) at regular intervals to induce tolerance. AIT is currently the only therapeutical strategy with curative potential, reduction of drug use and long-term symptom control. AIT is available for patients suffering from IgE-associated diseases such as allergic rhinitis and asthma.

➤ Oral immunotherapy (OIT) is recommended as a treatment option for children with persistent cow's milk, egg and peanut allergies.

Consider Referral If:

➤ The symptoms do not respond to a single-allergen elimination diet.
➤ The child has confirmed IgE-mediated food allergy and concurrent asthma.
➤ Tests are negative but there is strong suspicion of IgE-mediated food allergy.
➤ There is faltering growth.
➤ The child has had one or more acute systemic or severe delayed reactions.
➤ There is significant atopic eczema with food allergy.
➤ There are possible multiple food allergies.
➤ There is persistent parental concern.
➤ Advice is needed on whether an allergic reaction is sufficiently severe to require an EpiPen.

FOOD ALLERGY

General

➤ Food allergy (FA) is defined as an adverse health effect to foods arising from an immunologically mediated reaction, mainly IgE-mediated. There has been a dramatic increase in the prevalence of FA in the last 20 years. As many as 8% of young children and up to 10% of adults in Western countries have an allergy, and the prevalence is also rising in developing countries.
➤ Normally food proteins are broken down to peptides and amino acids by digestive enzymes, which render them non-allergenic. However, a small amount of intact food protein may be absorbed through the intestinal tract and elicit an immunological response. This occurs frequently in infants because of the increased permeability of the intestinal mucosa and deficiency of secretory IgA (this immunoglobulin inhibits abnormal immune response), which explains the increased FA in infants.
➤ Adverse food reaction (AFR), an abnormal clinical response following food ingestions, is often misinterpreted as allergy. Lactose intolerance is one example, which causes bloating and diarrhoea but is not an allergy. Other non-allergic AFRs include food poisoning and metabolic and pharmacological causes.
➤ Risk factors for severe allergic reactions include atopic dermatitis (AD), which is a major risk factor for food sensitization, ranging between 33% and 39%. Other risk factors include asthma, previous allergic reaction and IgE sensitization. Absence of prior allergic reaction does not exclude future risk of FA.
➤ A new and exciting development to manage FA is the use of allergen immunotherapy, which is a disease-modifying therapy consisting of oral introduction of the culprit food at regular intervals to induce tolerance and reduce the risk of life-threatening allergic reaction.

➤ *Food allergy is classified into (Box 5.3):*

  ➤ **IgE-mediated allergies** are rapid and may occur within a few minutes to 2 hours following food intake. Symptoms range from minor oral or gastrointestinal symptoms to more severe reactions such as anaphylaxis. IgE-mediated reactions involve degranulation of mast cells. Diagnosis is established by a clinical history and supported by SPT or serum-specific IgE-testing.

  ➤ **Non-IgE-mediated allergies** have a slower onset over hours or days. Symptoms often differ from IgE-mediated symptoms. Diagnosis is difficult and relies on clinical history supported by excluding and reintroducing suspected foods (oral food challenge [OFC]).

  ➤ **Mixed food allergies:** Up to 40% of children experience mixed symptoms combining acute IgE-mediated symptoms and cell-mediated slow symptoms such as exacerbation of AD.

➤ *Almost any food is capable of inducing an allergy, but eight foods account for most FA diagnoses:* Cow's milk, peanuts, tree nuts, eggs, fish, shellfish, soy and wheat. Sesame has recently been added to the eight foods as number nine. Allergy to cow's milk and eggs has a prevalence of 2–4% in infants. Fortunately, the prevalence of most FA declines with age, and approximately 80% of children are no longer allergic to foods by the age of 4–6 years.

BOX 5.3 Signs and symptoms of food allergy

IgE-Mediated (Few Minutes to 2 Hours)	Non-IgE-Mediated (2–72 Hours)
Skin	**Skin**
• Pruritus	• Pruritus
• Erythema	• Erythema
• Acute urticaria	• Atopic eczema
• Acute angioedema (lips, face and eyes)	
	Gastroenterology
Gastrointestinal	• Gastro-oesophageal reflux
• Oral pruritus	• Loose or frequent stools, with blood or mucus
• Angioedema (lips, tongue and palate)	• Enteropathy, esophagitis
• Nausea, vomiting, diarrhoea, colicky abdominal pain	• Constipation
	• Perianal redness
Respiratory	• Infantile colic, persistent crying
• Upper respiratory symptoms (nasal itching, sneezing, rhinorrhoea or congestion)	• Food refusal or aversion
• Lower respiratory symptoms (cough, chest tightness, wheezing or dyspnoea)	• Pallor and tiredness
	• Faltering growth
Cardiovascular: Tachycardia, Hypotension	
• Neurological: Dizziness, alteration of mental status	

Diagnosis

➤ An **allergy-focused history** should be taken and can often be diagnostic (Box 5.4).

➤ **OFC** is the gold standard for diagnosing FA. The procedure can be associated with the risk of serious allergic reactions and family anxiety. OFC is indicated when the clinical history, combined with results of SPT and/or IgE testing, are equivocal.

➤ Specific IgE test. IgE is an important antibody in host defence against parasites and a clinical marker of atopy. Many non-allergic conditions can be associated with high levels of IgE (Box 5.3). The test is usually requested along with an 'allergen-specific IgE test,' which measures different IgE antibodies to help diagnose FA.

➤ **SPT** evaluates the presence of IgE for specific allergens. In infants <1 year of age, a positive reaction is significant because IgE is not commonly detectable at this age, whereas a negative test result does not exclude allergy. In older children, the reverse is true: A positive SPT does not necessarily indicate that a specific food is the cause of symptoms. Results of these tests should always be interpreted in the context of the clinical history. Patients taking antihistamines should discontinue the medication 24 hours (for second-generation antihistamines) and 4–5 days (for first-generation antihistamines) before SPT testing.

➤ **Basophil activation test (BAT)** has the potential to measure activation markers (mainly CD63 or CD203c) on the basophil cell membrane following an IgE allergen–antibody reaction. The test is mainly used for suspected egg, milk and peanut allergies and in a situation where OFC cannot be performed because of parental anxiety, for example, or if there is a possibility that it may cause a severe reaction.

BOX 5.4 Food allergy–focused clinical history

- Any personal or family history of atopic disease?
- Feeding history (breast or formula) and age of weaning?
- Any foods suspected of allergy and those avoided and why?
- Age of first onset, speed of onset and setting of reaction? Who has raised the concern and suspected the food allergy?
- Duration, severity and frequency of symptoms?
- Cultural and religious dietary factors that affect the child's diet?
- Details of previous treatments, including any medications?
- Any response to the elimination and reintroduction of foods?

Management

➤ The child and parents should receive information that is relevant to the type of allergy, including the risk and management of severe allergic reactions.

➤ Allergy tests should not be offered without first taking an allergy-focused clinical history. Some tests, particularly OCT, should only be undertaken by competent healthcare professionals and where there are facilities present for resuscitation.

➤ There are currently no curative or disease-modifying treatments for FA. The standard care in treating FA is avoidance of known food allergens and rescue medications in case of an allergic reaction. Problems associated with food avoidance include reduced food diversity, social restrictions, potential risk of nutritional deficiency, stress and anxiety.

➤ Until 2008, clinical practice guidelines recommended delaying the introduction of allergenic foods. For children considered to be at high risk of developing food allergies, there is currently strong evidence for the early introduction of allergenic foods, particularly peanuts and eggs. There is now a clear consensus that not only should such foods not be delayed but that they should be introduced at approximately 4–6 months of age to minimize the risk of severe adverse reactions in the future.

➤ Children with a history of severe or frequent allergies should be supplied with injectable adrenaline and antihistamine. (See section on severe allergic reactions and anaphylaxis later.)

➤ Probiotics do not have an established role in the prevention or treatment of allergy, and probiotic supplement has not influenced the course of any allergic disease. Until there is evidence, supplementation with probiotics remains empirical.

Prevention

➤ The World Health Organization (WHO) recommends the 'introduction of nutritionally adequate and safe solid foods at 6 months of age with continued breastfeeding up to 2 years of age or beyond'. If breastfeeding is not possible, a hypoallergenic formula (see the section on milk allergy later) is to be given. Mothers should avoid eating allergen foods while breastfeeding if symptoms persist.

➤ The introduction of solid foods before the age of 4 months has been associated with the development of cow's milk allergy (CMA) and atopic diseases. Solid foods should be added one at a time, with an interval of several days before introducing the next solid food.

➤ It is best to start with iron-fortified rice cereal mixed with breast milk then cooked, puréed and strained fruits and vegetables. Allergy to kiwifruit has increased, and it should be avoided during the first few years of life.

➤ Most children grow out of a CMA, and the prognosis is far better in children than in adults. Young children with the most common causes of allergy (milk, eggs, wheat and soya) are expected to grow out of their allergy by the age of 4–5 years. Allergy to fish, shellfish, peanuts and tree nuts may continue into adulthood. These foods constitute about 90% of all FAs.

RED FLAGS

- Young children with an anaphylactic reaction may present with mild symptoms that can be misinterpreted as something harmless, e.g., repeatedly sticking out their tongue because of tingling or itching in the mouth.
- Certain foods, such as shellfish and wheat products, can trigger severe allergic reaction and anaphylaxis following physical exercise. These foods are usually tolerated without exercise. Symptom onset is usually urticaria followed by other anaphylactic shock symptoms.

SPECIFIC FOOD ALLERGY

Milk Allergy

➤ FA, defined as an immune-mediated adverse reaction to otherwise harmless food protein, is an increasing problem worldwide. FA affects 1–3% of adults and 6–8% of young children. CMA is the top of nine foods (cow's milk, peanut, tree nut, egg, soy, wheat, fish shellfish, sesame) that are responsible for more than 90% of all allergic reactions. CMA affects up to 3.8% of young children, usually before 6 months of age. The incidence of CMA is much lower (about 0.5%) in babies who are exclusively breastfed.

➤ CMA refers to an immune-mediated reaction induced by exposure to cow's milk and includes three types of reactions: IgE-mediated, non-IgE-mediated and mixed form.

➤ Clinical manifestations are variable, ranging from mild acute urticaria or exacerbation of AD to anaphylaxis (Box 5.5).

➤ CMA is responsible for 10–19% of all food-induced anaphylaxis cases and is the third cause of anaphylactic reactions after peanuts and tree nuts.

➤ Fortunately most children (about 80%) with CMA will grow out of their allergy by acquiring a tolerance to cow's milk by the age of 4–5 years, but some keep it for life.

BOX 5.5 The three types of CM reactions

	Symptoms	Onset of Symptoms
IgE-mediated	• Urticaria, angioedema, anaphylaxis	• Few minutes to 1–2 hours
Non-IgE-mediated	• Vomiting, regurgitation, diarrhoea, rectal bleeding, persistent crying, feeding difficulty, sleep disturbance	• 2–4 hours, up to 72 hours
Mixed CM reaction	• The earlier noted IgE-and non-IgE-mediated reactions	• Few hours to a few days

---

Diagnosis

➤ Diagnosis of IgE-mediated allergy is easy because of the clear time relation between ingestion of the offending food and the appearance of symptoms. Specific IgE and SPT can confirm the diagnosis. A positive SPT showing wheals ≥6 mm in diameter in children below the age of 2 years has a 100% specificity, and OCT is then not recommended.

➤ The diagnosis of non-IgE and mixed CMA is based on typical signs and symptoms that improve after withdrawal of the suspected trigger of CM protein. Oral food challenge and the skin atopy patch test can be used in non-IgE-mediated allergy to confirm the diagnosis.

➤ OCT. This procedure should be performed in a hospital with a resuscitation facility: A drop of the formula is put on the infant's lips. If no reaction occurs after 15 minutes, the formula is given orally and the dose is increased stepwise: 0.5, 1.0, 3.0, 10, 30, 50, to 100 mL, every 30 minutes. The infant is observed for 2 hours thereafter.

Management

➤ Strict dietary elimination of CM protein from the infant's diet and continued breast-feeding whenever possible (Box 5.6).

➤ In a breastfed infant with persistent symptoms, a 2- to 4-week maternal elimination diet without milk and dairy products is recommended. Without symptoms, there is no need for a maternal elimination diet during lactation.

➤ When breast milk is not available or insufficient, most guidelines recommend hypoallergenic formulas with extensively hydrolyzed formulas (eHFs) as a first choice for mild-to-moderate CMA, moving to amino acid formulas (AAFs) if eHF fails. Children receiving a hypoallergenic formula should be evaluated every 2–3 months.

➤ OIT consists of administration of progressively increasing amounts of baked milk to induce tolerance to milk and reduce the allergic symptoms. OIT has shown promising results in improving a child's quality of life and inducing long-term tolerance. Milk baking alters the structure of milk allergens, decreasing their allergenicity and changing their stability.

BOX 5.6 Summary of management of CMA

Exclusively Breastfeeding

● Elimination of CM from the maternal diet if the baby is still symptomatic.
● Supplementation of maternal diet with calcium, vitamin D and milk substitute
● Mothers to be supported to continue breastfeeding.
● Refer to local paediatric allergy service.

Formula-Fed Infants

● Strict elimination of CM protein from the diet.
● Encourage breastfeeding whenever possible.
● Consider a trial of an AAF.
● Refer to local paediatric allergy service.
● Cow's milk–free diet to continue until 9–12 months of age and for at least 6 months.

Peanut Allergy

Core Messages

➤ Peanuts (*Arachis hypogaea*) and tree nuts (almonds, walnuts, cashew and hazelnuts) have strong antioxidant and anti-inflammatory effects and are rich in unsaturated fats. Children with no eczema or food allergy may consume peanuts when age appropriate.

➤ Peanut allergy (PA) is an IgE-mediated hypersensitivity which develops early in life and is typically lifelong. PA affects around 2% of the general population of Western countries, possibly because of a general increase in atopy and increased consumption of peanuts by pregnant and nursing mothers. In contrast with other food allergies (milk, egg, wheat, soy):

➢ PA persists into adulthood in approximately 80% of children, while most children with other food allergies outgrow them by the age of 4–6 years.

➤ PA is associated with higher rates of accidental exposure, severe reactions and potentially fatal anaphylaxis. The widespread availability of peanuts in variable foods makes it particularly difficult to avoid peanut exposure. The anaphylaxis rate in children with PA is about 14% compared with 8% in children with other food allergies.

➤ Symptoms of PA can be triggered by tiny amounts of allergens and can manifest as anaphylaxis.

➤ Risk factors for developing a sensitization to peanuts include family history of atopy and the presence of eczema. Children with severe eczema and/or egg allergy should undergo evaluation for allergic sensitization to peanuts through a specific IgE test and/or SPT and, if necessary, an oral food challenge.

Diagnosis

➤ A history of acute reaction within 2 hours, more often within minutes, after peanut ingestion suggests the diagnosis of PA. A positive SPT or specific IgE test with total IgE level confirms the diagnosis.

➤ An oral challenge test is required if the history and earlier tests are inconclusive.

Management

➤ Ensuring that parents and anyone else who looks after the child is fully educated about the condition of PA. They should be instructed to carefully read labels of foods. Patients must carry and be able to self-administer an EpiPen at the first sign of allergic reaction. Antihistamines are usually used for mild allergic reactions.

➤ Previous UK and US guidelines have recommended a strict avoidance of peanuts and the use of rescue medication of adrenaline and oral or injected antihistamines to prevent the development of PA. This approach can cause stress and anxiety for the patient and for caregivers and may interfere with quality of life. In addition, despite these guidelines, the prevalence of PA has continued to increase. Therefore, there is growing evidence favouring early introduction of peanuts rather than early avoidance.

➤ Peanut OIT has recently shown effectiveness in inducing desensitization and establishing tolerance to peanuts. Oral introduction of peanuts early in life, aged 4–6 months, has shown a 75–80% reduction in PA prevalence of high-risk infants. Allergen powder from *A. hypogaea* is the first standardized oral drug recently approved in the United States and Europe to mitigate allergic reactions that may occur with accidental exposure to peanuts. Following treatment, patients demonstrated an increased ability to tolerate peanut protein. The IgE levels gradually returned to normal at the end of 12 months of treatment.

Egg Allergy

Guidelines on Management

➤ Egg allergy (EA) has a prevalence of approximately 2% in children aged 1–2 years and 0.1% in adults. It is the second most common allergy after cow's milk allergy. Egg white is a trigger for 7–12% of paediatric anaphylaxis episodes.

➤ A clear clinical history suggestive of EA and the detection of egg white–specific IgE (by SPT or specific IgE test) will confirm the diagnosis in most cases.

➤ Children with EA can tolerate baked eggs in 60–80% of cases. Baked egg can increase tolerance to egg by inducing immunological desensitization.
➤ Until recently, the management approach to EA has been strict avoidance of eggs. However, this is impractical due to the use of eggs in processed foods and pharmaceutical products, including vaccines. Oral and sublingual immunotherapy have shown to be effective ways to treat and relieve symptoms of EA.
➤ All children with EA can receive measles–mumps–rubella (MMR) vaccination.
➤ Influenza and yellow fever vaccines contain egg protein and should only be considered under the supervision of an allergy specialist if there has been a severe allergic reaction to egg previously.

Consider Referral to a Paediatric Allergy Specialist If:

➤ Symptoms do not respond to a single-allergen elimination diet.
➤ The child has confirmed IgE-mediated food allergy and concurrent asthma.
➤ Tests are negative but there is strong suspicion of IgE-mediated food allergy. There is faltering growth with one or more of the gastrointestinal symptoms shown in Box 5.3.
➤ The child has had one or more acute systemic or severe delayed reactions.
➤ There is significant atopic eczema where multiple or cross-reactive food allergies are suspected by the parent or carer.
➤ There are possible multiple food allergies.
➤ There is persistent parental concern about food allergy (especially where symptoms are difficult or perplexing).
➤ Advice is needed on whether an allergic reaction is sufficiently severe to require an EpiPen.

ALLERGIC RHINITIS

Definition
➤ Allergic rhinitis (AR) is an immune response to IgE-mediated inflammation of the nose resulting from allergen introduction in a sensitized individual. T-helper lymphocytes initiate a systemic IgE-driven reaction. AR indicates a symptom combination of nasal itching, sneezing, rhinorrhoea and nasal blockage.
➤ AR is the most common immunological disorder in the general population with a prevalence of 10–40%, depending on geographical location, with the highest incidence occurring in children. AR is nearly absent in infants and typically does not manifest until the second year of life at the earliest.

Clinical Manifestations

➤ AR is either seasonal, resulting from outdoor allergen exposure (hay fever), or perennial throughout the year triggered by indoor allergens such as house dust mites, moulds, animal dander or cockroaches.
➤ Within minutes of exposure to an allergen, patients experience nasal obstruction, nasal itching and sneezing, which are frequently paroxysmal and associated with congestion and profuse clear rhinorrhoea. After 4–8 hours symptoms ensue including nasal blockage, partial anosmia and increased mucus secretion.
➤ The nasal mucosa may be pale, blue or pink. Nasal turbinates are usually oedematous.

➤ Associated eye symptoms include redness, itching and watering eyes.
➤ Nasal polyps may occur in association with asthma and allergic rhinitis. Symptoms related to polyps include nasal blockage and nasal discharge.

Diagnosis

➤ The history of atopy and the symptoms and signs (as noted earlier).
➤ AR has three main symptoms: Sneezing, nasal obstruction and mucus discharge. Physical examination may reveal:
  ➢ Dark discolouration beneath the lower eyelids (allergic shiners), caused by venous plexus engorgement.
  ➢ Open-mouth breathing as a result of nasal blockage.
  ➢ Horizontal nasal crease (allergic salute sign) at the junction of the cartilaginous and bony bridge of the nose as a result of frequent upward rubbing of the nose.
  ➢ ENT examination is likely to show bilateral clear, mucoid secretions blocking the nasal passage with bluish, pale and swollen mucous membranes and positive nasal deviation and/or polyps.
➤ The diagnosis is confirmed by allergen-specific IgE test or by SPT. Results of the tests must be interpreted in the context of the clinical history.

Conditions that should be differentiated from AR are shown in Box 5.7.

BOX 5.7 Differential diagnosis of allergic rhinitis

Infectious rhinitis (IR)	• Seen mostly in infancy and during the early years of life, while AR is diagnosed at a later age in life. History of atopy is absent. • History is short for a few days in contrast to a more persistent history in AR. • Occurs mostly in winter months, and there is often a family history of an upper respiratory tract infection. • Sneezing and eye symptoms may occur in both types of rhinitis, but these are more persistent in AR.
Adenoid hypertrophy	• May coexist with AR. • Persistent nasal discharge. • Mouth breathing, which is worse at night when the child is lying supine. • Mouth may be kept open during the daytime as well. • Snoring during sleep; muffled voice; malodorous breath. • Irritating cough at night.
Ciliary dyskinesia (immotile cilia syndrome)	• Chronic nasal discharge and congestion, sinusitis. About one in five patients have nasal polyps. • Recurrent otitis media or chronic serous otitis media. • Recurrent respiratory infections leading to bronchiectasis. Cough is productive. Often the initial diagnosis is asthma. An associated situs inversus in 50% of cases.
Foreign body	• Young children may introduce a small object into the nose. • Unilateral blockage of the nose followed by discharge, which is often associated with pain, purulent nasal discharge and bleeding.

Management

➤ There is no evidence to support the use of nasal decongestants.
➤ Education on allergen avoidance should be provided, including educating parent/carer and the child about the nature of the disease and how to avoid areas with a high pollen count.
➤ Initiating measures to reduce house dust mites and moulds, such as washing bedding frequently, using dust-proof covers for pillows and mattress and removing bedroom carpets.
➤ Elimination of exposure to pet dander and feathers is essential for a child with perennial AR. Books or leaflets for the prevention of allergy should be offered.
➤ The use of nasal saline can reduce some nasal symptoms and the need to use other medications.
➤ Antihistamine treatment reduces nasal discharge (rhinorrhoea), sneezing and itching, while its effect on nasal blockage is minimal. First-generation sedating antihistamines (Table 5.2) should not be used (except for acute symptoms of allergy and when insomnia is present), as they cause sedation and impaired concentration and reduce academic performance. Most of the sedating antihistamines are relatively short-acting, but promethazine may be effective for up to 12 hours.

TABLE 5.2 Antihistamines licensed in the UK

From Age	Non-Sedating (Effect Onset/Duration)	Sedating
≥1 month		• Chlorphenamine
≥1 year	• Desloratadine (2–6 hours/>24 hours)	• Hydroxyzine hydrochloride
		• Chlorphenamine
≥2 years	• Cetirizine (<1 hour/<24 hours)	• Cyproheptadine hydrochloride
		• Promethazine
	• Loratadine (1–3 hours/24 hours)	
≥6 years	• Fexofenadine (1–3 hours/>24 hours)	
≥12 years	• Acrivastine = Benadryl (<1 hour/4–6 hours)	
	• Mizolastine (<1 hour/< 24 hours)	

➤ Second-generation antihistamines are the treatment of choice in children with mild seasonal AR and perennial AR. They are often weakly effective in controlling the symptoms of AR. If one oral antihistamine fails to control symptoms, trying a different one is not indicated.
➤ If symptoms of AR are not controlled by an oral antihistamine, the patient should be switched to an intranasal antihistamine (INA) or intranasal corticosteroids (INCs). A topical INA acts rapidly, within 15 minutes, and is often more effective than oral ones. Azelastine or olopatadine is effective in relieving nasal symptoms.
➤ INCs are more effective than antihistamines and leukotriene receptor antagonists and are the most effective therapy in children with AR.
   ➤ INCs are the first-line treatment for moderate-to-severe persistent symptoms, nasal polyposis and treatment failures with antihistamine. Table 5.3 shows some topical steroids used for AR.

- ➤ Starting treatment 2 weeks before the allergen season begins improves efficacy.
- ➤ Onset of action is 6–8 hours after the first dose; clinical improvement may not be apparent for 2 weeks.
- ➤ Side effects are minimal (local irritation, rarely epistaxis) even when taken for many weeks.
- ➤ The initial dose should be high: Two sprays in each nostril twice daily. Once the symptoms are controlled, the dose can be reduced to a spray once daily.
- ➤ Long-term growth studies in children using corticosteroids provide reassuring safety data. Regular high doses of beclomethasone may cause a slight reduction in height velocity. For this reason, regular checks of height and weight are indicated when this drug is used.
- ➤ A combination of INCs and antihistamines is superior than each group alone because of the synergic effect of antihistamines on corticosteroids.

TABLE 5.3 The main intranasal corticosteroids used for the treatment of AR

Age Recommended	Drug Name	Dose
• 2 years	• Triamcinolone	• I puff daily
• 3 years	• Mometasone	• 1 puff BD
• 4 years	• Fluticasone	• 1 puff BD
• 6 years	• Budesonide	• 1 puff OD
• 6 years	• Beclomethasone	• 1–2 puffs BD

- ➤ Systemic steroids are rarely indicated, except:
  - ➤ For severe nasal obstruction.
  - ➤ As short-term rescue medications for symptoms uncontrolled by conventional medications.
- ➤ Oral steroids should be used briefly and always in combination with topical nasal steroids. A suggested regimen for children is prednisolone 1 mg/kg for 5–7 days.
- ➤ Hyposensitization. This method of treatment (performed only in specialized allergy clinics) is mostly used when patients are not responding to the previous treatments. It involves frequent injections and the use of increasing quantities of allergenic extracts. Maintenance treatment may last as long as 3–4 years. Satisfactory results of hyposensitization have been obtained in cases of combined rhinoconjunctivitis if the allergens are clear-cut, like pollens. The most serious side effect of this method is systemic anaphylaxis. Oral immunotherapy (Grazax or grass pollen allergen extract) has recently been licensed for those aged 5–18 years. One sublingual tablet (75 000 units) is to be taken daily for 4 months before the hay fever season starts and should be continued for 3 years. The first dose should be taken under medical supervision. The drug is expensive, and there is insufficient evidence for its routine use.

INSECT STING ALLERGY

- ➤ Stinging insects causing an allergic reaction include the honeybee, wasp, yellow jacket, hornet, mayfly, caddis fly, moth and fire ant. Anaphylactic reaction may be immediate (IgE mediated) or delayed (T-lymphocytic mediated). Allergy to bees is most common among beekeepers. Risk factors to predict future reactions following an initial sting are summarized in Box 5.8.

➤ About 0.4–0.8% of children and up to 3% of adults are at risk of potentially life-threatening systemic reaction after an insect sting. On average, four people die in the UK every year from anaphylactic reactions to wasp and bee stings.

BOX 5.8 Risk factors which predict future severe allergic reactions to bee sting

- History of atopy
- History of previous reactions to insects
- Short time of reaction onset following the bee sting
- Absence of cutaneous manifestations
- Known to have high specific IgE or tryptase levels
- Beekeepers and their family members
- Adult age

Symptoms and Signs

➤ Insect stings can induce IgE-mediated hypersensitivity reaction in venom-allergic patients ranging from mild local reaction to severe systemic reactions and even fatal anaphylaxis.

➤ There are three grades of severity:
  ➤ A mild local reaction due to irritative and toxic venom components and causing transient pain, itching and swelling.
  ➤ Large local reaction (LLR) that peaks after 1–2 days after the sting and resolves 3–10 days later. LLRs are defined by oedema, erythema, pruritus and swelling of a diameter of greater than 10 cm. The reaction is either immediate IgE mediated or delayed cell mediated.
  ➤ Systemic reaction, which usually starts within a few minutes of a sting. It may manifest as generalized pruritus, urticaria, angioedema, dyspnoea (due to laryngeal swelling), bronchospasm, hypotension and shock. A whole limb may be involved, with marked swelling and blister formation. If the insect bite was on the lip, tongue or inside the mouth, severe and life-threatening laryngeal oedema may ensue.

Diagnosis

➤ Detailed history including previous stings reactions and severity.
➤ Detection of venom-specific IgE antibodies can confirm the diagnosis and may identify the insect responsible for the sting.
➤ The SPT and IDT are available and are more sensitive than specific IgE testing.
➤ Basophil activation test is recommended if all other tests show equivocal results despite a strong history of allergy to insect venom.

Management

➤ Plants and areas of the countryside which attract stinging insects should be avoided by those at high risk of anaphylaxis. Children should wear appropriate clothing and footwear when visiting areas known to have these insects.

➤ Patients with local reaction are treated with cold compresses, oral antihistamines and analgesics. An adrenaline auto-injector (EpiPen) should be used for severe reactions.

➤ Venom-specific immunotherapy using venom extracts is highly effective and usually well tolerated. It is indicated for patients who have a history of a severe venom reaction or anaphylaxis.

➤ In the case of anaphylaxis, see the section later on severe allergic reactions and anaphylaxis.

➤ Children with inhalation allergy should be treated with bronchodilators, steroids and oxygen (see the later section on anaphylaxis). VIT is not used for patients with a history of local cutaneous manifestations only, nor for those with venom-negative skin reaction and RAST results, as it is difficult to know which venom should be used.

➤ A summary of sting allergy is shown in Box 5.9.

BOX 5.9 Summary of insect sting reactions

● The severity of the sting reaction depends on the patient's sensitivity, the amount of venom injected and the site of the sting.

● In general, children are at lower risk of anaphylaxis than adults.

● Families of children with a history of insect allergy should keep antihistamine medicine at home for use in case of an allergic reaction. Adrenaline injection (such as EpiPen) should be considered for those with a history of a severe reaction.

● Although the severity of the reaction does not correlate well with the size of skin reaction or level of IgE, a negative skin reaction and undetected IgE level suggest that allergic reaction is very unlikely.

● Venom immunotherapy (VIT) can be an effective form of therapy in individuals at risk of insect sting anaphylaxis.

DRUG ALLERGY

General

➤ Drug allergy (DA) is an immunological IgE-mediated response to a drug or its metabolites, which disappears after discontinuation of the drug, with no other causes explaining the event after a careful history taking, physical examination and laboratory investigation. Drug hypersensitivity is the term used for any drug reaction that might be immunologically mediated by a non-IgE-dependent reaction.

➤ It is important to distinguish between an adverse drug reaction (ADR) and DA (Box 5.10). ADR is defined as any noxious and unintended response to a medication that occurs at a normal dose used for prophylaxis, diagnosis and/or treatment.

➤ Primary care physicians (PCPs) are usually the first to be consulted after an ADR event, and they have a key role in deciding whether to manage the case within the practice or to refer to the patient to a specialist. *If it is a B-type reaction, patients require further evaluation and potential referral.* In addition, PCPs need to recognize the common patterns of clinical features caused by drug reactions (Table 5.4).

➤ An A-type reaction is the most common non-immunological reaction, accounting for about 80–90% of drug reactions occurring in otherwise normal patients, and is the consequence of drug properties and its effects. They are dose dependent and predictable. The B-type reactions are less common (around 10–20%) and are usually immunological reactions occurring in individuals with a genetic predisposition.

➤ Immediate B-type reactions usually manifest within an hour after drug exposures as isolated urticaria, angioedema, allergic rhinitis, conjunctivitis, bronchospasm, nausea, vomiting, diarrhoea or anaphylaxis. Non-immediate type A reactions usually occur after 1 hour (likely several hours or days) and are characterized by variable cutaneous manifestations, particularly maculopapular eruption (Table 5.5).

BOX 5.10 Types of adverse drug reactions

ADR is a reaction that is drug-related, unintended when administered at standard dose resulting in noxious dose and unwanted consequence to the patient

Side effects represent unintended but generally foreseeable outcomes known before medication taken

Adverse drug events occur after administration of a drug at any dose and may or may not harm the patient

---

TABLE 5.4 Clinical manifestations that can be caused by commonly used drugs

Clinical Manifestation	Possible Drugs
Anaphylaxis	• Antibiotics (penicillin, amoxicillin), neuromuscular blocking agents, fluoroquinolone (ciprofloxacin) and proton pump inhibitors (e.g., lansoprazole).
Angioedema, urticaria	• Penicillin, muscle relaxants, insulin, NSAIDs (particularly ibuprofen)
Toxic epidermal necrolysis	• Antimicrobials, sulphonamide
Stevens–Johnson syndrome	• Antimicrobials, anticonvulsants (lamotrigine, phenytoin), NSAIDs (especially ibuprofen, piroxicam)
Various skin rashes	• Antiepileptic drugs, various antibiotics, allopurinol
	• (almost any other drug can cause skin rashes)
Serum sickness	• Antibiotics, thiazides, vaccines, phenytoin
SLE-like	• Procainamide, isoniazid
Photodermatitis	• Griseofulvin, tetracycline, furosemide
Contact dermatitis	• Topical antibiotics, topical antihistamines
Scleroderma-like	• Bleomycin

NSAIDs = non-steroidal anti-inflammatory drugs; SLE = systemic lupus erythematosus.

TABLE 5.5 Classification of drug reactions

Type of Reaction	Mechanism	Symptoms	Time after Exposure
Immediate • Type 1, IgE	• Mast cells and basophil angioedema, hypotension	• Anaphylaxis, urticaria	<1 hour, cell mediated
IgE-Non-Immediate • Type II, cytotoxic reaction	• Macrophage and lymphocyte IgG and/or IgM mediated	• Drug-induced haemolytic anaemia, thrombocytopenia	>6 hours to 1–2 weeks
• Type III, immune complex	• Antibodies (IgG/IgM) bind to soluble drug or its metabolites	• Serum sickness, vasculitis	1–2 weeks
• Type IV, delayed	• T cells react with a drug or its metabolites	• Benign skin rashes	1–7 days

Diagnosis

➤ A careful relevant drug history is an essential first step towards an accurate diagnosis and is often sufficient to identify the offending agent (Box 5.11). Diagnosis is suggested by complete or partial disappearance of symptoms after discontinuation of the offending drug and confirmed by tests (Box 5.12).

➤ For suspected immediate reactions, SPK and/or IDT is indicated. Risk factors for developing drug allergic reactions are listed in Box 5.13.

➤ The common manifestations of urticaria are indistinguishable in both immediate and non-immediate reactions, and the only distinguishing feature is the time interval between the drug intake and the onset of symptoms.

BOX 5.11 Information that should be recorded in patient with ADR

- Date and time of the ADR.
- Name of the offending drug and reason for prescribing.
- The number of doses taken.
- Time interval for recovery between the last dose and symptom onset.
- Detailed description of the symptoms.
- Other medication recently taken.
- Underlying conditions such as atopy.

BOX 5.12 Diagnostic tests used for drug allergy

- *Skin prick test* provides high diagnostic value for immediate IgE-mediated sensitization but has low sensitivity for non-immediate ones.
- *Intradermal test* using various allergens has a strong predictive value in patients with a history of penicillin allergy. The intradermal test may trigger a systemic ADRs and therefore should be carried out under supervision.

- *Patch test* is carried out by placing potential allergens on the patient's back for about 48 hours. It provides evidence for a delayed T-cell-mediated reaction and is the most useful test for the diagnostic evaluation of contact dermatitis.
- *Challenge test.* When the SPT or IDT cannot be performed and the diagnosis remains in doubt, a challenge test can be performed by an experienced physician under close supervision.
- *Specific IgE test* is used for a limited number of drugs such as beta-lactam antibiotics and chlorhexidine. It has a low sensitivity compared to SPT.

BOX 5.13 Risk factors for developing drug allergy

- Adults > children.
- Chemical potency of the drug, e.g., antibiotics (particularly beta-lactam), radiocontrast media, NSAIDs.
- The route of drug administration (topical > IV > oral route).
- High dose and frequent exposure to the drug.
- Concomitant diseases such as infection with HIV, cancer, graft-versus-host.
- Family history of drug allergy (genetic factors).
- Atopic (self or family history), particularly atopic dermatitis.

Management

➤ A safe and alternative drug is given if there is a history of allergy to a particular drug. If there is no alternative drug, the allergy should be excluded by IDT or SPT before giving the drug.

➤ Avoidance and alternative drugs are the mainstay of treatment. If the patient still needs the drug, an alternative drug is to be prescribed.

➤ Other options include desensitization, which is available for many drugs, including penicillin, insulin and aspirin.

BETA-LACTAM ANTIBIOTIC (PENICILLIN) ALLERGY

➤ The most frequently used members of this group are penicillins and cephalosporins (Box 5.14). Penicillin is the most common drug causing allergy, which is more common in adults than in children; its incidence in adults is 10%. The incidence of cephalosporin allergy is 1–2%.

➤ The basic structure of all beta-lactams is a common beta-lactam ring, and over 90% of allergic reactions are due to antibodies against the beta-lactam ring. Therefore, there is a risk of cross-reaction due to the similarity of the ring between these groups. The risk of cephalosporin allergy in a patient with proven penicillin allergy is 10%. If there is a confirmed drug allergy, the responsible drug and cross-reactive one should be avoided as a precaution.

➤ Many patients are erroneously labelled as 'penicillin allergic' after the occurrence of a non-specific rash seen in the course of a viral or bacterial infection.

About 90–98% with a reported or suspected reaction to beta-lactam antibiotics are actually not allergic.

➤ Reporting a history of penicillin allergy can result in a choice of a less effective antibiotic, which may cause adverse effects and increase the risk of antibiotic resistance.

➤ The SPT has a high sensitivity and specificity and has a good accuracy to confirm the diagnosis.

➤ If a patient has experienced a reaction to penicillin or a cephalosporin that was not IgE mediated and was not serious, cephalosporin administration is probably safe.

BOX 5.14 Commonly used beta-lactam antibiotics

- Penicillins (benzylpenicillin G, phenoxymethylpenicillin V)
  › Amoxicillin
  › Amoxicillin-clavulanic acid
  › Ampicillin
  › Flucloxacillin
- Cephalosporins
  › Ceftriaxone
  › Cefuroxime

› Imipenem

› Carbapenem
› Monobactam
› Piperacillin/tazobactam

Diagnosis and Management

➤ Diagnosis is confirmed by a drug skin test and provocation test. A positive skin test does not need a drug provocation test. In general, the safety of beta-lactam antibiotics has been confirmed.

➤ When an allergy to beta-lactam antibiotics is confirmed, another group of antibiotics with similar efficacy should be used. If this is not possible, skin testing should be carried out to confirm or exclude the allergy.

➤ Although IgE-mediated anaphylaxis can occur after penicillin use, such a reaction has become less frequent in recent years, mainly because penicillins have been prescribed more commonly orally than parenterally for bacterial infections.

➤ When an IgE-mediated allergy is excluded by proper testing, future antibiotic use is considered safe. However, some children (around 10%) with negative IgE testing may develop a benign delayed cell-mediated reaction upon exposure to the drug.

➤ When a previous doubtful or minor (e.g., cutaneous) reaction has occurred, a negative skin test makes the use of beta-lactams safe.

URTICARIA

General

➤ Urticaria is characterized by recurrent transient, erythematous, pruritic, raised skin lesions (wheals) and/or angioedema. Urticarias are a heterogeneous group of disorders which have in common a pathway system involving the release of histamine and the degranulation of mast cells. Angioedema indicates oedema of deeper subcutaneous tissues, and therefore the oedema is more extensive. Angioedema presents as a painful, tingling or burning sensation rather than itch and should resolve in 1–3 days.

➤ An estimated 20% of the population in Western countries have experienced at least one episode of urticaria in their life. About 50% of patients with urticaria present exclusively with wheals, 40% present with wheals plus angioedema and 10% with angioedema only.

Clinical Forms of Acute Urticaria

Spontaneous Urticaria

➤ **Acute urticaria.** This is usually self-limiting, rapidly occurring urticaria (within 5–30 minutes). Symptoms may last up to 6 weeks. IgE-mediated reaction is uncommon. Common causes include viral infections, bee and wasp stings, drugs (particularly beta-lactams and NSAIDs) and foods.

➤ **Chronic urticaria (CU).** This is defined as either persistent or episodic urticaria lasting longer than 6 weeks. Around 1.4% of urticaria sufferers experience CU. Infection (viral, bacterial, parasitic) may be the cause. In about 50%, CU is due to associated autoimmune diseases, and autoimmune antibodies may be positive.

Inducible Urticaria

➤ Cold urticaria is IgE mediated, and histamine is the most important released mediator. Within a few minutes following exposure to cold air, cold liquid or cold food, typical urticarial skin lesions appear. This type of urticaria often resolves within a few years.

➤ Solar urticaria is characterized by diffuse pruritic erythema and wheal formation on exposed areas of the skin occurring within minutes of exposure to ultraviolet radiation from sunlight or an artificial light source that emits ultraviolet radiation. It disappears within few minutes after removing the light exposure.

➤ Cholinergic urticaria is triggered by sweating occurring in response to exercise, a hot shower and even after eating spicy food. Acetylcholine is the important mediator in this type of urticaria. The diagnosis is made by reproducing the urticaria through exercise or raising the body temperature.

➤ Vascular urticaria results from inflammatory injury to small blood vessels of the skin. In addition to urticaria, patients often have arthralgia, glomerulonephritis and gastrointestinal and CNS vasculitis. In contrast to other forms of urticaria, this type of urticaria is often prolonged and lasts more than 24 hours.

➤ Urticaria pigmentosa mostly affects infants and is characterized by an accumulation of mast cells in different sites of the body. Brownish or erythematous patches occur typically on the chest and may blister on rubbing (Darier's sign). The lesions are often confused with insect bites. However, the lesions in urticaria pigmentosa may persist and increase in number for several months.

➤ Hereditary angioedema is inherited as an autosomal dominant condition and is characterized by a painless, non-erythematous, non-pruritic swelling which affects predominately the extremities and the face. The swelling can also affect the intestine, causing episodic severe abdominal pain with vomiting. Swelling in the pharynx and larynx may occur and lead to choking and asphyxiation. Bronchospasm causes wheezing, coughing and dyspnoea. The condition is usually triggered by trauma and emotional stress and lasts 2–3 days.

Management

➤ Most cases of urticaria are benign and self-limiting and do not usually require a diagnostic workup. Urticaria should be investigated if it is caused by a type 1 food allergy. The SPT and allergen-specific IgE test can establish the diagnosis. In about 80–90% of cases there is no apparent cause.
➤ Education is based on the known trigger. Avoid any cause if identified (e.g., foods, drugs, cold or sunlight).
➤ Medications to treat urticaria are shown in Box 5.15.
➤ For hereditary angioedema, a complement C1 esterase inhibitor (C1-INH) concentrate is given. Fresh frozen plasma can abort angioedema by replacing plasma C1-INH.

BOX 5.15 Current guidelines on the management of urticaria

- *Second-generation non-sedating antihistamines* (cetirizine, desloratadine, fexofenadine) are the first choice of treatment to alleviate pruritus and reduce the rash. Treatment should continue until symptoms have subsided. If there is a poor response, the dose of antihistamine should be increased.
- *First-generation antihistamines* (diphenhydramine, promethazine) are rapidly acting and effective for parenteral use in emergency situations. The oral use of this group is not recommended because of their numerous side effects (drowsiness, dryness of the mouth and inhibition of micturition).
- For prolonged and more persistent urticaria, a short course of *oral steroids* (e.g., prednisolone 1–2 mg/kg) is helpful in controlling the symptoms and shortening the course.
- For severe cases, *IM adrenaline* should be used (see the next section).

SEVERE ALLERGIC REACTIONS AND ANAPHYLAXIS

➤ Anaphylaxis, a term used for the first time in 1902 to describe a reaction opposite from prophylaxis, is common, and up to 5% of the US population has experienced it. The WHO defines anaphylaxis as 'a serious systemic hypersensitivity reaction that is usually rapid in onset and may cause death'. Both IgE-mediated and non-IgE-mediated reactions may occur; the former is the most common type of reaction leading to anaphylaxis.
➤ The risk of non-fatal incidence of anaphylaxis from insect stings is about 1% in the United States, while the risk of non-fatal anaphylaxis from penicillin there ranges from 0.7–10%. In the United States, approximately 100–500 deaths due to anaphylaxis are estimated to occur per year.

➤ Anaphylaxis is increasing worldwide, mainly due to foods. The estimated incidence of anaphylaxis in Europe is 1.5–7.9 per 100,000 person/per year, with a lifetime prevalence of 1:300. There are approximately 20–30 deaths caused by anaphylaxis each year in the UK mainly due to food anaphylaxis such as milk and nut allergies.

➤ Anaphylaxis has different grades of severity (Box 5.16). Severe anaphylaxis is characterized by potentially life-threatening compromise in airway, breathing and/or circulation and may occur without typical skin features or circulatory shock being present.

➤ Drugs (beta-lactams and neuromuscular blocking agents) and foods, such as peanuts, are the most common causes of anaphylaxis in children. In around a third of cases, the cause of anaphylaxis remains unknown.

➤ Anaphylaxis usually begins within 30 minutes of exposure to some allergens such as IV antibiotics. Food allergy often begins 2 hours after food ingestion. The more rapid the reaction after the allergen exposure, the more serious the reaction.

BOX 5.16 Severity grades of anaphylaxis

- **Grade 1** • Generalized skin symptoms (urticaria, angioedema)
- **Grade II** • Mild-to-moderate symptoms of pulmonary, cardiovascular and/or gastrointestinal systems
- **Grade III** • Shock, loss of consciousness
- **Grade IV** • Cardiac arrest, apnoea

Diagnosis

➤ The diagnosis of anaphylaxis is made clinically and is based on the history, symptoms and signs at presentation. Anaphylaxis is diagnosed when the following criteria are present:

➢ Exposure to a known or at least a suspected antigen. Factors that increase the risks of anaphylaxis are shown in Box 5.17.

➢ Sudden onset and rapid progression of the following symptoms: Cutaneous features are the most common clinical presentation (warmth or tingling, urticaria, angioedema, pruritus, periorbital oedema) followed by respiratory (noisy breathing, wheeze, hoarse voice), cardiovascular (pale, floppy, hypotension, tachycardia) and/or gastrointestinal features (nausea, vomiting, abdominal cramps and diarrhoea).

➤ There are no specific laboratory tests to establish the diagnosis of anaphylaxis except tryptase, which is a marker of mast cell activation. During anaphylaxis, tryptase can be detected in serum 30 minutes after the onset of symptoms, peaks within 30–60 minutes and returns to normal levels within 24–48 hours.

➤ These clinical features of anaphylaxis should be differentiated from conditions of similar presentation (Box 5.18).

BOX 5.17 Factors which increase the risk of anaphylaxis

- Previous anaphylaxis.
- Atopy: Asthma, peanut allergy, insect stings, particularly high number of stings.
- Delayed use of adrenaline.
- Presence of atopy (personal or family history).
- Drugs (beta-lactam, neuromuscular blocking agents).
- No adherence to dietary exclusion.
- Older age.

BOX 5.18 Differential diagnosis of anaphylaxis

- *Septicaemia* with high fever, possible non-blanching rash, usually slow progress.
- *Vasovagal syncope*, which may resemble anaphylaxis because of the sudden appearance of pallor, sweating and collapse, with possible impairment of consciousness. However, in syncope, improvement is rapid; there is usually bradycardia, in contrast to the tachycardia usually present in anaphylaxis. In addition, in syncope, there is an absence of laryngeal spasms or respiratory symptoms.
- *Urticaria*: Clinical symptoms progress slowly in contrast to the rapid symptomatology in anaphylaxis. Urticaria lacks the diffuse warmth, flushing and vascular collapse seen in patients with anaphylaxis.

Emergency Treatment

➤ Effective steps include those shown in the algorithm in Figure 5.1. Patients should be treated using the airway, breathing, circulation, disability, exposure (ABCDE) approach:
  ➣ Oxygenation (high flow) with monitoring of O_2 saturation.
  ➣ Support for circulation and tissue perfusion: Normal saline 20 mL/kg to be infused within 20–30 minutes.
  ➣ Adrenaline (Table 5.6) is the most important drug for the treatment of anaphylaxis, and early administration is essential. The IM route is the route of choice. Intravenous and subcutaneous routs are not recommended on the basis that higher plasma levels are achieved by the IM route. Recent guidelines emphasize a repeated adrenaline dose after 5 minutes if symptoms of anaphylaxis do not resolve rapidly.
  ➣ The use of antihistamines can cause sedation and precipitate hypotension, which can confound symptoms of anaphylaxis. Furthermore, antihistamines do not lead to resolution of respiratory or cardiovascular symptoms of anaphylaxis or improve survival. Recent guidelines relegate antihistamine to a second- or third-line intervention.
  ➣ The use of corticosteroids in treating anaphylaxis lacks strong evidence and may distract from the need to administer adrenaline. The routine use of

corticosteroids may be harmful and associated with increased morbidity and mortality. Their primary action is downregulation of the late phase of inflammatory response.

➤ The beta-2-agonist salbutamol may be helpful as an adjunct treatment for bronchospasm caused by anaphylaxis.

Anaphylactic Reaction?
↓
　　　　Airway, breathing. circulation, disability, exposure (ABCDE)
　　　　↓
Call for help, call 999
　　　　Assess area for safety
　　　　↓
　　　　Airway: Establish airway; high-flow oxygen
Breathing (assess breathing for 10 seconds: Rapid breathing, wheeze, cyanosis?)
　　　　Circulation: Pale, clammy, low BP, faintness, drowsiness?
　　　　Cardiac compression: Breathing rate 15:2

FIGURE 5.1 Simplified algorithms for anaphylaxis reaction outside a hospital.

TABLE 5.6 Usual medications used for treating anaphylaxis

Age (Years)	Adrenaline	Chlorphenamine	Hydrocortisone	Salbutamol (IV)
<6	0.15 mg (0.15 mL)	2.5 mg	50 mg	0.1–0.15 mg/kg
6–12	0.3 mg (0.3 mL)	5 mg	100 mg	
>12	0.5 mg (0.5 mL)	10 mg	200 mg	

CHAPTER 6

Haematology and Immunology

ANAEMIA

Core Messages

➤ Iron is an essential nutrient for all living organisms due to its oxygen-carrying capacity on haemoglobin, its key function in tissue oxygenation, DNA synthesis and enzyme activities.

➤ The World Health Organization (WHO) estimates that approximately a quarter of the world's population has anaemia, and almost half of preschool children are anaemic. Iron deficiency anaemia (IDA) is by far the most common form of anaemia, affecting 20% between newborn and 4 years old and almost 6% between 5 and 14 years old in Western countries. The classification of anaemia is shown in Table 6.1.

➤ In neonates, high haemoglobin (Hb) is due to active erythropoiesis in response to low arterial oxygen saturation (AOS) during fetal life. This erythropoiesis ceases abruptly at birth with the rise of AOS. Low erythropoiesis continues for the first 6–10 weeks of a child's life, causing a decline of Hb to 100–110 g/L in full-term and 70–90 g/L in preterm infants. This decline is termed physiological anaemia that is exaggerated by prematurity.

➤ IDA is defined as a decreased number of circulating red blood cells (RBCs), carriers of oxygen, which are insufficient to meet metabolic demands. In practice, IDA is defined as an Hb level of less than 110 g/L, a serum iron level of <14 μmol/L or serum ferritin <30 mcg/L.

➤ IDA is either due to reduced dietary intake (the most common cause), increased need for iron (e.g., growth), reduced absorption (e.g., malabsorption) or iron loss (e.g., intestinal haemorrhage). Premature babies are at high risk of anaemia because 80% of iron is acquired by the fetus during the last trimester of pregnancy.

➤ A child with mild-to-moderate anaemia is often asymptomatic or presents with fatigue, poor tolerance for exercise, poor school performance, pica, stomatitis and/or frequent infections.

➤ This section will only discuss anaemia relevant to primary care practice.

Recommended Investigations

➤ **Full blood count (FBC):** Hb <110 g/L indicates anaemia; low corpuscular volume, mean corpuscular volume (MCV) (<70 fL) and mean corpuscular haemoglobin

DOI: 10.1201/9781032642888-6

(MCH) (<26 pg) suggest microcytic, hypochromic anaemia. Table 6.2 shows normal levels of these indices.

➤ **Coombs test** for suspected autoimmune haemolysis.

➤ **Serum ferritin**: Low in IDA, normal or high in haemolytic anaemia.

➤ **Liver function tests**: Hyperbilirubinaemia suggests acute or chronic haemolysis.

➤ **Reticulocyte count**: Normal count >1 week of age is about 1%, higher in haemolytic anaemia.

➤ **Vitamin B12 and folate** to exclude the two most common causes of megaloblastic anaemia.

➤ Spherocytosis can be confirmed by the *osmotic fragility test*.

➤ **Hb electrophoresis**: HbS in sickle cell anaemia; high level of HbF can confirm thalassaemia.

➤ **Enzyme estimation** in G6PD deficiency.

TABLE 6.1 Classification of anaemia

Microcytic (MCV < 70)	Normocytic (MCV 70–90)	Macrocytic (MCV > 90)
• IDA	• Chronic disease	• Vitamin B_{12}
• Thalassaemia	• Acute haemorrhage	• Folate deficiency
• Lead poisoning	• Haemolytic anaemia	• BM failure
• Sideroblastic anaemia	• Haemoglobinopathy	○ Aplastic anaemia
	• Metabolic defects	○ DB syndrome
	• RBC membrane defects	• Copper anaemia
		• Hypothyroidism

BM = bone marrow; DB = Diamond–Blackfan syndrome; IDA = iron deficiency anaemia; MCV = mean corpuscular volume; RBC = red blood cell.

TABLE 6.2 Normal blood indices of FBC

Index	Age				
	0–2 weeks	6 months	12 months	1–6 years	6–12 years
• Hb	140–200	110–140	120–140	115–140	115–155
• MCV	90–105	76–84	72–84	74–77	77–88
• MCH	32–34	25–29	24–28	24–29	25–33
• Hct	40–65	28–42	33–40	34–40	35–40

FBC = full blood count; Hb = haemoglobin; Hct = haematocrit; MCH = mean corpuscular haemoglobin; MCV = mean corpuscular volume.

Diagnostic Tips

➤ Any anaemia (even mild) should be investigated, as it may indicate a serious underlying disorder. By far the most common cause of anaemia is nutritional iron deficiency, which can be easily diagnosed by low Hb, MCV, MCH and ferritin levels.

➤ In districts or localities with a high rate of socio-economic deprivation, IDA is very common. An Hb check should be considered in any child with prolonged feeding or dietary problems or fatigue.

➤ It can be difficult to distinguish thalassaemia from IDA, and IDA may coexist with thalassaemia. Both have low MCV and MCH. Ferritin is normal or high in thalassaemia. HbA_2 >3.4% is diagnostic of thalassaemia trait.

➤ In cases of iron deficiency unresponsive to iron therapy, the following possibilities should be considered:

 ➣ Incorrect diagnosis of IDA.

 ➣ Poor compliance with therapy.

 ➣ There may be another underlying disease such as thalassaemia trait, coeliac disease, inflammatory bowel disease or blood loss.

Management (Box 6.1)

BOX 6.1 Guidelines on treatment and prevention of anaemia

- Dietary iron deficiency is the leading cause of anaemia worldwide. Preventing and treating anaemia are crucial components of a public health strategy. Iron supplementation activates the immune system and response to vaccination, while iron deficiency leads to depressed immune and neurodevelopmental functions and impaired cognitive and academic performances.
- A normal singleton pregnancy requires 500–800 mg of iron from the mother. Iron supplements should be offered during the antenatal period to pregnant women. This leads to improved birth outcomes and improved maternal and infant health.
- Infants <1 year of age should be provided with breast milk or iron-fortified formula. At 6 months of age, foods rich in iron, e.g., iron-fortified cereals and foods can be given (Table 6.3).
- Iron supplements should be given to all preterm infants until the end of the first year.
- Treatment with oral iron should be given to all children with Hb <110 g/L for 4–6 weeks. Suitable preparations include 3 mg/kg of ferrous sulphate given once between meals without milk or dairy products which inhibit absorption. Ferrous sulphate preparations are the first-line choice due to their good bioavailability and efficacy.
- In macrocytic anaemia:
  - › Folic acid is given orally in a dose of 5 mg/day for 4 months.
  - › Vitamin B_{12} can be administered IM: 1 mg every 2–3 months as prophylaxis.
- Oral iron should not be offered to patients with gastrointestinal disorders including gastroenteritis, inflammatory bowel disease and intestinal malignancies.
- Unabsorbed iron in the intestinal lumen becomes an essential growth factor for nearly all pathogenic bacteria and neoplastic cells, leading to symptom deterioration.

Referral should be considered for:

➤ Unexplained anaemia or any type of haemolytic anaemia.

➤ IDA with Hb <70 g/L.

➤ IDA not responding to iron therapy.

➤ Secondary anaemia due to blood loss.

TABLE 6.3 Iron content in common foods

Foods (100 g)		mg
Meat	Calf, bovine	2–4
	fish (sea bass, cod)	0.4
		0.9
Eggs	Egg yolk	4.9
	whole egg	1.5
Vegetables, fruits	Spinach, lettuce, fresh fruits,	0.4–1.3
		0.4–0.5
	olives	1.6
Legumes	Fresh/	2.3
	dry	6–8
Cereal	Bread	2.5
	pasta	2.5
	rice	2.9

RED FLAGS

- Iron preparations are common and important cause of accidental overdose. Ensure that the drugs are kept out of the reach of children. Parents should also be told about common side effects of iron therapy including gastrointestinal irritation, constipation and loss of appetite.
- Although anaemia is easy to diagnose by using Hb levels, it is crucial and challenging to understand the disease and its complex aetiologies to develop appropriate interventions and search for the specific cause of anaemia.
- Although ferritin <30 micrograms/L indicates IDA, it can be normal or high in the case of comorbid inflammation even in the presence of IDA.

HAEMOLYTIC ANAEMIA (BOX 6.2)

BOX 6.2 Simple classification of the main causes of haemolytic anaemia

- Hereditary
  - Haemoglobinopathy
    - Thalassaemias (alpha and beta)
    - Sickle cell anaemia
  - Membrane defects
    - Hereditary spherocytosis
    - Hereditary elliptocytosis
  - Enzymopathy
    - G6PD
- Acquired
  - Autoimmune
  - Infections
  - Drugs

Homozygous Beta-Thalassaemia (Thalassaemia Major)

➤ **Characteristics**
  ➣ It is a chronic haemolytic anaemia characterized by a genetically defective production of the beta chain of Hb, which leads to hypochromic, microcytic anaemia, with HbF as the predominant haemoglobin present. Ineffective erythropoiesis, haemolysis and iron overload are the key points of this disease.

➤ **Presentation**
  ➣ Severe anaemia causing pallor, jaundice, splenomegaly and decreased growth. Cardiac failure may rapidly occur unless therapy ensues.
  ➣ Expanded bone marrow, causing thickening of the cranial bones and maxillary hyperplasia.
  ➣ The clinical course is dominated by regular transfusions (usually from between 6 months and 2 years) and subsequent absorptive iron overload, causing cardiomyopathy, liver diseases (e.g., cirrhosis, portal hypertension) and endocrinopathies (e.g., diabetes, hypothyroidism, hypoparathyroidism, hypogonadism, and growth hormone deficiency).

➤ **Diagnosis and management**
  ➣ Pregnant women are advised to undergo a screening test for thalassaemia between 10 and 12 weeks of pregnancy. If positive, a partner is advised to undergo the screening test as well.
  ➣ Laboratory findings include hypochromic microcytic anaemia, with a large number of nucleated erythroblasts, target cells and basophilia. Hb electrophoresis reveals elevated HbF (70–90% of the total haemoglobin). Serum iron, ferritin and unconjugated bilirubin are also elevated. Gene testing for thalassaemia mutation is recommended.
  ➣ Management includes blood transfusion and iron chelating. Curative treatment is based on haematopoietic stem cell transplantation and gene therapy.

PRACTICE POINTS

Patients with thalassaemia require regular monitoring, including:

➤ Every 1–3 months: Physical examination to check weight, clinical evidence of anaemia, looking for any sign of jaundice, any hepatosplenomegaly, any tachypnoea, cranial and facial bone changes.
➤ Every 1–3 months: FBC with iron level.
➤ Every 3 months: Ferritin level, liver function test, glucose and HbA1C, vitamin D level.
➤ Every year: Hepatitis profile (hepatitis A, B and C serology), ECG.
➤ Every 1–2 years: Liver ultrasonography, bone mineral density.
➤ Every 1–2 years: Testing for endocrinopathies (thyroid function test, parathyroid).
➤ Every 1–3 years: Echocardiography, cardiac MRI.

Alpha-Thalassaemia

➤ Due to a defect of alpha-globin peptide chain synthesis in haemolytic anaemia.
➤ The mild form, resulting from one alpha-globin deletion, presents with mild anaemia, while the severe form, resulting from an absence of alpha-globin chain synthesis, presents with hydrops fetalis.

Thalassaemia Trait (Minor Thalassaemia)

➤ **Characteristics**: Carrying the gene mutations that cause the thalassaemia.
➤ **Presentation**: Children are usually asymptomatic and do not require blood transfusion. Occasionally, there may be tiredness and fatigue. Mild haemolysis may cause iron overload.
➤ **Diagnosis**: Hb levels are usually 2–3 g/dL lower than normal, with an MCV of <70 fL and an MCH of <30 pg. Iron levels are either normal or elevated (unless there is associated IDA). Diagnosis is established by an elevated HbA of 3.4–7%.

RED FLAGS

● Children with thalassaemia traits are often misdiagnosed as having IDA and may be inappropriately treated with iron. Therefore, thalassaemia always has to be considered in any microcytic, hypochromic anaemia before iron is commenced.

SICKLE CELL DISEASE

Core Messages
➤ The haemoglobinopathies are a heterogeneous group of more than 1000 genetic disorders. The basic pathophysiological defect of sickle cell disease (SCD) is a substitution of valine for glutamic acid at position 6 of the beta-chain, leading to the production of a defective form of haemoglobin known as HbS. The RBCs are too fragile to withstand the mechanical trauma of circulation, leading to haemolysis. The life span of RBCs in sickle cell anaemia is 10–20 days (normal RBC life span is 120 days).
➤ SCD is now the most common serious genetic condition in the UK, affecting approximately 1 in 79 born with sickle cell trait. About 350 babies with SCD are born each year in the UK. About **15,000** people have sickle cell disorders.
➤ Universal newborn screening (at 5–8 days of life) for SCD and thalassaemia has been established in England since 2006 as part of the newborn dried blood spot screening programme.
➤ Life expectancy has improved considerably over the last decades, and mortality is now about 1–2% directly due to the disease, with a current median survival is between 67 and 52.6 years in people with SCA.

TABLE 6.4 Summary of presentations of SCA

Presentation	Clinical Findings
Anaemia	• Aged 2–4 months, pallor and lethargy, usual Hb 60–90 g/L, coinciding with the replacement of the majority of HbF by HbS. Peripheral target cells, sickle cells, poikilocytes.
Dactylitis	• Painful, symmetrical swelling of the hands and feet.
Infection	• Increased risk of bacterial infections (pneumococcal and *Salmonella*).
Spleen	• Acute splenic sequestration, enlarged spleen.
Gastrointestinal	• Intra-abdominal vasoocclusion causes intestinal infarcts, repeated pain.
Neurological	• Stroke, hemiplegia, cerebral infarction, cognitive impairment.
Parvovirus B19 infection	• Severe pallor due to aplastic crisis with acute severe anaemia.
Priapism	• Painful penile erection.
Heart/lung	• Dyspnoea, cardiac failure, dilated cardiomegaly, acute chest syndrome.
Hepatic	• Cholelithiasis, cholecystitis, pancreatitis.
Renal	• Albuminuria, urinary tract infections, sickle nephropathy.

Presentation

➤ Chronic haemolytic anaemia and intermittent acute pain episodes are the two hallmark characteristics of SCD. An abnormal HbS leads to increased blood viscosity, deoxygenation and reduced RBC deformability (Table 6.4).

Laboratory Findings

➤ SCA is characterized by normocytic, hypochromic anaemia (usual Hb 60–90 g/L, RBC 2–3 million per L), leukocytosis, thrombocytosis, hyperbilirubinaemia, and hyperplastic bone marrow.
➤ The marrow may become aplastic during a sickling crisis or severe infection.
➤ Hb electrophoresis shows mainly HbS with a variable amount of HbF. Blood tests can fail to detect HbS under the following circumstances:
  ➢ Blood transfusion within 3–4 months before testing.
  ➢ Coexisting iron deficiency anaemia, hyperglobulinaemia, hyperlipidaemia.
  ➢ Hb variants such as Hb-D Punjab.

Management

Management includes:

➤ Education of parents, which includes the need to bring the child to hospital at the onset of acute illness such as fever or sudden pallor.
➤ Ensuring that affected babies have been referred to the local paediatric unit for multidisciplinary management.
➤ Physical examination should include checking for pallor, jaundice, enlarged spleen and cardiac murmur.
➤ Assessment of growth using centile chart.

➤ Children with SCD should be offered annual transcranial Doppler scans from the age of 2 years.
➤ Ensuring lifelong penicillin prophylaxis of phenoxymethylpenicillin (penicillin V):
➤ 62.5 mg orally BD in children <1 year old.
➤ 125 mg orally BD in children 1–5 years old.
➤ 250 mg orally BD in children >5 years old.
➤ Medication: Analgesics (paracetamol and ibuprofen) are used to control mild pain in a child who is otherwise well and afebrile or with mild fever. Children with fever and a temperature >38.5°C who appear to be in severe pain or seriously ill should be promptly transferred to hospital for IV antibiotics (such as ceftriaxone). Hydroxyurea (hydroxycarbamide) 10–20 mg/kg once daily taken orally reduces the frequency of painful crises by 50%. Deferasirox is an effective oral iron chelator to treat transfusional iron overload.
➤ Transfusion is urgently required for acute problems such as stroke, acute chest syndrome (ACS), sickle cell crisis and parvovirus infection. Regular blood transfusion for mild anaemia is generally discouraged to avoid iron overload.
➤ Hydroxyurea was approved for use in 1998 and is used to decrease the rate of vaso-occlusive crises.

New and Emerging Therapies

There are several new drugs for SCD:

➤ Deferiprone (Ferriprox) is a new iron chelator.
➤ L-Glutamine (Endari) was approved in 2017 to help sickle RBCs tolerate oxidative damage, which is an important complication of SCD. The main side effects include nausea, abdominal pain and constipation.
➤ Voxelotor (Oxbryta) acts by increasing oxygen affinity of the HbS, thus reducing haemolysis.
➤ Crizanlizumab (Adakveo) prevents RBCs from sticking to the inside of blood vessels, thus minimizing the vasoocclusive crises.

Sickle Cell Trait

➤ This is a heterozygous HbS disorder (HbS is between 20% and 45%) which usually follows a benign clinical course and normal life expectancy. Under conditions of severe hypoxia (e.g., high altitude or general anaesthesia), symptoms of vasoocclusive crisis may occur such as bone pain, splenic infarction and haematuria.
➤ The disorder occurs when an individual inherits one gene for normal HbA and one gene for HbS. If both parents have SCT, 50% of their children will inherit the SCD.

RED FLAGS
● Any child with SCD who presents with cognitive impairment or learning difficulties should have an MRI scan to exclude silent stroke. This occurs in about 20% of patients by the age of 20 years.

GLUCOSE 6-PHOSPHATE DEHYDROGENASE DEFICIENCY

➤ G6PD is the most common enzyme deficiency worldwide (Box 6.3).

➤ Screening for G6PD deficiency in newborns, as recommended by WHO, helps prevent severe haemolysis, hyperbilirubinaemia and bilirubin encephalopathy.

➤ The presence of a high number of reticulocytes may interfere with the diagnosis of G6PD deficiency because reticulocytes contain a higher amount of this enzyme than mature RBCs.

➤ Later in life, individuals with G6PD deficiency are generally asymptomatic unless exposed to certain bacterial and viral infections, foods such as fava beans and drugs (Table 6.5) that can trigger a haemolytic anaemia that may require blood transfusion.

➤ There is increasing evidence that SAR-CoV-2 enhances susceptibility to haemolytic triggers in G6PD-deficient individuals.

➤ In recent years there has been huge interest in the role of G6PD in certain tumours (e.g., urinary tract cancer, breast cancer). The levels of the enzyme seem to be related to the overall of survival of patients with these tumours.

BOX 6.3 Summary of G6PD

- **Characteristics**
  - An X-linked recessive inborn error affecting primarily males because the enzyme is located on the X chromosome.
- **Presentation**
  - Neonatal hyperbilirubinaemia on day 2–3 of life, acute haemolytic anaemia after consuming fava beans (favism) or drugs (Table 6.5) and chronic haemolytic anaemia.
- **Diagnosis**
  - Neonatal screening test.

PURPURA AND BLEEDING DISORDERS

Core Messages

➤ Blood clotting mechanisms are complex, but primarily based on vascular response (vasoconstriction and retraction of blood vessels), decreased blood flow to the affected area, platelet clot formation and activation of coagulation factors to form fibrin and stabilize the clot.

TABLE 6.5 Drugs capable of causing haemolysis in patients with G6PD deficiency

Drugs with definite risk of haemolysis in most patients
- Dapsone
- Quinolones (including ciprofloxacin)
- Nitrofurantoin
- Methylene blue
- Primaquine
- Sulfonamides (including co-trimoxazole)

Drugs with possible risk of haemolysis in some patients
- Aspirin
- Quinine
- Chloroquine

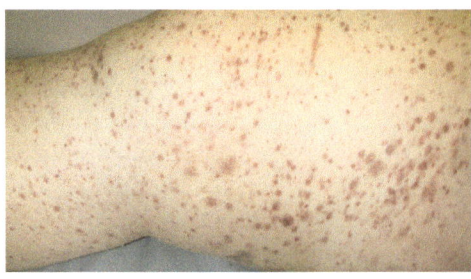

FIGURE 6.1 Extensive purpuric lesions on the leg.

➤ Purpura indicates extravasation of blood into the skin or mucosal membranes. Lesions are not raised. Purpura is due to vasculopathy, thrombocytopathy or coagulopathy or a combination of these mechanisms (Box 6.4).

➤ Depending on their size, purpuric lesions are either petechiae (pinpoint haemorrhages usually <1 cm) or ecchymoses (>1 cm in diameter).

➤ In contrast to exanthem and telangiectasia, purpura does not blanch on pressure (Figure 6.1). It may be a benign condition or an indication of a serious underlying disorder.

➤ In neonates, petechiae are commonly observed on the presenting part during delivery, particularly if the delivery was traumatic. In late infancy and toddlerhood, bruises frequently occur over bony prominences such as the shins, knees and forehead.

BOX 6.4 Classification of purpura

Non-thrombocytopenic purpura
- Henoch–Schönlein purpura
- Physical abuse, trauma, vomiting
- Infection (e.g., meningococcal septicaemia [MCS])
- Vascular purpuras (e.g., von Willebrand's disease)
- Drugs

Thrombocytopenic purpura
- Idiopathic thrombocytopenic purpura (ITP)
- Bone marrow infiltration/failure (e.g., leukaemia)
- Wiskott–Aldrich syndrome
- Haemolytic uraemic syndrome
- Kasabach–Merritt syndrome (thrombocytopenia with haemangioma)

Coagulation disorders (bleeding disorders)
- Hereditary coagulation defects (haemophilia A and B)
- Liver disease
- Ehlers–Danlos syndrome (an inherited connective tissue disease)
- Malabsorption

Investigations

➤ Urine to screen for renal involvement in Henoch–Schönlein purpura (HSP).

➤ FBC to confirm isolated thrombocytopenia; on blood film, blasts suggest leukaemia.

➤ Liver function test (LFT) and urea and electrolytes (U&E) for underlying renal and liver disease.

➤ Coagulation screen: Bleeding and clotting time; partial thromboplastin time (PTT; screen for factor VIII; haemophilia); prothrombin time (PT; for factors VII, V, X); clotting factors (e.g., VIII and IX); von Willebrand factor (vWf).

PRACTICE POINTS

● Baseline tests for most purpuras should include FBC, peripheral blood smear, PT and PTT. Additional tests should be performed according to baseline screening test results.

● Infants up to the age of 3–4 months have physiological prolongation of PTT. Normal values for screening tests are shown in Table 6.6.

● Distribution of the purpura can offer important clues to the diagnosis. In meningococcal septicaemia (MCS), lesions are often on the neck and chest; in HSP, the lesions are predominately on the shins, feet and buttocks; in idiopathic thrombocytopenic purpura (ITP), there is bruising and bleeding from the gums and mucous membranes.

● *Of all diseases with purpura, those caused by sepsis and meningococcal disease are the most serious and require urgent referral.*

● Whenever there are unexplained bruises, non-accidental injury (NAI) should always be suspected. Lesions are suspicious when they are found in areas of the body not normally subjected to injury (trunk, buttocks and cheeks). Additional clues for NAI should be sought: Inflicted cigarette burns, retinal haemorrhages and intraoral injury and skeletal examination should be performed. *Referral for radiological skeletal survey may be indicated.*

● *Any purpura with pallor is likely to be serious: Urgent referral is required to exclude leukaemia.*

● ITP typically affects children 1–4 years old with sudden generalized petechiae and bleeding from the gums and mucous membranes in response to a viral infection 1–4 weeks previously.

● Haemophilia A and B are the most common clotting factor deficiencies that can be diagnosed by prolonged PTT. PT, platelets and bleeding time are normal.

● Von Willebrand's disease is the most common hereditary bleeding disorder, with a prevalence of around 1% of the population. It is characterized clinically by excessive bruising, recurrent epistaxis and menorrhagia. Laboratory findings include prolonged bleeding time and PTT (often), normal PT and thrombocyte count and abnormal assay of vWF.

TABLE 6.6 Normal values for screening tests in an infant with bleeding*

Test	Preterm Infant	Term Infant	Child >2 Months Old
Platelets × 10⁹/L	15000–40000	15000–40000	15000–40000
Prothrombin time (seconds)	14–22	13–20	12–14
Partial thromboplastin time (seconds)	35–55	30–45	25–35
Fibrinogen 1.5–3.0 g/L	150–300	150–300	150–300

* Note that these normal values may vary from one laboratory to another.

IMMUNITY

➤ Immune responses are classified broadly into innate and adaptive immune responses (Figure 6.2).

➤ Skin is the first line of innate cells in host defence to provide immediate and non-specific response against foreign pathogens and toxins. The next barrier includes blood protein, dendritic cells, macrophages, phagocytic cells and neutrophils.

➤ T-cell development occurs in the thymus and mainly generates CD4 and CD8 T-cell subsets. CD8 T cells kill infected cells. CD4 T-helper cells (Th) differentiate into several subsets, including Th1 cells, which protect the host against intracellular bacteria and viruses by inducing proinflammatory cytokines such as interferon (IFN)-γ. Th2 cells protect the host against helminth infections, facilitate tissue repair and contribute to chronic inflammation such as asthma and allergy.

Immunodeficiency Disorders

➤ Immunodeficiency disorders include a variety of diseases that cause increased susceptibility to infection, malignancies and autoimmune diseases. About 5–10% of children with recurrent infections have immunodeficiency. Box 6.5 shows a broad classification of these disorders.

➤ The overall incidence of immunodeficiency is about 1:10,000 children.

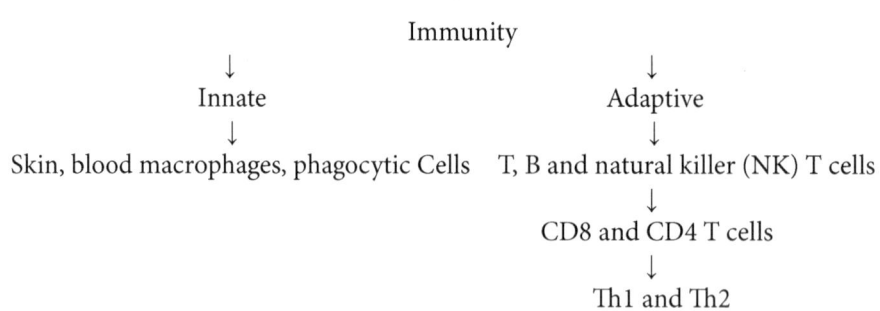

FIGURE 6.2 Broad classification of immunity.

BOX 6.5 Classification of immune deficiencies with examples of disorders

- Primary B-cell immune deficiency (50–75% of cases)
  - ❯ Congenital (mostly inherited), secondary agammaglobulinaemia and hypogammaglobulinaemia
  - ❯ Selective IgA deficiency
- Combined B- and T-cell immune deficiency (about 25%)
  - ❯ Ataxia telangiectasia
  - ❯ Wiskott–Aldrich syndrome
- T-cell immune deficiency (about 5%)
  - ❯ Thymic hypoplasia (DiGeorge's syndrome)
  - ❯ Defective cytokine production
- *Phagocytic cell immune deficiency* (Primary deficiency: About 1%)
  - ❯ Neutrophil defects
  - ❯ Chronic granulomatous disease
  - ❯ Spleen dysfunction/asplenia
- Complement immune deficiency (about 1–2%)
  - ❯ Hereditary angioedema

➤ **B-cell immunodeficiency disorders** are the most common, inherited as X-linked or autosomal recessive. Children commonly present after the age of 6 months with increased rate of infections, typically by encapsulated bacteria (e.g., otitis media, pneumonia) and poor growth (Box 6.6). The condition is characterized by loss of immunoglobulins and/or antibody production and decreased or absent B cells. IgA and IgG are typically reduced or absent with normal/elevated IgM. Agammaglobulinaemia is characterized by an absence of all types of immunoglobulins with an absence of B-cells.

➤ **Selective IgA deficiency** affects as many as 1 in 143 people and is asymptomatic in two-thirds of cases. Symptomatic patients suffer from allergies, recurrent sinopulmonary and mucosal infections, gastroenteritis and gastrointestinal and lymphoid malignancies. It is defined as a serum level of <7 mg/dL and normal levels of IgG and IgM. This primary IgA deficiency must be distinguished from secondary causes of IgA deficiency due to medications such as anticonvulsants (e.g., carbamazepine), and NSAIDs.

➤ **Children with combined B- and T-cell immunodeficiency** suffer from recurrent infections during the first 2 years of life, including:
  - ➤ Sinopulmonary infections, which are by far the most common infections and can be associated with an abscess formation.
  - ➤ Gastrointestinal infections with frequent or persistent diarrhoea.
  - ➤ Mucocutaneous infections caused by opportunistic organisms, *Candida albicans* and generalized molloscum infections.

Initial evaluation of a child with frequent infections includes a detailed history, thorough examination and appropriate screening tests (Box 6.7).

BOX 6.6 Clinical presentation of a child with immunodeficiency

- Healthy child with mild forms of immunodeficiency not detected until adulthood.
- Serious infections and/or long-lasting infections which respond poorly to conventional treatment.
- Two or more bacterial infections such as pneumonia, sepsis or meningitis.
- More than three episodes of otitis media, cellulitis or lymphadenitis in 1 year.
- Recurrent tissue or organ abscess.
- Infection with an opportunistic organisms such as *Pneumocystis carinii*.
- Recurrent muco-cutaneous candidiasis.
- Autoimmune diseases.
- Poor growth, failure to thrive.
- Persistent lymphopenia.

BOX 6.7 Screening tests for a child with recurrent infections

Immunological Tests	Likely to Exclude
1. FBC, peripheral film, CRP	
● Normal neutrophil count	● Neutropenia, leukocyte adhesion defect, phagocytic cell defect, T-cell defects
● Normal lymphocyte count	● T-cell defects
● Normal platelet count	● Wiskott–Aldrich syndrome
● Normal CRP or ESR	● Bacterial or fungal infections
● Absent Howell–Jolly bodies	● Asplenia
2. Screening tests for B cells	
● Normal immunoglobulin	● B-cell defects (e.g. IgA deficiency)
● Normal antibody titres to tetanus or *Haemophilus influenzae*	
3. Screening tests for T cells	
● Normal lymphocyte count	● T-cell defects (e.g. DiGoerge syndrome)
● Positive *C. albicans* skin test	
Normal thymic shadow (chest x-ray)	

RED FLAGS

If a child is suspected of having immunodeficiency, particular attention should be given to the following:
- Immunization history, which should include any adverse effects from vaccination, particularly live virus vaccination, as well as vaccine failure, such as the occurrence of chickenpox in a varicella-vaccinated child.
- Medications: Current and past history should also be noted, particularly immunosuppressive drugs such as corticosteroids.

NEUTROPENIA

Core Messages

➤ Neutrophils are the largest group of leukocytes in peripheral blood and are part of innate immunity, which plays an important role in the initial defence of the host against infections, particularly bacterial and fungal infections.

➤ Neutropenia is defined as an isolated (without anaemia or thrombocytopenia), absolute neutrophil count (ANC) of less than 1500 mm^3 resulting from either impaired cell production of bone marrow or increased peripheral utilization (Box 6.8). *It is a common cause of referral to paediatric and adult haematologists.*

BOX 6.8 Severity of degrees of neutropenia

- Mild   1500–1000 cells
- Moderate   1000–500 cells
- Severe   <500 cells
- Agranulocytosis <200 cells

➤ Neutropenia is classified into congenital and acquired (Box 6.9).

➤ Following the correct diagnosis of neutropenia, it is vital to differentiate between benign and severe forms of neutropenia to assess the risk of infection (Box 6.10). Any type of anaemia with an ANC of less than 500 should be regarded as serious. In addition, it is important to ensure that the neutropenia is isolated, with no other FBC abnormalities.

BOX 6.9 Classifications of neutropenia

Congenital

- Genetic
  - Mutations in the *ELANE* gene or other genes
  - Benign ethnic neutropenia (BEN)
  - Fanconi anaemia, Shwachman–Diamond syndrome
  - Barth syndrome (X-linked disease associated with cardiomyopathy)

Acquired

- Infection   Viral, bacterial or parasitic infections
- Drugs   Chemotherapy, antithyroid medications
- Autoimmune   Primary and secondary
- Cyclic neutropenia   Genetic, often autosomal dominant inheritance
- Hypersplenism   Thalassaemia
- Bone marrow failure   Malignancy, infection
- Chronic idiopathic   Not attributable to drugs, genetic or inflammatory causes

---

➤ **Congenital causes of neutropenia** are rare and include hereditary groups (predominately autosomal recessive) that are characterized by intermittent or persistent moderate-to-severe neutropenia. Patients usually present with sepsis and invasive bacterial infections such as pneumonia and skin infections. Bone marrow examination reveals maturational arrest of myelopoiesis. BEN is a common chronic neutropenia in individuals of African, Middle Eastern and West Indian descent. There is no increased risk of infection in BEN patients.

➤ **Viral infections** are by far the most common cause of acquired neutropenia, usually a mild leukopenia (WBC count <4000, ANC <1500–1000) occurring frequently in response to viruses such as influenza A and B, adenovirus and respiratory syncytial virus (RSV). The infection is of short duration, and recovery of the neutrophils within a few weeks is usually the rule.

➤ **Autoimmune neutropenia (AIN)** is an antigen–antibody reaction resulting from a sensitization by a specific antigen to neutrophils. Diagnosis is confirmed by the presence of anti-neutrophil antibodies. Primary AIN often affects infants, who usually have a benign course and a recovery of over 90% within 24–36 months. Secondary AIN occurs in association with rheumatoid arthritis and systemic lupus erythematosus.

➤ **Chronic benign neutropenia** is a common cause of neutropenia, affecting infants 7–9 months of age. Spontaneous remission occurs usually in all cases with recovery of neutrophils to normal levels.

➤ **Drugs**: Neutropenia may occur after intake of NSAIDs, antiepileptics and antibiotics.

➤ **Cyclic neutropenia** is caused by mutations in the gene encoding neutrophil elastase (*ELANE*). It is characterized by mild, self-limiting neutropenia recurring every 3 weeks, each episode lasting 3–6 days. The diagnosis is established by checking the blood count twice weekly for 6 weeks.

BOX 6.10 Risk factors for infections in patients with neutropenia

High Risk
- Neutropenia <500 mm^3
- Neutropenia associated with recurrent infections
- History of splenectomy
- Secondary to cytotoxic therapy
- Febrile neutropenia
- History of bone marrow transplantation

Low Risk (Usually Benign)
- Isolated postviral infection (without anaemia and/or thrombocytopenia)
- Benign ethnic neutropenia
- Drug induced
- Primary autoimmune
- Cyclic
- Chronic benign

> **RED FLAGS**
> - *Neutropenia in association with an unwell/febrile child requires urgent referral.*
> - If the patient is well and afebrile and there is no associated anaemia and/or thrombocytopenia, FBC may be repeated in 24–48 hours; if neutropenia persists, the child may require an *urgent outpatient appointment.*

LYMPHOPENIA

➤ Lymphocytes are important elements of the adaptive immune system. They are divided into T lymphocytes (T cells), B lymphocytes (B cells) and natural killer (NK) cells.

➤ Lymphopenia (or lymphocytopenia) is defined as blood lymphocytes <1000 × 10^9/L. Lymphopenia is physiological during the prenatal and neonatal periods. The proportion of lymphocytes increases rapidly during infancy, reaching an average of 60% of white blood cells (WBCs) by 2 years of age. Lymphopenia is usually associated with a reduction in the number of CD4 cells that are responsible for activation of the innate immune system and B lymphocytes.

➤ Inherited causes of lymphopenia include cases with severe combined immunodeficiency and ataxia telangiectasia and autoimmune diseases; acquired causes of lymphopenia include HIV infection, treatment with cytotoxic drugs, azathioprine, corticosteroids and systemic lupus erythematosus (SLE). Malnutrition is a common cause of lymphopenia globally.

➤ Viral infections are by far the most common cause of transient benign lymphopenia. While most viral infections (e.g., glandular fever, cytomegalovirus [CMV], varicella) cause relative lymphocytosis, a few other viruses, such as SAR-CoV-2 infection, lead to lymphopenia.

➤ Lymphopenia is a reliable predictor of infection severity and increased mortality in sepsis, pneumonia and SAR-CoV-2 infection. Pre- and post-treatment lymphopenia is an indication of poor prognosis in patients with cancers such as lymphoma and head and neck malignancy.

CHAPTER 7

Malignancy

INTRODUCTION

➤ Cancer is the second most common cause of death in children 0–14 years of age (after accidents). Around **400,000** children are diagnosed with cancer annually globally. The definitions of terms are shown in Table 7.1.

➤ There are over 200 different cancer types affecting about a third of a million people. In the paediatric population, the incidence of malignancy is approximately 1500 children <15 years annually; in other words, 1 in 550–600 children will be affected by cancer by the age of 15 years in the UK. Acute leukaemia accounts for one-third and CNS accounts for one-quarter of all childhood cancers (Figure 7.1).

➤ The outcome for children with cancer has dramatically improved over the past few decades, mainly because of more effective chemotherapy. Today, nearly 90% of children with cancer are surviving at least 5 years after diagnosis, and >70% will survive >10 years. Chemotherapy is used more often in children than in adults because childhood malignancy is more responsive to chemotherapy and because children can better tolerate its adverse effects. Radiotherapy, on the other hand, is not often used in children because they are more vulnerable than adults to its late adverse effects.

➤ Recurrence of primary cancer is still the leading cause of death in childhood cancer patients up to 15 years after diagnosis, followed by death due to secondary malignant neoplasm (SMN). The incidence of SMN after a cancer diagnosis is between 8% and 9% at 20–30 years. SMN is associated with significant morbidity and mortality. Therapeutical radiation (TR) has been associated with the highest risk for SMN.

➤ Recent meta-analysis and systematic reviews indicate that breastfeeding has a potential role in preventing childhood cancer growth, especially leukaemia and cancer of the nervous and urinary systems. Breast milk has components not found in formula, including active hormones and peptides, in addition to beneficial stimulation of the immune system. On the other hand, obesity is a risk factor for many types of cancers, including lymphoma.

Risk Factors for Cancer

In most cases, no risk factor can be identified. It is likely that development of cancer involves both genetic and environmental factors. Known risk factors are shown in Table 7.2.

DOI: 10.1201/9781032642888-7

TABLE 7.1 Definitions of terms

• Children	• Birth to 15 years
• Young people	• 16–24 years
• Not urgent	• Referral or investigation that is not considered to be very or urgent.
• Urgent	• Referral/investigation within 2 weeks
• Very urgent	• Referral/investigation within 2 days
• Malignancy	• The presence of cancerous cells that have the ability to spread to different sites (metastasis) and destroy tissues
• Cancer cure	• Complete remission (all signs and symptoms of cancer have disappeared) for ≥5 years

The most common cancers diagnosed in children aged 0–14 years in the UK, based on cancers registered between 1997 and 2016

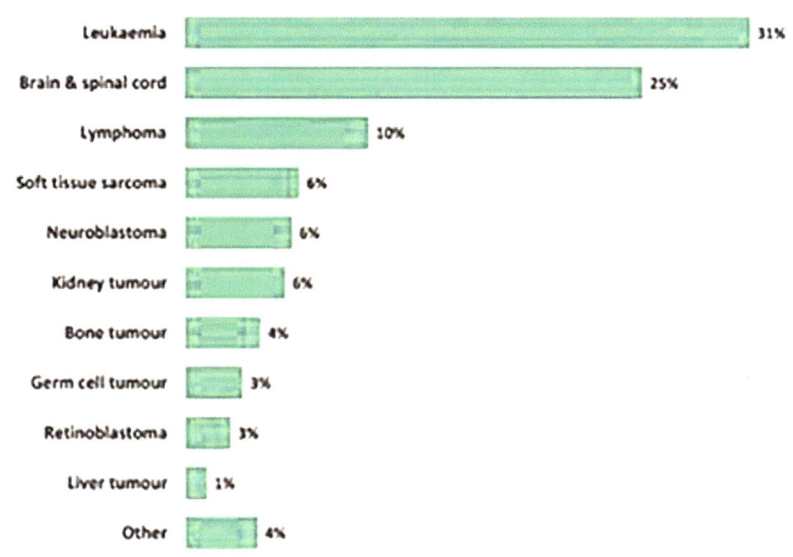

Leukaemia	31%
Brain & spinal cord	25%
Lymphoma	10%
Soft tissue sarcoma	6%
Neuroblastoma	6%
Kidney tumour	6%
Bone tumour	4%
Germ cell tumour	3%
Retinoblastoma	3%
Liver tumour	1%
Other	4%

FIGURE 7.1 Percentages of childhood cancers.

Note: Relative distribution of main cancer groups among children aged 0–14 years in Great Britain, 2001–2005, based on data provided by the National Registry of Childhood Tumours.

TABLE 7.2 Some risk factors for developing cancer

• Genetic susceptibility (e.g., Down's syndrome)	• Leukaemia, retinoblastoma
• Environmental causes (ionizing radiation, benzene, nickel, traffic emissions)	• All cancers
• Immunodeficiency	• Lymphoma
• Drugs (immunosuppressive)	• Non-Hodgkin's lymphoma
• Infections (hepatitis B and C viruses, Epstein–Barr [EB] virus, HIV)	• Hepatoma

Non-Cancerous Signs That May Trigger Referral by Primary Care

➤ **Reactive lymphadenopathy**. A common finding in children around the age of 2–7 years is several small (<1 cm), firm and mobile lymph nodes that are not attached to the underlying tissues and are palpable mainly in the cervical and inguinal regions. Although this is usually a benign finding, it can cause parental worry, particularly in families with a history of cancer. Parents need to be reassured. A worrying sign is a firm or hard mass more than 1 cm in diameter of a lymph node that is matted or fixed to the skin or underlying structures or if a lymphadenopathy is associated with lingering fever, weight loss and decreased appetite. These features suggest malignancy. Full blood count (FBC), ultrasonography and a chest x-ray are essential investigations. *The referral should be urgent.*

➤ **Headaches** are a common childhood complaint, occurring in about 50% of children aged 7 years and 80% of children aged 15 years. Although most causes of headaches in children are benign, it is essential to consider some headaches may be due to underlying pathology. *Worsening headaches presenting in the morning that are exacerbated by stooping or straining suggest increased intracranial pressure (ICP) requiring urgent referral for neuroimaging.*

➤ **Petechial rash** can be a serious sign of infection and malignancy such as leukaemia, it is more often due to a physical trauma causing bruises on the shins in young children. Some petechial rashes may appear on the face and neck resulting from severe coughing or vomiting. History and physical examination, presence or absence of fever or pallor are clues necessary to exclude serious illness.

Childhood Cancer Survivors

As survival rates are increasing, cancer is now regarded as a chronic rather than a fatal condition. The management is covered by the following interventions needed to maintain a good quality life (Box 7.1).

BOX 7.1 Interventions to manage cancer survivors

- General support
- Pain management
- Mouth care
- Treatment of nausea and vomiting
- Treatment for constipation
- Sleep and anxiety management
- Advice with reproductive function
- Advice for growth and endocrinopathy

General Support

➤ Once a childhood cancer survivor (CCS) is discharged from hospital, a posttreatment management plan should be available and carefully explained to the parents.

Children should be given as much information as they can understand. Effects of treatment, e.g., loss of hair during chemotherapy, must be fully explained.

➤ CCSs commonly experience cognitive, emotional and psychological problems, such as anxiety, PTSD, depression and fatigue. Fatigue is a debilitating late effect and is defined as a distressing, persistent physical, emotional and/or cognitive tiredness or exhaustion related to cancer or to its treatment and is not proportional to recent activity.

➤ Adequate emotional and financial support is invariably needed for the family. Relationships within the family may become disturbed, and siblings may be neglected. Parents and children will need help expressing their feelings of anxiety, guilt, anger or depression. Tutoring should be encouraged, and children should try not to fall behind in their schooling. In the UK, Sargent Cancer Care and a number of local charities provide invaluable support by funding specialist nurses and social workers, as well as offering financial assistance. They provide practical support during treatment in hospital and at home.

➤ Owing to a growing number of children and young people with cancer currently surviving, awareness of short- and long-term adverse effects of cancer treatment is increasing. CCSs are likely to need further therapeutical interventions at some point (Box 7.1).

Pain Management

➤ Pain is one of the most common symptoms reported by cancer patients. Insufficient pain relief can affect the emotional wellbeing and lead to increased anxiety, depression and possible reluctance to cooperate with further cancer treatment.

➤ Pain measurement can be assessed using pain scales (Revised Face Pain Scale, visual analogue and numerical rating scales), where 0 is no pain and 10 is the worst pain.

➤ Pain should be managed in a stepwise manner as recommended by the World Health Organization (WHO; paracetamol, NSAIDs and opioids; Table 7.3). Opioids remain the mainstay of severe cancer pain management. Fentanyl causes less constipation and sedation than morphine.

➤ Unfounded fear of addiction can lead physicians to administer opioids only as a last resort. Therefore, children may not receive the potent analgesics required to relieve severe cancer pain (Tables 7.4 and 7.5).

TABLE 7.3 WHO pain relief guidance

● **WHO step 1**	● Paracetamol and NSAIDs for mild pain
● **WHO step 2**	● Weak opioids, Paracetamol and NSAIDs for moderate pain
● **WHO step 3**	● Potent opioids, Paracetamol and NSAIDs for severe pain

Mouth Care

➤ CCSs are an increasing population who are at risk for oral and dental decay complications. Around 30–40% of CCSs experience oral health disorders including hyposalivation, xerostomia, oral blisters, dental caries and enamel hypoplasia.

➤ All children should undergo a dental assessment at the time of cancer diagnosis and, preferably, before cancer treatment commences. CCSs should undergo a dental examination every 3–4 months.

TABLE 7.4 Opioid dosage guidelines

Opioids	Route	Dose	Frequency
Weak opioids			
● Codeine	● Oral: tablets, drops	● 0.15–0.3 mg/kg/dose	● 4 h
● Codeine-paracetamol		● 10 mg/5 mL	● 4 h
● Tramadol	● Oral	● 100–150 mg (soluble tablet)	● Once daily
Potent opioids			
● Morphine	● Oral solution	● 0.2 mg/kg/dose	● As required
		● Modified-release-preparation	● 12 h
		● Modified-release-preparation	
● Fentanyl	● Sublingual	● Buccal route (lozenges)	● 24 h
	● Patches	● 0.2 mg over 15 min	● As a single dose
	● Intranasal	● Transdermal	

TABLE 7.5 Adjuvant drugs for specific pain types

Group	Drugs	Indication
● Anticonvulsant	● Gabapentin	● Neuropathic pain
	● Tegretol	
	● Pregabalin	
● Antidepressant	● Amitriptyline	● Neuropathic pain
● Corticosteroids	● Dexamethasone	● Bone pain, e.g., metastasis
● Benzodiazepine	● Lorazepam	● Anxiety, insomnia

➤ Communication between primary care clinicians (PCCs), paediatric dentists and the oncologist is crucial to ensure proper care. PCCs play key roles in facilitating referrals to paediatric dentists.

➤ Management consists of good general dental care including the use of fluoride toothpaste and mouth rinses, flossing and limitation of sweets. Alcohol-free chlorhexidine mouth rinse is recommended in case of gingivitis or periodontitis. The common symptom of xerostomia should be monitored, and a saliva substitute or moistening agent should be considered.

➤ In the case of neutropenia (<1000 mm^3) and/or thrombocytopenia ($<$**50,000**), dental procedures should not be undertaken.

Nausea and Vomiting

➤ Two of the most common side effects of cancer therapy are chemotherapy-induced nausea and vomiting (CINV), estimated to occur in up to 70% of cases. CINV can have profound physical and psychological consequences, e.g., electrolyte imbalance, anorexia and weight loss.

➤ Although pharmacological therapy for CINV has advanced over the past 15 years, nausea and vomiting continue to be persistent during paediatric cancer treatment, causing a major distress and affecting the quality of life of children.

➤ The development of 5-hydroxytryptamine (5-HT$_3$) receptor antagonists, such as ondansetron and palonosetron, and the wider use of corticosteroids have greatly improved CINV. The antiemetics used are listed in the Table 7.6.

TABLE 7.6 Antiemetics used for CINV in cancer patients

5-HT3 Ondansetron + Dexamethasone	IV or s.c. infusion Oral	0.1–0.15 mg/kg/dose 1–12 years: 4 mg 12–18 years: 8 mg	 BD/ TDS	Effective as post-chemotherapy and radiotherapy
Prochlorperazine	Tab/syrup Buccal (3 mg) IM	2.5–12.5 mg	TDS BD/ TDS	Severe dystonic side-effects may occur
Metoclopramide	Syrup (5 mg/mL) (Tab: 10 mg)	0.1–0.15 mg/kg/dose	BD/ TDS	Extrapyramidal side-effects may occur
Domperidone	Tab/syrup	0.25 mg/kg/dose 10 mg tablets, 1 mg/ mL suspension	TDS	Less effective than metoclopramide but less risk of extra-pyramidal side-effects
Cyclizine	Oral/IV rectal	0.5–1 mg/kg/dose 25–50 mg	TDS	Particularly effective if symptoms due to vestibular disorders

Constipation

➤ Constipation occurs commonly in patients undergoing cancer treatment. It is defined according to Rome lV criteria: Three or fewer bowel movements per week in association with straining and lumpy or hard stools.
➤ Risk factors for developing constipation in cancer patients include:
   ➣ Immobility, decreased fluid intake, dehydration, hypercalcaemia.
   ➣ Medications: Iron supplements, opioids, antihistamines, anticholinergics, diuretics, antiemetics.
➤ Of all medications, opioid-induced constipation is the most significant factor in causing constipation. Management of constipation for patients receiving opioids is shown in Box 7.2.

BOX 7.2 Management of constipation in childhood cancer survivors

- CCSs should be informed that opioids are necessary to treat bad pain and they may cause or worsen constipation and that laxatives will likely be needed.
- Supplemental fibre, exercise and adequate fluids are recommended.
- *First-line treatment* is an osmotic laxative such as polyethylene glycol (known as macrogol).
- Anthraquinones such as docusate, senna, picosulfate and bisacodyl are effective laxatives in chronic constipation.
- The stool softener lactulose undergoes fermentation by microflora causing bloating and flatulence and therefore is not recommended.
- *Second-line treatment* includes an opioid receptor antagonist such as methylnaltrexone (subcutaneous), naloxegol (oral) and naldemedine (oral) to reverse some of the side effects of opioids.

Sleep Disturbance

➤ A diagnosis of cancer is one of the most distressing pieces of news for patients and negatively affects their life. Around 30–50% of patients with cancer have sleep disturbance characterized by delayed sleep onset, sleep maintenance and reduced total sleep time.

➤ Evidence-based non-pharmacological measures include cognitive behavioural therapy (CBT), exercise and mindfulness-based stress reduction. Exercise interventions have been shown to reduce sleep–wake disturbance and improve mental health in cancer patients.

➤ If these measures fail, medications may be used:
  ➢ Melatonin up to 10 mg/day is safe and effective, particularly for children with delayed sleep-onset.
  ➢ Anxiolytic medication such as benzodiazepines.

Reproductive Function

➤ Cancer treatment may cause infertility, which does not become apparent until puberty or years after. The presence of normal pubertal development does not guarantee adequate gonadal function.

➤ In females, cancer treatment may cause premature ovarian insufficiency. Regularity of menstrual cycles and serum follicle-stimulating hormone (FSH) concentration can evaluate gonadal function.

➤ In males, FSH serum levels >10 IU/l and/or inhibin B levels of <100 ng/L may indicate damage to spermatogenesis. In contrast, the measurement of serum luteinizing hormone (LH) and testosterone is a marker of fertility.

CCSs and Growth

➤ Radiotherapy to the part of the brain that includes the hypothalamic-pituitary axis can cause neuroendocrine abnormalities. Growth hormone (GH) secretion is particularly sensitive to radiotherapy. The production of thyroid-stimulating hormone (TSH) can also be affected. In addition, cranial radiotherapy can increase the risk of obesity and diabetes. Therefore, regular monitoring of height, weight, body mass index (BMI) and HbA1c should be done.

CANCER TYPES

Leukaemia

➤ Leukaemia is the most common paediatric malignancy in high-income countries, and acute lymphoblastic leukaemia (ALL) is the most common paediatric malignancy, accounting for around 80% of childhood acute leukaemia and 20% of all cancers diagnosed in children <15 years of age. Peak age: 2–4 years.

➤ Children usually present in primary care with non-specific symptoms or signs evolving over days and weeks. They initially do not indicate a serious illness and could mimic a viral illness (Table 7.8).

➤ As nearly all leukaemias have abnormal FBCs, diagnosis can easily be made through blood tests in primary care once the disease is considered.

TABLE 7.7 Common cancer types in children, their incidence (UK) and referral urgency

Malignancy (No. of Cases p.a.)	Leading Symptoms	Urgency for Referral
Leukaemia (650)	• Unexplained petechiae, hepato-splenomegaly, pallor, infection, bleeding, fatigue, lymphadenopathy	• V. urgent (within 48 hours)
Brain tumour (400)	• Progressive headaches, vomiting, ataxia, behavioural problems	• V. urgent (within 48 hours)
Lymphoma (160)	• Unexplained lymphadenopathy, hepatosplenomegaly, fatigue, pallor bone pain, pruritus, fever, weight loss	• V. urgent (within 48 hours)
Neuroblastoma (100)	• Palpable abdominal mass or enlarged abdominal organ	• V urgent (within 48 hours)
Nephroblastoma (80)	• Palpable abdominal mass, haematuria	• V. urgent
Retinoblastoma (40–50)	• Visual defect, white reflection of the eye pupil	• Urgent (within 2 weeks)

➤ Advances in the treatment of leukaemia are responsible for an improved 5-year overall survival from only 10% in the 1960s to 90% in recent years.

➤ Intake of vitamins and folate supplement during the preconception period of pregnancy, breastfeeding and exposure to routine childhood infections can reduce the risk of leukaemia, while environmental pollutants, e.g., air pollution, solvents, tobacco smoke, ionizing radiation and traffic emissions, increase the risk.

➤ *The presence of the following signs requires immediate referral (within few hours):*
  ➢ Unexplained petechiae or bleeding
  ➢ Hepatosplenomegaly

➤ Offer a very urgent FBC (within 48 hours) to assess for leukaemia with pallor, persistent fatigue, unexplained fever, persistent infection, generalized lymphadenopathy and/or bone pain.

➤ Discussion with a specialist (e.g., by telephone) if there is uncertainty about interpretation of symptoms/signs or symptoms are not classical as to whether a referral is needed.

TABLE 7.8 Uncommon symptoms/signs in children with leukaemia

Physical	Behavioural
• Unexplained fever	• Bad mood
• Loss of appetite	• Irritability/quiet
• Nosebleeds	• Grumpy
• Tachycardia/palpitation	• Tiredness/apathy
• Night sweats	• Lack of normal activity
• Bone and joint pain	• Weight loss
• Shortness of breath	

Brain Tumours

➤ Brain tumours (BTs) are the most common malignancy after leukaemia, accounting for about 25% of all childhood cancers. About 450 children are diagnosed with BT each year in the UK, localized predominately in the infratentorial area (Table 7.7).

➤ Headache is a common complaint in children, which is usually benign, and it is a prominent and frequent symptom of BT (see Red Flags).

BOX 7.3 Clinical symptoms/signs of CNS tumours

● **Supratentoria**   ● Convulsion, headache, loss of vision., vomiting ataxia, papilloedema

● **Infratentorial cerebellar**
  ● Cerebellar   ● Increased ICP: headaches, vomiting, abnormal gait, Eye movement dysfunction, squint, papilloedema
  ● Brainstem   ● Focal neurological signs, incoordination, abnormal gait, cranial nerve dysfunction

---

Supratentorial area includes cerebrum, lateral and third ventricle, hypothalamus, pituitary gland, and optic nerveInfratentorial area includes cerebellum, fourth ventricle and brain stem.

RED FLAGS IN CHILDHOOD HEADACHE

Refer immediately children with headache if they have a:

● Headache that wakes them at night.
● Headache that is present on awakening in the morning.
● Headache that progressively worsens.
● Headache that is triggered or aggravated by coughing, sneezing, defecating or bending down.
● Headache that is associated with vomiting, ataxia, impaired consciousness, or neurological focal signs or occurs within 5 days of a head injury.

➤ Although diplopia is a common symptom in posterior fossa tumour, children rarely complain of double vision; instead, children present with a head tilt in an attempt to align the two images. However, any diplopia warrants prompt evaluation, as it may signal the onset of a serious intracranial disease.

➤ Risk factors for BT are shown in Table 7.9. Cellular phone technology was introduced in the 1980s and since then has increased rapidly all over the world. When held against the head, phones emit a radio-frequency field, and the brain absorbs the largest dose. However, most publications have found no association between cellular phones and BT.

➤ BTs are graded from I to IV according to WHO classification. Most BTs are non-malignant, including meningiomas and pituitary adenomas. The most malignant (WHO III and IV) include gliomas such as glioblastoma (Table 7.10).

TABLE 7.9 Factors that increase or decrease the risk for BT

Increased Risks	Decreased Risks
• Largely unknown	• Vitamins
• Maternal smoking	• Aspirin
• Maternal exposure to benzene, insecticide	• Vegetables
• Age	• Statins
• Genetic (small around 5%)	• Allergy
• High socioeconomic status	
• Ionizing radiation, cranial radiation	
• Syndromes, e.g., neurofibromatosis	
• Cellular phones?	

TABLE 7.10 WHO grades of BT types

WHO Grade	Brain Tumour	Median Survival Rate
1	Pilocytic astrocytoma	96% for 10 years
2	Oligodendroglioma	11.6
	Glioma: Astrocytoma	5.6
3	Anaplastic astrocytoma	1.6
4	Glioblastoma multiforme	0.4

LYMPHOMA

➤ This is a malignant lymphoproliferative tumour, primarily involving B-cells and commonly found in cervical lymph nodes. The annual incidence is around 160 childhood cases in the UK, with a peak age of occurrence of 10–14 years.

➤ The common initial presentation of Hodgkin lymphoma (HL) is usually a painless lymph node observed in about 80% of patients. The lymph node is typically firm, rubbery, non-tender, matted or fixed to the underlying tissue and >2 cm in diameter, often involving the cervical, supraclavicular and/or axillary regions. In addition to lymphadenopathy, about 75% of patients present with a mediastinal mass causing dyspnoea and dysphagia. Non-Hodgkin lymphoma has much more varied presentations, more frequently involving the abdomen.

➤ Another presentation in a patient with HL is B symptoms, which consist of high fever, night sweats and/or >10% weight loss occurring in 40% of presentations. It may occur with cervical lymphadenopathy.

➤ Obesity is a risk factor for many types of cancers, including lymphoma. There is an increased incidence rate of both obesity and lymphoma over the past few decades, and obesity is associated with poor clinical outcomes and responses to treatment in patients with lymphoma.

➤ Enlargement of the left supraclavicular node suggests malignancy such as lymphoma or rhabdomyosarcoma arising in the abdomen. Enlargement of the right supraclavicular node suggests intrathoracic lesions.

➤ Treatment is combined chemotherapy, radiation and, more recently, immunotherapy. The dose of radiation has been reduced in the paediatric population because of the high rate of long-term side effects. Box 7.4 shows the four stages of lymphoma on which the prognosis depends.

➤ *Arrange a very urgent referral (within 48 hours)* to a specialist for children who present with unexplained lymphadenopathy or splenomegaly, taking into consideration other symptoms such as fever, night sweats, shortness of breath, pruritic and weight loss.

BOX 7.4 Stages of lymphoma

- **Stage 1**   Disease limited to a single lymph node region
- **Stage II**   Disease involvement of two or more lymph node regions
- **Stage III**   Involvement of lymph node region on both sides of the diaphragm
- **Stage IV**   Disseminated involvement

NEUROBLASTOMA

➤ Neuroblastoma arises from the sympathetic nervous ganglion, most often from the adrenal medulla, and, less commonly, from other sympathetic ganglions.

➤ It is the most common extracranial solid tumour in children, with about 100 cases annually in the UK and accounting for 8% of paediatric cancer cases. Over two-thirds of cases occur during the first 5 years of life (peak age: <4 years, mean: 2 years).

➤ The clinical presentation can be very heterogenous (Box 7.5). Most cases develop in the abdominal region arising from adrenal medulla and causing an abdominal mass which extends beyond the midline of the abdomen. An abdominal plain x-ray or ultrasound scan may detect stippled calcification in the adrenal gland.

➤ Metastases are present at diagnosis in about 50%, particularly bone marrow, liver and CNS involvement.

BOX 7.5 Presenting signs of neuroblastoma

- Skull
- Involvement of the neck
- Thoracic
- Adrenal medulla
- Liver involvement
- Pelvic area
- Skin metastases
- Bone marrow
- Systemic

- Eye proptosis
- Horner's syndrome
- Dyspnoea, cough
- Abdominal distension
- Hepatomegaly, coagulopathy
- Bladder dysfunction
- Subcutaneous nodule
- Aplastic anaemia with low Hb and platelets
- Fever of unknown origin, weight loss

➤ Diagnosis is established by imaging and urine estimation of catecholamines.

➤ Therapy includes surgery, chemotherapy and immunotherapy. In infants less than 6 months of age, a large proportion of neuroblastomas will regress spontaneously. Close monitoring of these infants is required.

NEPHROBLASTOMA

➤ This is the most common paediatric renal cancer, with a total number of new cases in the UK estimated at about 80/year. It accounts for 5% of paediatric cancers. The majority of cases are sporadic; only about 10–15% are genetic.

➤ The most common presentation is an incidental palpable, asymptomatic abdominal mass in a young child (median age 3 years), often detected by a parent (in over 80% of cases). Other presentations include fever (reported incidence 25–50% of cases), gross haematuria and hypertension (caused by renin secretion). Cough and dyspnoea may occur due to pulmonary metastasis.

➤ The current survival rate is >90%. The prognosis depends on the stage of the tumour at presentation (Box 7.6).

BOX 7.6 Stages of nephroblastoma

- **Stage 1** Tumour confined to the kidney with intact capsule.
- **Stage II** Tumour extends beyond the kidney or penetration of renal capsule; can be completely resected.
- **Stage III** Tumour extends to or beyond resection.
- **Stage IV** Haematogenous or distant lymph node metastasis.
- **Stage V** Bilateral involvement at the time of initial diagnosis.

RETINOBLASTOMA

➤ There are 40–50 new cases of retinoblastoma annually in the UK – an incidence of 1 in every 18,000 live births, and it accounts for 3% of all childhood cancers. It is the most common malignant intraocular tumour in children, mostly diagnosed before the age of 5 years.

➤ Retinoblastoma, familial and sporadic, mostly results from a mutation of the retinoblastoma *RB-1* gene located on chromosome 13. Offsprings and siblings of affected patients require regular screening examination.

➤ The survival rate in countries with high incomes is higher than 95%. It is curable if diagnosed at early stages and is often lethal if not treated timely.

➤ The most common presenting feature is a white pupillary reflex (leukocoria "cat's eye reflex" Figure 7.2), often recognized by parents, in addition to a sudden squint (detected by performing cover tests) and decreased visual acuity. Ocular ultrasonography and MRI are important to confirm the tumour.

➤ Current therapy includes intravenous, intra-arterial (current first-line therapy) and intraocular chemotherapy. Enucleation is rarely performed nowadays unless the tumour is too advanced.

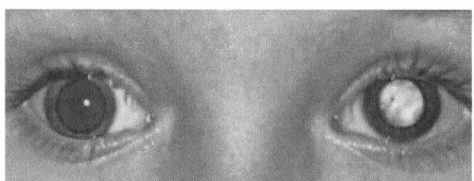

FIGURE 7.2 Abnormal red reflex in the left eye, caused possibly by congenital cataract or retinoblastoma. (Image courtesy of the Childhood Eye Cancer Trust.)

GRIEF AND BEREAVEMENT

Grief and bereavement reflect a state of deep and intense sadness and mourning after the loss of a loved one. The grief process depends on the relationship with the person who died. Unlike adults, some bereaved children do not experience continual and intense emotional grief reactions, although this is age dependent:

➤ Children before the age of 6 years see death as a kind of sleep. The child cannot fully separate death from life. Although children often know that death occurs physically, they think it is temporary, reversible and not final
➤ Children aged 6–9 years may react differently. They often react with learning difficulties, develop antisocial or aggressive behaviour and tend to withdraw from others.
➤ After the age of 9 years, children will have increased anxiety over their own death. Physical reactions are more intense than in younger children and include sleeping disturbance and a change in appetite.

Breaking bad news is best achieved by:

➤ The parent or someone known to or trusted by the child telling them of the death as soon as possible, using touch to comfort and console. Children can handle sad news much better than they are given credit for by adults.
➤ Using simple factual words such as "dead" or "has died" rather than "going to heaven" or "slipping away", which is confusing.
➤ Preparing them gently to make choices about whether they want to say "goodbye", place a favourite toy or flowers in or on the coffin or write a letter of farewell.
➤ Informing the child's school of the death and asking for the support of teachers.

Children need support, most of which comes from friends and family. Doctors, nurses and charity organizations are an important source of support. This is best given by people who have been trained in bereavement work and have expertise with children. Such people are found in charity organizations which include:

1. *Child Bereavement Charity (CBC)* which provides specialized support, information and training to all those affected when a child dies or when a child is bereaved. In addition, the charity provides books, DVDs, videos and a confidential listening service to anyone affected by the death of a child or who is caring for a someone who is bereaved.
2. *Childhood Bereavement Network,* which is a national, multiprofessional organization providing help for bereaved children and young people.

CHAPTER 8

Gastrointestinal Diseases

MOUTH ULCERS

Core Messages

➤ Mouth ulceration is common in children and estimated to affect 9% of all children attending the A&E department. It may be caused by trauma (physical or chemical), viral infections, aphthous ulcers, dermatological or haematopoietic disorders, gastrointestinal disease, nutritional deficiency and side effects of certain drugs (Box 8.1).

➤ In young children, most oral ulcers are caused by viral infection, such as acute herpetic gingivostomatitis (AHG). AHG has no tendency to recur, in contrast to aphthous stomatitis occurring in older children and adults.

➤ Ulcers that last more than 2 weeks are considered chronic.

BOX 8.1 Causes and clinical characteristic of oral ulcers

Trauma	• Including oral signs of child abuse, chemical burns.
Viral Infections	
• Herpetic gingivostomatitis	• AHG presents with fever and widespread superficial mouth vesicles, which rapidly break down as ulcers. Typical age: 6 months to 5 years.
• Hand–foot–mouth disease	• This affects the front of the mouth, tongue and buccal mucosa. It affects children <5 years.
• Herpangina	• Presents with sudden throat pain; fever; multiple oral ulcers on hard palate, tonsils, and uvula.
• Other viruses	• For example, varicella and EB viruses cause oral ulcers.
Inflammation	
• Erythema multiforme	• Causes multiple painful shallow ulcers with red margins.
• Gastrointestinal	• CD and UC can cause oral ulcers, dental enamel defects and recurrent aphthous stomatitis.
• SLE	• Oral ulcers are a frequent finding, affecting 70–75% of cases.
Haematological	
• Neutropenia	• Mouth ulcers are common and may be the first symptom.
• Leukaemia	• Oral symptoms include mouth ulcers, mucositis, bleeding, petechiae and xerostomia.

DOI: 10.1201/9781032642888-8

Medications	• Chemotherapy, NSAIDs, antiepileptic drugs.
Lichen Planus	• Causes painful buccal mucosal erosions and ulcers.
Nutritional	• Deficiency of vitamin B complex, folic acid
Periodic Fever (e.g., PFAPA)	• Causes recurrent aphthous stomatitis.
Stevens–Johnson Syndrome	• Mucocutaneous ulcers of the mouth, eye and genital areas.
Reiter's Syndrome	• Consists of urethritis, conjunctivitis and reactive arthritis.
	• Oral lesions include buccal ulcerations, gingiva and lips.

AHG = acute herpetic gingivostomatitis; CD = Crohn's disease; EB = Epstein–Barr; NSAID = non-steroidal anti-inflammatory drug; PFAPA = periodic fever, aphthous stomatitis, pharyngitis, adenitis; SLE = systemic lupus erythematosus; UC = ulcerative colitis.

Investigations

➤ Full blood count (FBC): Neutropenia in cyclic neutropenia; anaemia likely in Crohn's disease (CD); leukopenia, anaemia and thrombocytopenia are common findings in systemic lupus erythematosus (SLE).

➤ C-reactive protein (CRP): Elevated in bacterial infectious diseases.

➤ Serological tests for HIV infection if clinically indicated.

➤ Scraping for culture in suspected fungal infection.

PRACTICE POINTS

- Differentiating herpangina from AHG is usually easy: Herpangina has more oral posterior lesions (tonsils, tonsillar pillars, uvula, pharyngeal wall and soft palate), while AHG affects the lips, gingiva and tongue and cheek mucosa.
- Children with atopic dermatitis who may become infected with herpes simplex virus (HSV) resulting in eczema herpeticum. This is a very serious manifestation of herpes virus, which may lead to a fatal outcome.
- Mouth ulcers are common in coeliac and CD, but rare in ulcerative colitis (UC). The mouth lesions may precede the intestinal manifestations. They may be the first signs of neutropenia or aplastic anaemia.
- Episodes of fever, aphthous stomatitis, pharyngitis and cervical adenopathy (PFAPA) are characterized by attacks of unprovoked systemic inflammation with periodic fever. Each episode is followed by a symptom-free interval lasting from weeks to months. Steroids are effective therapy. Tonsillectomy may be indicated.
- Oral manifestations of child abuse include bruises on lips and gums, loosened or broken teeth, lip injury and/or tears of the lingual frenum. Abuse should be considered if the explanation by the parents or carer does not match the injuries. These injuries could be a safeguarding issue and need to be reported.
- Oral gels, often used to treat oral ulcers, may contain salicylate salts. They should not be given to children below 12 years of age, as they may cause Reye's syndrome.

ACUTE ABDOMINAL PAIN

Core Messages

➤ Acute abdominal pain (AAP) is a common complaint seen frequently at the A&E and accounts for 5–10% of visits. It is defined as pain of non-traumatic origin with a duration of <5 days.

➤ The main objective in dealing with a child with abdominal pain is to differentiate between non-surgical benign and self-limited conditions, such as constipation or gastroenteritis (>90% of cases), and more life-threatening surgical conditions, such as volvulus or appendicitis (<10% of cases).

➤ Pain originating from the liver, pancreas and upper intestine is typically felt in the epigastric area; pain originating from the small intestine or appendiceal inflammation is felt typically in the periumbilical area (because the pathway is at the T10 level); and pain from the distal colon and urinary tract is felt in the suprapubic area.

➤ Extra-abdominal conditions of AAP, such as pneumonia or pharyngitis, are important causes of referred abdominal pain in children.

Diagnosis

➤ AAP remains a major diagnostic challenge despite the increased availability of diagnostic imaging and laboratory use. This is due to non-specific symptoms and difficulty to perform a thorough and reliable examination in children.

➤ Obtaining a detailed history, assessing vital signs and the patient overall appearance help triage between ill children who require immediate attention and treatment (urgent including surgical cases) and those who are clinically stable and not critically ill.

➤ An early and correct diagnosis of AAP results in better outcomes and lower risk of morbidity and mortality.

➤ Classification of AAP based on age can narrow the differential diagnosis (Table 8.1).

TABLE 8.1 Age-related differential diagnosis of AAP

	Surgical	**Medical**
● Age <1 year	● Incarcerated IH	● Gastroenteritis
	● Intussusception	● GO reflux
	● Malrotation	
● Age >1 year	● Appendicitis	● Tonsillitis
	● Malrotation	● UTI
	● Volvulus	● SCA
	● Incarcerated IH	● Renal calculus
		● Trauma
		● IBD (Crohn's disease)
		● Functional AP
		● Pancreatitis

AP = abdominal pain; GO = gastro-oesophageal; IBD = irritable bowel disease; IH =; SCA = sickle cell anaemia; UTI = urinary tract infection.

Recommended Investigations

➤ Urinalysis is essential in every child with abdominal pain, with or without fever.
➤ Gastroenteritis: Stool culture, ova, parasites, antigen, e.g., for adenovirus.
➤ FBC, CRP.
➤ Upper AP/epigastric pain: Liver function test (LFT), stool for *Helicobacter pylori* and for calprotectin.
➤ Pancreas enzymes such as amylase and lipase.
➤ Ultrasonography may confirm constipation or renal or gallbladder stones.

PRACTICE POINTS

- Abdominal examination should be performed with extreme gentleness and compassion, with careful hands-off inspection being the first step, followed by the non-intimidating position of sitting down or kneeling to be at the same level as the child. A young child is best examined in the parent's arms or lap. Distracting the child while palpating the abdomen is helpful. It is worth asking the child to point with a finger to the area 'where it hurts most'.
- A student or a postgraduate doctor in an examination who hurts the child while examining the abdomen should expect a failure mark as a result.
- The primary objective of managing a child with AAP is to exclude a surgical condition. The closer the pain is to the umbilicus, the less likely it is to be a surgical condition.
- The typical abdomen in gastroenteritis is non-distended, soft and mildly tender but with little or no guarding. Gastroenteritis can present with abdominal pain only prior to developing diarrhoea. Gastroenteritis may mask appendicitis, and abdominal pain in diabetic ketoacidosis may mimic appendicitis.
- We should always ask whether the pain was followed, not preceded, by vomiting. This is suggestive of appendicitis. Perforation of the appendix presents as acute abdomen, and children typically have a longer history of pain, greater systemic effect, high fever, more generalized tenderness and minimal or absent bowel sounds.
- When a diagnosis of mesenteric adenitis is made, stool culture for the bacteria *Yersinia* should be performed.
- Extra-abdominal causes of AAP are important, as tonsillitis, spine or hips (synovitis) or lower lobe pneumonia can produce abdominal pain and mimic abdominal emergencies, e.g., appendicitis. Thorough examination of these sites is essential.
- A young child with mild abdominal pain and vomiting who has clinical signs of dehydration but no ketones in the urine should be suspected of having an inborn error of metabolism.

RECURRENT ABDOMINAL PAIN

Core Messages

➤ Recurrent abdominal pain (RAP) is a common symptom estimated to affect at least 10% of school-age children. Irritable bowel syndrome (IBS) has been recognized as an important cause of RAP. Although many causes in non-surgical cases of RAP are largely unknown, higher rates of detecting pathologies have been achieved by recent imaging technology.

➤ RAP is defined as pain severe enough to interfere with normal activity, recurring at least three times over a 3-month period with symptom-free intervals (Apley's criteria). The current diagnosis of RAP is made using Rome criteria and only after excluding organic causes and alarming signs and symptoms (Box 8.2).

➤ RAP is significant because it is responsible for a high rate of morbidity, missed school days, high use of health resources and parental anxiety.

➤ Most children with RAP have no organic diseases (functional abdominal pain [FAP], also termed functional gastrointestinal disorders [FGIDs]) and present typically as a central abdominal pain, with no guarding, rebound or rigidity and without abnormal physical signs or investigations. Parasites, such as *Giardia*, are a common and important cause of RAP in low-income countries (Table 8.2).

➤ There is an increasing recognition of an altered intestinal microbiome and interrupted intestinal barrier having an important role in FAP pathogenesis.

BOX 8.2 Rome criteria for functional AP

Functional Dyspepsia

1. Postprandial fullness
2. Early satiation
3. Epigastric pain not associated with constipation

Irritable Bowel Syndrome

1. AP associated with at least one of the following:
   - Related to constipation
   - A change in stool frequency and form
2. With constipation, the pain is unresolved with resolution of the constipation

Abdominal Migraine

1. Paroxysmal episodes of intense periumbilical midline or diffuse AP lasting at least 1 hour
2. At least two episodes for at least 6 months, and episodes separated by weeks and months
3. Episodes of stereotypical pattern and symptoms that interfere with normal activities

Functional AP

1. Episodic or continuous AP that does not occur during eating or menses
2. Insufficient criteria for IBS, functional dyspepsia or abdominal migraine

---

TABLE 8.2 Main causes of RAP

Non-Organic Causes	Organic Causes
• Infantile colic (evening colic)	• GO reflux
• FGID (e.g., psychogenic)	• IBD (Crohn's disease)
• Food intolerance/allergy	• Parasites (e.g., *Giardia*)
• Abdominal migraine	• Sickle cell anaemia (SCA)
• IBS	• Renal/gallbladder calculi
• Familial Mediterranean fever	• Constipation

Recommended Investigations

➤ Urinalysis: Haematuria may suggest renal stones; leukocytes and nitrites suggest urinary tract infection (UTI).
➤ Stool for calprotectin, *H. pylori*, parasites and culture.
➤ FBC and CRP: Useful in some cases.
➤ Blood for LFTs to diagnose hepatitis and Gilbert's disease, amylase and lipase.
➤ Coeliac screening tests in blood, particularly in association with weight loss and anaemia.
➤ Abdominal ultrasound scan: Will confirm renal or gallbladder stones.
➤ Endoscopy: In case of high suspicion of an organic cause.

PRACTICE POINTS

- The history should provide the basis for diagnosis and investigation. Most diagnoses can be made by careful history, through examination and minimal investigation.
- The closer the pain is to the umbilicus, the less likely it is to be significant, while pain away from the umbilicus (e.g., flanks, upper or lower abdomen) can suggest an organic cause.
- In contrast to AAP with about 10% having organic causes, RAP has much fewer organic causes. Psychogenic factors (e.g., school phobia) are a significant cause of RAP. These psychogenic causes need to be diagnosed on positive grounds, not simply by excluding organic disease.
- For a child with RAP thought to have a psychogenic cause, it is not a good practice to tell the parents 'the cause is psychological'. It is of great comfort to support the parents by offering reassurance that their child is healthy and the abdominal pain will not affect their wellbeing.
- Pain in constipation is often overrated as a diagnostic entity. It should not be made only because no other cause apart from constipation is elicited from the history and examination.
- Food intolerance/allergy is an important cause of RAP in young children. Eliminating the suspected food item (e.g., milk or wheat) for about 2 weeks is the best diagnostic and therapeutic tool. Blood or skin testing can confirm the allergy.
- Alarming signs are listed in Box 8.3.

BOX 8.3 Alarming signs in RAP

- Weight loss
- Upper or lower AP
- Haematemesis
- Perianal abnormality, e.g., abscess, fistula, condylomas
- Unexplained fever or associated arthritis
- Dysphagia
- Delayed puberty
- Family history of inflammatory bowel diseases

Management

➤ Treatment of children with RAP should be directed at the underlying cause when it can be diagnosed. For those with FAP, non-pharmacological approach should be the first intervention. Counselling and reassurance that no serious pathologies are suspected are often effective, particularly when the clinician establishes a trustful relationship with the child and the family.

➤ There is a bidirectional relationship between RAP and depression and anxiety in adolescents. In young children, victims of bullying at school are at risk of RAP. Therefore, intervention to eliminate these underlying causes can greatly help the patient.

➤ Modification of diet can play a crucial role in the management of AP. This may involve excluding or reducing certain foods, e.g., fructose, gluten, monosaccharides, dairy and increasing other items such as fibre-rich foods such as soluble fibre (Box 8.4).

➤ FAP, particularly in older children, is frequently associated with anxiety, stress and depression. Cognitive behavioural therapy (CBT), a form of psychotherapy, aims at teaching patients to recognize and challenge distorted thoughts, engage in positive coping and change behaviours to promote wellbeing.

BOX 8.4 Summary of RAP management

- General
  - The diagnosis of FGID is based on excluding organic causes and alarming signs.
- Dietary
  - Modification of diet, which may involve excluding or reducing lactose or fructose, as malabsorption or intolerance can cause bacterial fermentation and gas production.
- Fibre
  - May have a beneficial effect on symptom control. A Cochrane review in 2017 showed no great improvement.
- Probiotics
  - Use a supplement particularly for children with FGID caused by IBS or symptoms that have occurred following gastroenteritis or after an antibiotic course.
- Psychosocial
  - Particularly CBT, which is effective by addressing dysfunctional emotion, stopping thoughts related to pain and replacing negative thoughts with positive ones, distracting oneself when pain arises.
- Exercises
  - These aim at promoting muscle relaxation and breathing exercises.
- Medication
  - Peppermint oil can have a positive effect on symptoms of IBS. Mebeverine has a special effect on smooth muscle causing relaxation. PEG 3350 (Macrogol) for patients with constipation-dominant IBS.

ABDOMINAL DISTENSION (AEROPHAGIA)

Core Messages

➤ Abdominal distension (AD) is defined as an increased girth of the abdomen caused by air or, rarely, by a mass. The condition must be evaluated carefully.

➤ Functional aerophagia (FA) is a gastrointestinal disorder characterized by abdominal distension, belching and gas accumulation. Pathological aerophagia (PA) in addition causes gastrointestinal symptoms such as abdominal pain and decreased appetite. The typical clinical presentation in both FA and PA is a non-distended abdomen in the morning followed by progressive AD during the day.

➤ The prevalence of aerophagia in children is 3.6% worldwide. About 70% of the abdominal air originates from air swallowing.

➤ Mild abdominal distension in a toddler who is thriving and well is common and normal. A long history of abdominal distension associated with underweight and loose bowel movements is highly suggestive of malabsorption. Disaccharidase deficiency and coeliac disease are other common causes.

➤ Other rare but important causes of AD in infants and toddlers are neuroblastoma and nephroblastoma.

Diagnosis

➤ Aerophagia is based on Rome III and IV criteria (Box 8.5). Aerophagia is included in the classification of FGIDs.

➤ The patient must be observed swallowing air.

Differential Diagnoses

AEROPHAGIA

➤ Physiological in toddlers (usually mild)

BOX 8.5 Definition of aerophagia based on Rome III criteria

Aerophagia must include at least two of the following:

- Air swallowing (causing AD during the day)
- Abdominal distension because of intraluminal air
- Repetitive flatulence and belching that are present for >12 weeks in a year
- Symptoms cannot be explained by another medical condition

➤ Functional aerophagia
➤ Pathological aerophagia
➤ Malabsorption (coeliac, cystic fibrosis [CF], *Giardia*)

MASS

➤ Constipation
➤ Abdominal mass (e.g., neuroblastoma)
➤ Glycogen storage disease
➤ Ascites (e.g., nephrotic syndrome)

➤ Intrabdominal congenital and hereditary cyst, ovarian cyst
➤ Kwashiorkor (in the tropics)

Recommended Investigations

➤ In general, investigations are determined by the history and clinical findings.
➤ Urine for VMA and HVA in suspected cases of neuroblastoma.
➤ FBC, CRP, and coeliac screen.
➤ Plasma protein/albumin, U&E for cases with malabsorption.
➤ A stool microscopy for *Giardia*, stool calprotectin and stool culture.
➤ Abdominal plain x-ray will show the extent of the aerophagia.
➤ Ultrasound scan to confirm intra-abdominal tumour, renal pathology or ovarian cysts.
➤ Sweat test for CF.

PRACTICE POINTS

- In contrast to aerophagia causing AD, bloating is an intra-abdominal sensation of fullness, heaviness, tightness and discomfort inside but without an increase of abdominal size.
- Bloating and AD occur in most patients with IBS and in nearly 9% of children with neurocognitive disorders and patients with anxiety and depression.
- A child who is failing to thrive with AD should not be considered physiologic; the most likely cause is malabsorption. In malabsorption and malnutrition, initial weight loss is typical; when the disease becomes chronic, deceleration in height ensues.
- A lower intestinal obstruction (e.g., Hirschsprung's disease) usually presents with AD and late vomiting, while an upper one presents with early vomiting and no distension.
- Causes of abdominal distension in the tropics differ from those in developed countries; parasites (e.g., *Giardia*, worms) and kwashiorkor are prevalent in the tropics.
- A summary of management is shown in Box 8.6.

BOX 8.6 Management of aerophagia

- Reassurance should be given, particularly for patients with stress.
- Children should be instructed to eat and drink slowly.
- Avoid foods producing gas (e.g., beans, cabbage, processed foods) as well as carbonated beverages. Lactulose is poorly absorbed in the small intestine and undergoes fermentation in the colon, producing gas and AD.
- Speech therapy can help patients with aerophagia.
- Patients should be screened for psychiatric illness such as anxiety and depression.
- Medications (simethicone or dimethicone) can reduce gas formation in the bowel and are used for more severe cases of aerophagia.

UNEXPLAINED VOMITING

Core Messages

➤ Vomiting is a forceful action accomplished by a downward contraction of the diaphragm along with tightening of the abdominal muscles against an open sphincter, propelling gastric contents out. Unlike vomiting, which is a forceful action, regurgitation indicates discharge of gastric contents without effort and nausea.

➤ Retching signals the beginning of vomiting. These steps are coordinated by the medullary vomiting centre, which receives afferent signals from GI tract, the bloodstream, equilibrium system of the inner ear and CNS.

➤ According to Rome IV criteria, the category of nausea and vomiting disorders consists of three subcategories (Box 8.7).

➤ Cyclic vomiting syndrome (CVS) is characterized by episodic bouts of uncontrollable vomiting separated by symptom-free intervals. The episodes are often associated with intense nausea, abdominal pain, headache, photophobia and phonophobia. Diseases associated with CVS include migraine, mitochondrial diseases and psychiatric comorbidities.

BOX 8.7 Rome diagnostic criteria for nausea and vomiting

Chronic Nausea and Vomiting

● Severe nausea occurring at least 1 day/week and/or 1 or more vomiting episodes/week
● The exclusion of self-induced vomiting, eating disorder, regurgitation and/or rumination
● No evidence of organic cause, systemic or metabolic diseases

Cyclic Vomiting Syndrome

● Stereotypical episodes of vomiting, less than 1 week, at least 3 episodes in the prior year and 2 episodes in the past 6 months occurring at least 1 week apart
● Absence of vomiting between the episodes
● Supportive evidence of history or family history of migraine

Cannabinoid Hyperemesis Syndrome

● Episodic vomiting resembling CVS, but vomiting occurs after prolonged use of cannabis.
● Cessation of vomiting occurs after cessation of cannabis.

Differential Diagnoses

INFANTS

➤ Gastro-oesophageal (GO) reflux

FOOD ALLERGY/INTOLERANCE

➤ Inborn errors of metabolism (e.g., galactosaemia)

➤ Systemic infection (e.g., urinary tract infection [UTI])
➤ Medications (e.g., antipyretics, antibiotics)

OLDER CHILDREN/ADOLESCENTS

➤ CVS
➤ Food allergy/intolerance
➤ Migraine
➤ IBD
➤ Subdural haematoma
➤ Renal or biliary colic

Recommended Investigations

➤ Investigations should be directed according to the history and clinical findings.
➤ Urine for reducing substance to diagnose galactosaemia; blood gases, amino acids and other metabolic screen tests are required for suspected inborn error of metabolism.

PRACTICE POINTS

- About 50% of neonates and infants regurgitate or vomit several times a day after feeding. If they are well otherwise and thriving and the vomit looks like milk, a diagnosis of GO reflux can be made.
- Pyloric stenosis is differentiated from GO reflux by vomiting (projectile) occurring in the first 2–3 weeks of life in a baby who is hungry with visible gastric peristalsis and a palpation of an 'olive' in the right upper quadrant. With reflux, children vomit during or immediately after feeding, and it starts soon after birth.
- Most infants with GO reflux do well by age 6–12 months; rare complications include oesophagitis, aspiration pneumonia and abnormal neck and head posturing (Sandifer's syndrome).
- Consider inborn errors of metabolism in the differential diagnosis of any unwell neonate who presents with poor feeding, lethargy, vomiting and convulsions in early life. The condition is often lethal unless prompt treatment is initiated.
- Vomiting usually causes metabolic alkalosis. The presence of metabolic acidosis is suggestive of gastroenteritis or inborn errors of metabolism. The latter possibility is high on the list in the presence of metabolic acidosis without diarrhoea.
- All children with unexplained vomiting should be referred to paediatrics.

UPPER GASTROINTESTINAL BLEEDING

Core Messages

➤ GI bleeding may originate anywhere from the mouth to the anus. It is much less common in children than in adults because of the rarity of GI cancers.

➤ Haematemesis usually indicates a bleed from a site proximal to the ligament of Treitz of the duodenum. Haematochezia refers to distal bleeding (Box 8.8).

➤ Upper gastrointestinal bleeding (UGIB) is uncommon but potentially serious. When haematemesis is caused by brisk bleeding, it usually indicates an arterial source, while coffee ground emesis results from bleeding that has slowed or stopped or from conversion of the red colour of Hb to brown haematin by gastric acid.

➤ The causes of haematemesis vary accordingly to the age of the child and whether there are other associated symptoms.

➤ Haematemesis (usually associated with nausea, vomiting, pain and possible tenderness of the abdomen) must be differentiated from haemoptysis (associated with cough, frothy colour, crackle noises on lung auscultation and evidence of pulmonary disease) and swallowed epistaxis (blood present in the nose, dripping into the posterior nasopharynx).

BOX 8.8 Terms and characteristics of GI bleeding

● UGIB	● GI bleeding proximal to the ligament of Treitz of the duodenum (oesophagus, stomach and duodenum).
● LGIB	● GI bleeding below the ligament of Treitz (small and large bowel).
● Haematemesis	● Vomiting of blood or coffee-like material from the upper GI tract.
● Haematochezia	● Passage of fresh red blood per anus, usually resulting from the colon (IBD, Meckel's diverticulum, juvenile polyps).
● Melaena	● Refers to black, tar-like and foul-smelling stools due to blood converted by intestinal enzymes. The bleeding usually originates from UGIB (peptic ulcer, gastritis, oesophageal varices).
● Occult blood	● Invisible blood from UGIB and LGIB, which can be detected by lab tests and presents as iron deficiency anaemia.

Differential Diagnoses

NEONATES/INFANTS

➤ Swallowed maternal blood (during birth) or from cracked nipple
➤ Oesophagitis (GO reflux)
➤ CMPA
➤ Coagulation disorders (vitamin K deficiency)

1–5 YEARS OF AGE

➤ Oesophageal varices (usually large haematemesis)
➤ Swallowed blood (e.g., epistaxis)
➤ Gastric erosion or ulcer
➤ Thrombocytopenia
➤ Meckel's diverticulum

5 YEARS

➤ Coagulopathy
➤ Drugs (NSAIDs)
➤ Mallory–Weiss syndrome

Recommended Investigations

➤ FBC: Anaemia suggests chronic blood loss or vomiting a large amount of blood; thrombocytopenia suggests a haematological cause of the bleeding.
➤ Coagulation tests (prothrombin time [PT], partial thromboplastin time [PTT], clotting factors) and liver function tests (LFTs) for bleeding or coagulation disease.
➤ Apt test to assess if the haematemesis is maternal (blood denatures with alkali) or fetal (blood does not denature with alkali) in origin.
➤ Abdominal ultrasound scan is the first line of imaging for suspected intussusception; if confirmed, an enema is used for reduction.
➤ Endoscopy for upper GI bleed.

PRACTICE POINTS

● Haematemesis is always a frightening experience for parents. There should be a low threshold to admit the child; this alone can relieve the parents' anxiety.
● The most common cause of haematemesis in a well full-term baby is swallowing of maternal blood during delivery or from the breast. Inspection of the mother's breast or expressing milk will suggest the diagnosis. Diagnosis can also be an Apt test performed on blood aspirated from the stomach.
● A history of passing blood mixed with toilet tissues is often due to a polyp that may be associated with abdominal pain.
● Haematemesis caused by medications, particularly NSAIDs, is underreported and underestimated; it is always worth taking a detailed history of recent intake of drugs. Aspirin should not be given to children (except in certain indications, e.g., Kawasaki's disease). Parents may not be aware that many over-the-counter (OTC) cough remedies and analgesics contain aspirin.
● Mallory–Weiss tear, described in 1929 in association with alcohol bingeing, is rare in children. GO reflux remains one of the most common causes of this tear. A Mallory–Weiss tear (linear laceration at the GO junction) may occur after a single episode of vomiting. Children with portal hypertension or hepatic insufficiency are at high risk of developing this tear.
● The proton pump inhibitors (PPIs) have shown benefit in the treatment of UGIB, particularly ulcer-related bleeding, and are superior to H2 antagonists. There are no differences (apart from price) between the five available PPIs (omeprazole, lansoprazole, pantoprazole, rabeprazole and esomeprazole) in clinical practice.

LOWER GASTROINTESTINAL BLEEDING

Core Messages

➤ GI bleeding is a fairly common, anxiety-provoking complaint. Massive bleeding, however, is rare.

➤ Damage to the GI mucosa is the most common cause of bleeding with the exception of few causes such as swallowed blood or bleeding due to polyps.

➤ Beyond the neonatal period, anal fissures resulting from constipation are the most common cause of rectal bleeding. The child presents with painful defecation and small blood streaks on the surface of the stool.

➤ Haematochezia, passage of bright red blood, usually indicates a bleed from a site below the ligament of Treitz of the duodenum, i.e., blood that has not been in contact with gastric juice.

➤ Bright blood mixed with loose stools suggests a bleeding site above the rectum (colitis, e.g., infectious or ulcerative colitis). Melena, the passage of black tarry stools, usually indicates an acute UGIB.

Differential Diagnoses

INFANTS

➤ Swallowed maternal blood
➤ Haemorrhagic disease (vitamin K deficiency)
➤ Polyps (juvenile colonic polyp)
➤ Anal fissure
➤ CMPA
➤ Coagulopathy

OLDER CHILDREN

➤ Polyp
➤ Intussusception
➤ Henoch–Schönlein purpura (HSP)
➤ Milk protein intolerance
➤ Drugs
➤ Meckel's diverticulum
➤ Sexual abuse causing proctitis, for example
➤ Colitis, e.g., allergic colitis
➤ IBD
➤ Familial adenomatous polyposis coli
➤ Hereditary haemorrhagic telangiectasia
➤ Peutz–Jeghers syndrome
➤ Haemorrhoids

Recommended Investigations

➤ FBC: Anaemia suggests chronic blood loss or acute massive bleeding and haemolytic uremic syndrome (HUS). Anaemia with high CRP suggests IBD. Low platelets in thrombocytopenia and disseminated intravascular coagulation (DIC).
➤ Blood grouping if bleeding is massive.
➤ LFTs may suggest liver cirrhosis. Renal function test (RFT) showing high urea and creatinine suggests HUS.
➤ Clotting study to evaluate coagulopathies such as haemophilia.
➤ Apt test to differentiate maternal from fetal blood.
➤ Stool testing for occult blood to confirm or exclude bleeding; culture will rule out infective colitis.
➤ Abdominal plain x-ray is useful in suspected cases of necrotizing enterocolitis (NEC) and intussusception.
➤ Sigmoidoscopy/colonoscopy indicated in suspected polyp.
➤ Air-contrast barium enema and nuclear scintigraphic imaging if the diagnosis remains unclear.

PRACTICE POINTS

● Red or black stools may be caused by ingestion of iron, charcoal, liquorice, blueberries and bismuth preparations, which can be mistaken as rectal bleeding.
● Rectal bleeding in a healthy neonate is most often maternal in origin through swallowed blood either during delivery or breast feeding.
● A neonatal peptic ulcer may be caused by hyperalimentation or drugs such as indomethacin used for patent ductus arteriosus (PDA) closure. Neonatal stress ulcers have often been linked with antenatal dexamethasone given for lung maturity in preterm infants.
● In paediatrics, anorectal disorders such as anal fissures, polyps and haemorrhoids are the most common causes of GI bleeding, producing fresh, bright red blood.
● Juvenile colonic polyps are the most common GI tumour in childhood, affecting 3–4%. The most common age at presentation is 2–8 years.
● GI bleeding is less common with CD than with UC. The former presents with the triad of anaemia, weight loss and abdominal pain.
● Dominantly inherited familial polyposis (familial adenomatous polyposis coli, Gardner's syndrome and Peutz–Jeghers syndrome) are premalignant polyps requiring resection (e.g., by snare cautery). Children with a positive family history need supervision and genetic counselling.
● Always consider child sexual abuse presenting as GI bleeding, e.g., perianal trauma, tags, irregular or dilated anal tone and contour or proctitis.

PERSISTENT DIARRHOEA

Core Messages

➤ Diarrhoea is common in children and is most often infectious in origin. It is defined as an increase in the daily fluid losses of stool and is usually associated with frequent stools (Box 8.9).

➤ Most diarrhoeal diseases in children living in high-income countries are viral, mild and self-limiting and do not require hospitalization or further laboratory evaluation. In middle- and low-income countries, diarrhoea is often infectious and severe, caused by bacteria or parasites. It causes a high rate of deaths, and up to 17% of under-5 child mortality is attributable to diarrhoea. Persistent diarrhoea (PD) causes up to 50% of the total deaths.

➤ The incidence of IBD has increased significantly during the past few decades. Diarrhoea (recurrent and bloody) is the hallmark symptom of IBD and occurs in almost 80% of all cases.

BOX 8.9 Definitions of diarrhoea-related terms

● Diarrhoea is three or more looser-than-normal stools in the preceding 24 hours.
● An episode of diarrhoea is a diarrhoea lasting >1 day and separated from another episode by ≥ 1 day without diarrhoea.
● Acute diarrhoea is an episode of diarrhoea that lasts <7 days.
● Prolonged diarrhoea is an episode of diarrhoea that lasts 7–14 days.
● PD is an episode of diarrhoea that lasts >14 days.

Differential Diagnoses

INFECTIOUS

➤ Infective enteritis (viruses, bacteria and parasites)

NON-INFECTIOUS

➤ Physiological in breastfed/toddler's diarrhoea
➤ Food induced (monosaccharide and disaccharide malabsorption, CMPA)
➤ Postinfectious
➤ Malabsorption (e.g., coeliac disease, CF)
➤ IBD
➤ Antibiotic induced (e.g., pseudomembranous colitis)
➤ Irritable bowel syndrome (IBS)
➤ Immunosuppression
➤ Induced illness

Recommended Investigations

➤ Blood U&E is indicated unless the diarrhoea is mild.

➤ Stool for culture (bacterial) and antigen for viral cause (adenovirus, rotavirus)

➤ Testing the stool with Clinitest tablets (reducing substances >0.5% indicate lactose or glucose malabsorption).

➤ Stool pH: In lactose intolerance, it is acidic (pH <5.5).

PRACTICE POINTS

- The principal complication from diarrhoea is dehydration. If a child is alert and playful, the degree of dehydration is insignificant (Table 8.3).
- Parents are usually good historians. Simply asking about urine frequency and colour can give an important estimate of the degree of dehydration: Concentrated urine (orange colour) suggests mild dehydration; infrequent and small amounts of urine suggest moderate dehydration. Anuria means severe dehydration.
- Toddler's diarrhoea is common and may be misdiagnosed as gastroenteritis. These children are healthy and thriving and passing three to five soft stools daily, often containing undigested food particles (e.g., carrots, whole peas).
- Large watery diarrhoea in association with central abdominal pain and vomiting is typical for enteritis (usually termed gastroenteritis), whereas small frequent stools and lower abdominal pain with blood in stool are highly suggestive of colitis.
- Diarrhoea persisting for >2 weeks is often due to milk lactose or protein intolerance. Temporary withdrawal of milk and dairy products is usually diagnostic and therapeutic.
- Laxative-induced diarrhoea (induced illness or Munchausen's syndrome) is rare but should not be missed. The diarrhoea is usually chronic or recurrent. There is an underlying psychiatric disturbance in the carer of the child.

TABLE 8.3 Rapid assessment of dehydration

	Normal	Dehydration
● Mental status	● Alert, playful, responds to appropriate questions and commands	● Inactive, not smiling and playing, drowsy
● Oral mucous	● Moist, visible saliva	● Dry
● Skin pinch	● Immediate flattening of skin fold after releasing	● Slow flattening after skin pinch >2 seconds
● Capillary refill	● Skin colour after pressing (e.g., finger) returns to normal <2 seconds; normal light colour	● Slow return to normal colour >2 seconds
● Urine output	● Normal light colour	● Concentrated dark urine, oliguria

CONSTIPATION

Core Messages

➤ Constipation is a common complaint and accounts for approximately 25% of visits to paediatric gastroenterologists.

➤ It is either functional (FC), occurring in 95% of cases, or organic (in 5% of cases). The latter often presents in the first few weeks of life.

➤ Constipation is defined according to Rome criteria (Box 8.10). It is important to remember that infrequent defaecation is common in breastfed babies, who may not have a stool for up to 10 days without needing further assessment. There should be no intervention as long as babies are thriving, feeding well, have no abdominal distension and pass stools without straining or blood. Mild straining during defecation can be normal.

➤ In older children, the most common reason for retentive posturing is withholding stool for fear of having a bowel movement. Parents may wrongly interpret withholding stool as pushing. Parents need to be taught about this posturing that is a behavioural issue.

➤ There is an increasing recognition of the role of cow's milk protein (CMP) allergy in children with constipation. CMP allergy has been reported in 4.6%. The diagnosis should be considered in children with concomitant atopic signs and symptoms or in those constipated children who are unresponsive to conventional therapy. There is currently no recommendation for routine testing in children with FC. An exclusion diet should confirm the diagnosis.

BOX 8.10 Diagnostic criteria of constipation

At least two of the following features in a child at least 4 years of age:

- Two or fewer defections in the toilet per week
- History of retentive postering
- History of painful or hard bowel movements
- Presence of a large faecal mass
- History of large-diameter stool which may obstruct the toilet
- It cannot be explained by another condition

Management

➤ Physical examination of a child with constipation should routinely include palpation of the abdomen for a faecal mass, anal and sacral areas for fissure and sacral anatomical abnormalities. Alarm signs and symptoms for organic diseases (Red Flags) should be excluded in all children with constipation as a first step. Rectal examinations in children are not performed in primary care.

➤ Toilet training: About 80–100% of all young children with FC exhibit features of stool withholding, and most refuse to pass stool in the toilet. Children should be instructed on proper seating on the potty or toilet for 5 minutes after waking, after lunch and after dinner while keeping the legs and perineum relaxed. Parents may need to reinforce positive behaviour with small rewards for sitting and passing a stool in the toilet.

➤ Dietary measures, including 5–10 g of fibre daily, e.g., corn fibre in addition to water.

WARNING SIGNS (RED FLAGS) IN CONSTIPATION

- Delayed passage of meconium
- Bilious vomiting
- Abdominal distension
- Failure to thrive
- Anal fissure in children >2 years of age
- Neurological abnormalities/lower limb weakness
- Developmental delay
- Hair tuft, haemangioma, scars on spine
- Abnormal anal/cremasteric reflex
- Suspected child sexual abuse
- Undue fear of anal examination

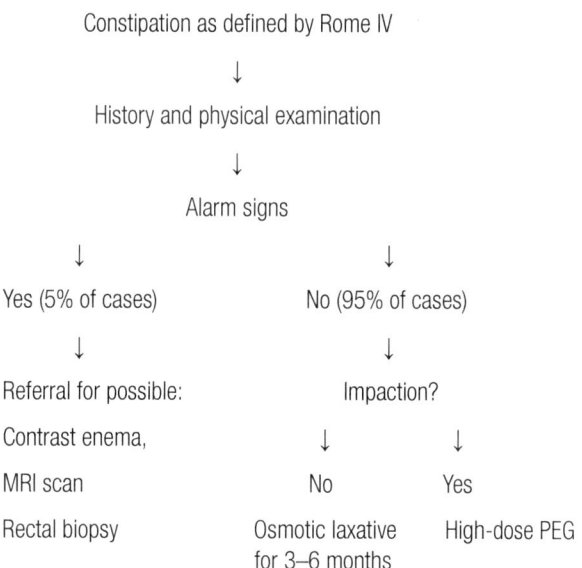

FIGURE 8.1 Summary of management of constipation.

➤ Laxatives include polyethylene glycol (PEG) as the most effective osmotic laxative for stool impaction in a high dose of 0.7 g/kg (Figure 8.1). Bisacodyl and senna are useful adjunct stimulants (prokinetic) in case of insufficient response with PEG.

➤ CMP can occasionally cause FC. Guidelines recommend a CMP-free diet only in laxative-resistant FC.

PRACTICE POINTS

- Over 90% of healthy neonates pass a stool in the first 24–48 hours of life, but delay in passing meconium after 48 hours is abnormal.
- By far the most common cause of constipation is functional. Organic diseases (Hirschsprung's disease, hypothyroidism, hypercalcaemia, renal tubular acidosis) are rare in practice and account for 5% only.
- Faecal soiling (involuntary seepage of a small amount of stool) is usually caused by chronic rectal retention. It is treated by evacuating the rectum. Faecal soiling may be mistaken for diarrhoea. Parents should receive information about the mechanism causing soiling.
- Routine radiography and anorectal manometry are not recommended for evaluation of children with constipation.
- Parents of constipated children should be told that long-term treatment is often required. While 60–70% of children with FC recover within 1–2 years, approximately 30% may expect longer treatment times with laxatives.

JAUNDICE

Core Messages

➤ Jaundice, defined as bilirubin levels ≥33 μmol/L (≥2 mg/dL), is most commonly observed during the neonatal period. Almost all neonates become jaundiced with indirect or unconjugated hyperbilirubinaemia (UH) in the first few days of life.

➤ The unconjugated bilirubin is fat soluble and can enter the brain tissue, causing kernicterus. Conjugated bilirubin is water soluble, not fat soluble, and therefore it does not damage the brain tissue to cause kernicterus. It is, however, associated with serious diseases such as biliary atresia (Box 8.11).

➤ Jaundice appearing after 4 or 5 days of life suggests an infection, e.g., UTI or sepsis. Jaundice after the first week of life suggests breast milk jaundice, biliary atresia, infection or metabolic disorders, e.g., galactosaemia.

➤ After the neonatal period, viral hepatitis remains the most common cause of jaundice worldwide and is characterized by conjugated hyperbilirubinaemia (CH) and elevated liver enzymes. Hepatitis A virus (HAV) used to be a common infectious disease, but its incidence has declined significantly in high-income countries. However, HAV continues to infect 200 million worldwide, with up to 30,000 deaths each year.

➤ The prevalence of hepatitis B virus (HBV), hepatitis C virus (HCV) and other hepatotropic viruses has increased worldwide causing chronic liver disease and primary hepatocellular carcinoma.

➤ Autoimmune hepatitis is characterized by hypergammaglobulinaemia and autoantibodies and may present as acute, fulminant or asymptomatic hepatitis.

BOX 8.11 Main causes of jaundice

Local (hepatic)

Unconjugated hyperbilirubinaemia

- Physiological
- Haemolytic (e.g., ABO incompatibility, G6PD deficiency)
- Breast milk
- Gilbert's syndrome
- Crigler–Najjar syndrome

Conjugated hyperbilirubinaemia

- Congenital hepatitis (e.g., cytomegalovirus [CMV])
- Autoimmune hepatitis
- Liver cirrhosis
- Drug-induced

Systemic

Unconjugated hyperbilirubinaemia

- Congenital spherocytosis
- Other haemolytic diseases, e.g., G6PD

Conjugated hyperbilirubinaemia

- Genetic liver diseases (Dubin–Johnson and Rotor syndromes)
- Mononucleosis
- Wilson's disease
- Metabolic (e.g., galactosaemia)
- Obstructive jaundice (e.g., by gallstones)
- Cystic fibrosis

PRACTICE POINTS

- Physiologic jaundice occurs in most neonates during the first few days of life. It is not a disease, it is not present in the first 24 hours, and it is always a UH. Breast milk jaundice is nothing else than physiologic jaundice, which may persist for weeks. It is not a disease, and mothers should be encouraged to continue breastfeeding.

- Gilbert syndrome (GS) is a common genetic cause (*UGT1A1* genotype) of UH (typically not exceeding 6mg/dL or 103 mmol/L), affecting 5–10% in Europe. Liver function tests are otherwise normal, including liver enzymes. The diagnosis is often made during routine health checks. The first description of GS was in 1901 and included Napolean Bonaparte and his mother.
- GS is the most common cause of UH in older children. The hyperbilirubinemia typically manifests during puberty, particularly after a period of fasting, dehydration or exertion. The diagnosis is based on genetic testing. Before the availability of the gene testing, It was a diagnosis of exclusion (e.g., excluding haemolytic anaemia) and based on calorie restriction (fasting) resulting in hyperbilirubinemia.
- Although infectious hepatitis is the most common cause of jaundice worldwide, jaundice is present in as few as 1 in 10 children with HAV, 1 in 4 in HBV and in less than 1 in 3 in HCV. The jaundice is characteristically due to CH and is defined as a conjugated bilirubin >1 mg/dL (17 mmoL).
- Acute HAV causes a mild self-limiting illness. Effective and safe inactivated HAV vaccines have been available since 1996, and two doses elicit seroprotection for an estimated period of 30–40 years. There is no need for a later booster.
- Acute HBV infection is a subclinical illness in two-thirds of cases, and one-third of patients develop symptomatic hepatitis. Infected blood or bodily fluid (e.g., vertical transmission from mother to child, IV drug use or sexual contact) is the usual route of transmission. Universal childhood vaccination is the best prevention.
- HCV evades the immune system to cause chronic hepatitis in most cases with this infection. Nearly all cases of HCV are asymptomatic, often causing later liver cirrhosis. IV drug use and sexual contact are the main modes of transmission. A new modality of treatment, 'direct-acting antivirals (DAAs)', is very effective.

CHAPTER 9

Respiratory Diseases

INTRODUCTION

➤ Respiratory diseases are a leading cause of morbidity and mortality worldwide. Of the 6.6 million children under the age of 5 years who die annually, respiratory diseases are the leading cause of death. Respiratory tract infections occur most frequently in early childhood.

➤ The microbiome, which consists of commensal, symbiotic and pathogen microorganisms living in the human body, plays an important role in host health and immunity. For example, when the microbiome in the upper airway becomes dysfunctional or imbalanced (dysbiosis), pathogens can spread and lead to development of otitis media, sinusitis and asthma.

➤ The history and systemic physical examination (Box 9.1) are the most important first steps in diagnosing respiratory diseases. The symptoms and the observed signs influence the direction of the subsequent investigation.

BOX 9.1 Approach to the respiratory system

Observation

- Abnormal chest shape?
- Audible respiratory sounds? (Table 9.1)
- Count of respiratory rate (RR)?
- Any signs of respiratory distress?
  - › Subcostal recession?
  - › Nasal flaring?
  - › Tachypnoea?

Palpation

- Mediastinal deviation (tracheal position)?
- Chest expansion?

Percussion

- Any dullness?
- Define the upper liver edge

Auscultation

- Breath sounds (using the diaphragm of the stethoscope) to detect bronchial breathing, which occurs with pneumonia.
- Wheezing (indicating bronchospasm) as heard in asthma. Crepitations (crackles) are normal if cleared by coughing; if not, they are suggestive of consolidation.

RESPIRATORY NOISES

➤ Respiratory noises are extremely common and often difficult to differentiate from each other. Children may also make multiple noises, be intermittent or change from one noise to another in a few minutes or depending on whether they are awake or asleep or change sleep position (polyphonic).

➤ Clinicians should be familiar with common noises, which include snuffle, wheeze, stridor, rattle, grunt and snore (Table 9.1). An error in recognizing specific types of noises will lead to diagnostic and therapeutic errors.

➤ Imitating a wheeze, stridor or whoop to parents can be helpful in identifying the right noise.

➤ Snuffles and stridor are caused by obstruction of the extrathoracic airways (nose, pharynx, larynx and the extrathoracic portion of the trachea), while wheezing is caused by intrathoracic obstruction.

TABLE 9.1 Summary of common respiratory sounds

Noise	Description
Extrathoracic	
• Snuffles	• Commonly due to blocked nose in children <6 months of age, usually caused by normal mucus collected in the nose and not by infection.
• Stridor	• Consists of a harsh inspiratory sound caused by extrathoracic airway obstruction. Acute stridor with involvement of the vocal cords (hoarseness) is usually caused by croup. Persistent stridor without vocal cord involvement is likely caused by laryngomalacia.
• Snore	• Inspiratory and irregular noise caused by partial obstruction of the naso-oro-pharynx area.
Intrathoracic	
• Wheeze	• Indicates intrathoracic airway obstruction, heard mainly during expiration, often with subcostal retraction.
• Rattle	• Coarse, irregular sound mainly heard in inspiration and is caused by secretions in the trachea or major bronchi subsequent to viral infection and, occasionally, gastro-oesophageal (GO) reflux.
• Grunt	• Short expiratory sound caused by partial closure of glottis during expiration. It is an important sign of pneumonia.

PRACTICE POINTS

- Acute snuffles are mostly caused by a viral infection, while persistent ones may be due to allergic rhinitis, adenoid hypertrophy or common snuffle noises of infancy. The latter is expected to disappear around the age of 4–6 months. In older children with persist entnasal snuffles, polyps need to be excluded.
- Expiratory grunts are usually associated with respiratory distress syndrome in neonates and pneumonia in older children.
- A rattle, if acute, is usually due to viral infection and occasionally bacterial infection. If persistent, it is often due to GO reflux or sputum retention, often found in neuromuscular diseases.
- The association of hoarseness and stridor suggests an obstruction at the vocal cords of the larynx such as viral laryngotracheobronchitis. Hoarseness is not present in laryngomalacia because the vocal cords are not involved. If a cough is present, it suggests the trachea is involved.
- Laryngomalacia is the most common cause of chronic stridor, noted usually soon after birth, and disappears at the age of 12–18 months. It does not require laryngoscopy unless there are atypical features such as failure to thrive, persistent cough, hoarseness of the voice or feeding problems.

STRIDOR

Introduction

➤ Stridor is a noisy respiration, usually produced in inspiration, resulting from a turbulent passage of air through a partial obstruction of the airway. The upper airway obstruction (extrathoracic) is commonly caused by viral infections (croup or laryngotracheobronchitis [LTB]) such as parainfluenza (>40% of cases), influenza, rhinovirus and adenovirus. Croup without apparent infection or fever is termed spasmodic croup, which usually occurs late at night. Bacterial causes include bacterial tracheitis caused by *Staphylococcal aureus* or epiglottitis caused by *Haemophilus influenzae* type B (Box 9.2).

BOX 9.2 Main causes of stridor

- Acute transient stridor
  - ❯ Laryngotracheobronchitis (LTB; viral croup)
  - ❯ Spasmodic croup
  - ❯ Aspiration of foreign body (FB)
  - ❯ Angioedema
  - ❯ Bacterial tracheitis (staphylococcal infection)
  - ❯ Epiglottitis
  - ❯ Laryngospasm (hypocalcaemia tetany)
- Persistent stridor
  - ❯ Laryngomalacia
  - ❯ Tumour, e.g., papilloma, haemangioma, nodule
  - ❯ Vocal cord paralysis

➤ Symptoms of viral croup and spasmodic croup are usually mild and transient, and recovery within few days is the likely outcome, in contrast with croup caused by bacterial infection (Table 9.2). Severe degrees of obstruction usually occur with bacterial infection (epiglottitis) and produce rapidly progressive respiratory distress, worsening cough, irritability, restlessness, nasal flaring, subcostal and intercostal recession and potential risk of death. Since the introduction of *H. influenza* type B vaccination in 1985, the incidence of bacterial epiglottis has significantly decreased.

➤ Management of croup is shown in Box 9.3.

TABLE 9.2 Assessing croup severity and typical presentation of LTB vs. bacterial infection

	Viral (e.g., LTB)	Bacterial (e.g., Tracheitis)
• Typical age	• 6 months to 3 years	• Preschool-aged children
• Appearance	• Normal, miserable	• Toxic
• Level of consciousness	• Good	• Agitated or tired/drowsy
• Preceding viral URTI	• Usual	• Possible
• Fever	• Mild or absent	• High >39°C
• Symptom occurrence	• At night	• Any time
• Symptoms/signs subsiding	• 1–3 days	• Longer unless receiving parenteral antibiotics
• Air entry/chest retraction	• No/mild	• Decreased/mild-to-moderate
• Prognosis	• Good	• Life-threatening

PRACTICE POINTS

- Croup is one of the most common causes of respiratory distress, affecting 5% of children aged between 6 months and 3 years. Nearly all cases of croup are caused by viral infections. Following 12–24 hours of non-specific symptoms of an upper respiratory tract infection (URTI), there is usually an abrupt onset of a barky cough with inspiratory stridor, hoarse voice and varying degrees of respiratory distress, occurring mostly at night. There may a mild degree of fever, but higher degrees of fever are found in cases due to influenza or parainfluenza viruses.

- Laryngomalacia is the most common cause of childhood persistent stridor due to a collapse of the supraglottic structures during inspiration (laryngoscopy finding). It typically presents in the first weeks of life with an inspiratory stridor that worsens with activity, crying and feeding. It has a high rate of resolution without intervention in about 90% of cases at an age of 8 months on average (range: 4–42 months).

- In contrast to viral croup, epiglottitis is a potentially lethal condition because of rapidly progressing obstruction leading to severe hypoxia. There is a high fever, and the voice is muffled with a mild stridor. Typically, the child has not been immunized against *H. influenza*. *Urgent referral is required.*

- Bacterial tracheitis is a rare but potentially life-threatening condition with a high mortality rate – up to 20%. Like epiglottitis, children appear toxic with high fever, stridor and hoarse voice. Infection progresses rapidly, leading to airway obstruction.
- In cases of viral croup or epiglottitis, throat inspection, including the use of a tongue depressor, may result in sudden cardiorespiratory arrest and therefore should be omitted.
- A young child (typically 6 months to 2 years) with sudden choking and coughing with or without stridor or hoarseness should be suspected of having an FB. The diagnosis requires a high index of suspicion, as FB occurrence is often unwitnessed and the child could be in the preverbal age group.

BOX 9.3 Management of croup

- Most children with acute viral croup/spasmodic croup can be managed at home.
- The child should be disturbed as little as possible. Care should be taken to keep the child calm, best achieved on the parent's lap. If admission becomes necessary, a parent should be allowed to stay with the child.
- At home (as in the hospital) the child should be observed carefully for worsening symptoms of respiratory distress.
- The use of steam from a shower or vaporizer at home is often effective.
- Antibiotic treatment is not indicated in viral croup.
- The Westley score system (Chapter 12) provides further management.
- *Dexamethasone:* 0.15 mg/kg one dose to be given before transfer to hospital, to be repeated after 12 hours (Dexamethasone soluble tablets: 2, 4 and 8 mg are available and as a solution 20 mg/5 mL).
- *Prednisolone:* 1–2 mg/kg (before transfer to hospital).
- Nebulized adrenaline is indicated for severe croup. This should not be administered in primary care; *urgent referral is essential.*
- *Referral is indicated in the case of:*
  - ❯ A croup with symptoms which do not improve 6–12 hours after dexamethasone treatment.
  - ❯ Suspected epiglottitis.
  - ❯ Progressive or severe stridor.
  - ❯ Tachypnoea, as this may be the first sign of hypoxia.
  - ❯ Severe respiratory distress (e.g., obvious suprasternal recession).
  - ❯ Restless or drowsy child.
  - ❯ High fever or toxic-appearing child.
  - ❯ Feeding or swallowing difficulty.
  - ❯ Poor air entry on auscultation.
  - ❯ Concerned parents.

ASTHMA AND UNEXPLAINED SHORTNESS OF BREATH

Introduction

➤ Dyspnoea is a common symptom of a variety of cardiopulmonary diseases (Box 9.4). Asthma is the most common cause for dyspnoea. Congestive cardiac failure is an important but a rare cause of dyspnoea at any age of childhood. Dyspnoea rarely occurs in isolation, and accompanying features include cough, wheezing, tachypnoea and subcostal recession.

➤ Young children may describe dyspnoea as 'getting easily tired' or 'can't keep up with other kids'. It may occur spontaneously or during certain activities such as exercise or during feeding in infants.

➤ The differentiation between cardiac and pulmonary causes of dyspnoea can be difficult. The presence of a murmur, liver enlargement and relative tachycardia favours cardiac causes. While oxygen supplementation does not significantly improve O_2 saturation in cardiac diseases, in pulmonary diseases, there will be rapid improvement of the O_2 saturation.

BOX 9.4 Main causes of severe dyspnoea

- Pulmonary
  - ❯ Undiagnosed asthma
  - ❯ Viral-induced wheeze/bronchiolitis
  - ❯ Pneumonia
  - ❯ Pulmonary oedema
  - ❯ Pulmonary embolism
  - ❯ Inhaled foreign body
  - ❯ Pleural effusion
  - ❯ Congenital malformations, including hypoplasia
  - ❯ Pneumothorax
- Cardiac
  - ❯ Congestive cardiac failure (CCF)
  - ❯ Myocarditis, pericarditis
  - ❯ Hypertrophic obstructive cardiomyopathy
- Metabolic acidosis such as diabetic ketoacidosis
- Neuromuscular diseases
- Psychogenic

Investigations

➤ Essential bedside observation and investigation:
  - ➣ Respiratory rate
  - ➣ Oxygen saturation monitoring (oximetry)
  - ➣ Peak expiratory flow rate

➤ Spirometry can differentiate between obstructive (decrease in flow) and restrictive (decreased lung volume) causes of dyspnoea.

➤ A chest x-ray is a helpful investigation. It may show hyperinflation (e.g., asthma), collapse or consolidation (pneumonia) or pneumothorax. However, a chest x-ray in the absence of a clinical indication should not be part of the initial diagnostic workup.

➤ Echocardiography and ECG in patients with suspected heart diseases.

ASTHMA

➤ Asthma is the most common chronic childhood respiratory disease, with a worldwide prevalence of 5–10%.

➤ Asthma is diagnosed in clinical practice by nonspecific symptoms and signs, usually triggered by exercise, viral infection, or inhaled allergens, due to chronic airway hyperresponsiveness and airway inflammation (Box 9.5).

➤ In young children, viral infections are the most common cause of asthma attacks. Other causes include air pollution, allergy (pollen, house dust mites), tobacco, exercise, stress, and drugs such as beta-2 blockers.

➤ Diagnosis of asthma in children <5 years of age is difficult and mainly based on the occurrence of cough and wheezing. The presence of atopy (own or family history) makes asthma more likely.

➤ Most individuals with asthma can be managed entirely in primary care, either face to face or remotely. Management aims to achieve a good control of symptoms of asthma (Box 9.6).

BOX 9.5 Clinical diagnostic features of asthma

● Symptoms of wheeze, cough, dyspnoea and chest tightness, particularly if these are frequent and recurrent; are worse at night; and are triggered by viral infections, exercise, pets, cold or damp air exposure or with emotions.

● Personal and family history of atopic disease.

● Symptom variation throughout the day and season.

● Substantial improvement of airway obstruction from an inhaled bronchodilator, with a positive bronchodilator reversibility >20% being positive.

Supporting Evidence

● Spirometry and peak expiratory flow rate (PEFR) monitoring are recommended to demonstrate variable airflow obstruction. *Referral is indicated if a patient presents with cough as the only symptom.*

● Fractional exhaled nitric oxide (FeNO). A positive test indicates the presence of eosinophilic inflammation and provides support for an asthma diagnosis.

BOX 9.6 Good asthma control

- No daytime or nighttime troublesome symptoms due to asthma.
- No asthma attacks or infrequent and mild attacks requiring occasional SABA.
- Normal physical activity, including exercises.
- Associated with little or no need for bronchodilator.
- Normal lung function (FEV_1 and/or 80% PEF >80% of predicted).
- No more than one canister of short-acting beta-2 agonist (SABA) per month.
- No or minimal side effects from medications.

MANAGEMENT OF ASTHMA IN PRIMARY CARE

Non-Pharmacological

➤ Growth measurement (weight and height centiles) and plot on a centile chart.
➤ Checking for any asthma exacerbations, oral steroid use, and absence from school.
➤ Concordance (engaging patients in shared decision-making to reach an agreement through communication, for example, by reviewing a "Self-management plan").
➤ Explain when and how to use inhalers.
➤ Avoidance of asthma triggers.
➤ Possession of and use of a self-management plan (Box 9.7).

BOX 9.7 Self-management plan

- Patients with asthma should be offered a self-management plan that focuses on individual needs and that is reinforced by a written personalized action plan. Useful action in this plan includes:
  - ❯ PEF <80% best necessitates increase of the inhaled steroid.
  - ❯ PEF <60% best necessitates commencing an oral steroid.
  - ❯ PEF <40% best necessitates seeking urgent medical help.
- Early use of steroid tablets can reduce the need for hospital admission. A suitable dose is 20 mg for children aged 2–5 years and 30–40 mg of prednisolone for those older than 5 years.

Pharmacological (>5–16 Years; for Children <5 Years, see Box 9.8)

➤ **SABAs**
  ➢ SABA (such as salbutamol) should be used as a metered dose inhaler (MDI) via a spacer to provide the best method of delivery SABA or ICS.
  ➢ SABA inhaler should be used for emergency for children <11 years of age who may be unable to activate a dry powder inhaler during an acute asthma attack.

➤ **Inhaled corticosteroids (ICSs)**
  ➤ Available preparations are beclometasone, budesonide, ciclesonide, fluticasone and mometasone.
  ➤ ICSs are the most effective medication for controlling asthma symptoms and treating the chronic airway inflammation, particularly in poorly controlled asthma treated with SABA alone (Box 9.9). Indications for ICS use include:
    ➤ Using SABA three times a week or more.
    ➤ Symptomatic three times or more per week.
    ➤ Waking one night per week.
    ➤ Asthma attack requiring treatment with oral corticosteroid in the last 2 years.
  ➤ Beclometasone is initially administered in small doses of 100–200 micrograms twice daily or budesonide 100–400 micrograms twice daily.
  ➤ If symptoms did not resolve during a trial period of 4–8 weeks, stop the ICS and check:
    ➤ For medication adherence, inhaler technique and trigger elimination.
    ➤ Whether an alternative diagnosis is likely (Box 9.10). Consider a referral for specialist assessment.
    ➤ Other options:
➤ **Add-on therapy** is to be considered with *leukotriene receptor antagonists (LTRAs)* in addition to the low dose of ICS. The LTRA *Montelukast* is not more effective than an ICS, but the drugs have an additive effect. Dose: 5 mg for 6- to 11-year-olds and 4 mg for 5-year-olds in the evening.
➤ If asthma is still uncontrolled, consider stopping the *LTRA* and offer a long-acting beta-2 agonist (LABA) in combination with a low dose of ICS.
➤ If asthma remains uncontrolled, consider maintenance ICS and *LABA* and reliever therapy (MART).
➤ For still uncontrolled cases, consideration should be given to an increased dose of ICS.

BOX 9.8 Management of probable asthma

- After an initial clinical assessment based on the occurrence of cough and wheezing, children are offered SABA inhalation for symptomatic relief.
- If the probability of asthma is high, ICS can be considered.
- If there is no response and the medication has been taken, asthma is unlikely, and the child should be referred for specialist assessment.

BOX 9.9 Uncontrolled asthma

- Three or more episodes per week with symptoms.
- Three or more episodes per week with required use of SABA.
- One or more nights per week with awakening due to asthma.

BOX 9.10 Summary of conditions mimicking asthma

Cystic Fibrosis

- Cystic fibrosis (CF) is second most common chronic airway disease after asthma (incidence: 1 in 2500).
- Persistent respiratory symptoms (cough, dyspnoea, expectoration of sputum).
- Symptoms and signs of malabsorption.
- Finger clubbing is an important diagnostic clue.
- Little or no response to a short course of bronchodilator and steroids.

Ciliary Dyskinesia

- Persistent cough almost since birth, persistent or recurrent otitis media.
- May present with purulent sputum production due to bronchiectasis.
- Situs inversus (Kartagener's syndrome) is present in about 50% of patients.

Post-Foreign Body Inhalation

- Typical age 1–3 years; child was previously asymptomatic with a history of sudden onset of respiratory distress with choking and cough.
- FB inhalation was unwitnessed, and the child could be in the preverbal age group. Symptoms may persist or disappear for a period to present later with cough and wheeze mimicking asthma attack due to bronchiectasis or pneumonia.

Hyperventilation (Psychogenic)

- Usually adolescents, often girls.
- Normal examination of the cardiopulmonary system, normal respiratory rate and normal lung function tests.

Immunodeficiency

- Recurrent pneumonia, often pyogenic; other recurrent infections.

Gastro-Oesophageal Reflux

- Reflux with repeated vomiting may cause aspiration with recurrent cough/wheezing.

MANAGEMENT OF AN ACUTE ASTHMA ATTACKS

➤ Assess the degree of severity (Table 9.3).
➤ Measurement of PEFR using peak flow meter in 1 second (spirometer) and pulse oximeter for oxygen saturation.
➤ Inhaled SABA either with an inhaler or nebulizer.
  ➢ A puff can be given every 30–60 seconds up to 10 puffs.
  ➢ Each puff should be given one at a time and inhaled within five breaths. Repeat the inhalation every 10–20 minutes according to the clinical response.
  ➢ Ipratropium (Atrovent) can be added in severe cases.
➤ Oral corticosteroid 1–2 mg/kg for 3–5 days.
➤ *Referral of children for specialist assessment may be indicated* (Box 9.11).

TABLE 9.3 The three degrees of severity of asthma

Symptom	Mild	Moderate	Severe
• General	• Looks well	• Mildly unwell	• Unwell
• Pulse rate	• <120/minute	• 120–170/minute	• >170/minute
• RR	• <40/minute	• 40–70/minute	• >70/minute
• Subcostal	• Mild	• Moderate	• Severe
• recession			
• SaO_2	• >94%	• 90–94%	• <90%
• FEP	• >70% predicted	• 50–70%	• <50%
• Alert	• Yes	• Yes	• Agitated or drowsy
• Speech in sentences	• Yes	• Yes	• Difficult/unable

BOX 9.11 Indication for specialist/hospital referral

- Moderate or severe asthma attack.
- Failure to respond to asthma treatment, particularly inhaled steroid over 400 mcg/day or frequent use of oral corticosteroids.
- Persistent cough without wheezing.
- Diagnosis unclear or in doubt.
- Symptoms present since birth, or symptoms related to perinatal problems.
- Persistent wet or productive cough.
- Excessive vomiting or posseting.
- Weight loss/failure to thrive.
- Nasal polyps.
- Unexpected clinical findings (e.g., focal signs, inspiratory stridor, dysphagia).
- Parental anxiety and their wish for referral to see a specialist.

PERSISTENT COUGH

Core Messages

➤ Cough is a reflex which is a vital physiological protective response aimed to clear airway irritation (e.g., inflammation and secretions) to maintain airway patency and prevent aspiration. It is defined as acute (<2 weeks), subacute (2–4 weeks) or chronic/persistent (>4 weeks). Box 9.12 lists the main causes of persistent cough.

➤ *Cough is the single most common reason for primary care visits and, if persistent, a frequent indication for specialist referral.* It is responsible for >50% of new patient attendances in the primary care setting. A viral URTI-associated cough is the most common cause of cough in children. Risk factors of cough are shown in Box 9.13.

➤ Children's cough is rarely productive, as children are unable to expectorate sputum, and, therefore, the term 'wet cough' rather than 'productive cough' is more appropriate. Cough is also divided into dry (e.g., asthma) and wet-moist (bronchiectasis).

BOX 9.12 Causes of persistent cough

Extrathoracic

● URTI (viral URTI, croup)

Pulmonary

● Asthma
● Infections (pneumonia, bronchitis, bronchiolitis, tuberculosis [TB])
● Ciliary dyskinesia
● Inhaled FB
● CF
● Bronchiectasis
● Alpha-1 antitrypsin deficiency
● Pertussis
● Allergy (dust or pollen inhalation)
● GO reflux

Psychogenic

BOX 9.13 Risk factors of exposure to infections and cough

● Children aged 1–3 years
● Winter months (January and February)
● Nursery attendance
● Lack of vaccination
● Cough in family members
● Atopic individuals
● Immunosuppression

Investigations

➤ Full blood count (FBC): White blood cells (WBCs) and C-reactive protein (CRP): Raised in bacterial infection and sometimes in asthma. Eosinophilia suggests an allergic condition (abnormal if >4%).
➤ Sputum for culture from children with productive cough.
➤ Lung function testing: Using spirometry or peak flow meter.
➤ Chest x-ray is very helpful in diagnosing pneumonia or FB. Also very useful in excluding pathology if the presentation does not suggest a clear diagnosis.

➤ CT scan of the lung if bronchiectasis is suspected (done in hospital).
➤ Sweat test if CF is suspected (done in hospital).
➤ Gastric pH study for cases suspected of GO reflux (done in hospital).

PRACTICE POINTS

- Cough for several days or weeks in otherwise healthy children usually occurs after a viral URTI. Other triggers include tobacco, smoke, pollutants, aerosols and dust.
- A child who presents with cough on exertion only is likely to have exercise-induced asthma. Performing peak expiratory flow measurements before and after exercise can help diagnose asthma. If the cough is persistent and a diagnosis is unexplained, a trial with a bronchodilator is justified. Improvement after salbutamol inhalation will support the diagnosis of asthma.
- FB can mimic symptoms of croup and asthma. In any child with abrupt onset of cough, particularly with choking/spluttering, FB should be excluded. If missed, chronic respiratory infections, such as bronchiectasis, are the likely consequences.
- A common cause of persistent cough is protracted bacterial bronchitis (PBB), especially in children <6 years. Diagnostic criteria are a history of persistent cough, positive bronchoalveolar lavage fluid culture for respiratory bacterial pathogens and cough resolution after a 2-week course of oral antibiotic (co-amoxicillin).
- An underweight child with chronic cough should undergo a sweat test to exclude CF.
- Pertussis (whooping cough), with typical paroxysmal cough often ending in a 'whoop' noise. The diagnosis is clinical. Antibiotic treatment (with erythromycin or azithromycin) is effective if it starts in the first 1–2 weeks of starting the cough and before coughing paroxysms occur.
- Ciliary dyskinesia is suspected if persistent cough begins in infancy in addition to recurrent otitis media. About 50% have situs inversus (Kartagener's syndrome).
- TB often causes persistent, unremitting cough associated with low-grade fever, fatigue, night sweating and weight loss/failure to thrive. Identification of *Mycobacterium tuberculosis* from sputum is diagnostic. A positive tuberculin test will support the diagnosis.
- A psychogenic cough is rare but may occur; typically it never occurs during sleep.

MANAGEMENT OF PERSISTENT COUGHS

➤ Treatment of cough depends on the correct diagnosis. Cough in infants and toddlers is usually caused by viral URTI and may persist for weeks.
➤ Cough is usually self-limited, and the focus should be directed at the cause. Parents should be educated that 'cough medicines' will unlikely help children with cough. Prescribing medications to suppress the cough is not part of paediatric practice; rather, finding the underlying cause of cough is essential.
➤ The use of over-the-counter (OTC) or prescribed cough medications (e.g., cough suppressant, mucolytic drugs, first-generation antihistamine) offers generally no

symptomatic relief for cough and places young children at risk for potential side effects and adverse reactions.

➤ Recent studies and a meta-analysis have demonstrated that honey-based syrup has a beneficial effect for symptomatic relief of URTI-associated cough, particularly nocturnal cough. Honey has antioxidant, anti-inflammatory and antibacterial activities. The World Health Organization (WHO) regards honey as a potentially valuable demulcent for treatment of URTI-associated cough.

➤ *Referral to paediatric services may be carried out if the cough:*
  ➣ Is significantly interfering with the child's sleep or daily activity.
  ➣ Persists and the cause is obscure.
  ➣ Is causing considerable anxiety to parents.

CHEST PAIN (SEE ALSO CHAPTER 10)

Introduction

➤ Chest pain is a common complaint in children caused by a variety of conditions (Box 9.14). It is the second most frequent cause of referral to paediatric cardiologists after cardiac murmur.

➤ The first clinical issue in a child with chest pain is to decide whether the history and clinical findings suggest an organic or non-organic cause.

➤ Chest pain can be acute or chronic. The latter lasts longer than 6 months. Chronic or recurrent chest pain is likely to be benign (mostly caused by anxiety). It often leads to numerous school absences, restriction of normal activities and considerable worry to patients and their parents.

BOX 9.14 Causes of chest pain

Non-Pulmonary

- Idiopathic (20–45%)
- Musculoskeletal (15–30%)
  - ❯ Costochondritis
  - ❯ Tietze's syndrome
  - ❯ Child abuse (fracture of the ribs)
- Cardiac (5–10%), including Marfan's syndrome
- Familial Mediterranean fever
- Gastrointestinal (4–7%)
- Anxiety (5–10%)

Pulmonary (12–20%)

- Asthma
- Pneumothorax
- Pneumonia
- Pleurisy
- Sickle cell disease (SCD), e.g., acute chest syndrome

PRACTICE POINTS

- Idiopathic chest pain is the most common cause, reported to occur in 20–45% of cases. The condition is defined by the absence of a cause after thorough history, physical examination, and laboratory testing. Diagnosis should be made only after excluding organic diseases. Management is summarized in Box 9.15.
- Chronic obstructive airway diseases, such as asthma, are characterized by chronic inflammation and constriction which lead to cough, dyspnoea and chest pain. If these symptoms occur in exertion, it may suggest exercise-induced asthma. The use of a bronchodilator before the exercise is likely to prevent these symptoms and suggests the diagnosis. Peak expiratory flow measurements before and after using a bronchodilator support the diagnosis of asthma.
- The hallmarks of SCD are vasoocclusive events, which are associated with acute and chronic pain caused by pulmonary thromboembolism, acute chest syndrome (ACS), pneumonia and pulmonary hypertension. ACS is an acute, life-threatening complication of SCD, defined by new pulmonary infiltrates in association with fever and other symptoms of respiratory distress.
- Musculoskeletal chest pain often follows physical exercise or trauma and presents as sharp, burning or stabbing. The pain may worsen with certain body positions, movements or deep breathing. While both costochondritis and Tietze's syndrome are caused by cartilage inflammation connecting the ribs with the sternum, the latter has localized inflammatory swelling of the affected cartilage of the costochondral, costosternal or sternoclavicular joints, mostly involving the second and third ribs.
- Patients with Marfan's syndrome require close attention because they are at risk of dilatation of the ascending aorta and dissecting aneurysm.
- Acid reflux can cause retrosternal or left-sided chest pain or epigastric pain. The pain often produces a burning sensation.
- Patients with cardiac disease present with a variety of symptoms including chest pain. These diseases include severe aortic stenosis, atrial myxoma (associated with tuberous sclerosis), hypertrophic cardiomyopathy, long QT syndrome and supraventricular tachycardia (SVT). History and a careful physical examination can detect these diseases.
- Chronic or recurrent episodes of chest pain >6 months without abnormal findings are likely to be psychogenic. This cause accounts for 5–10% of cases. Typical for psychogenic causes of chest pain: Dull or sharp, of short duration and unrelated to exercise. Teenagers are mostly affected. Possible causes include loss, a break-up with a friend or if a parent or close relative has had angina or a heart attack.

> **BOX 9.15** Management of chest pain
>
> - Management depends on the underlying cause of the chest pain, which mostly rests on the history and physical examination.
> - Benign causes of chest pain, e.g., idiopathic, psychogenic or musculoskeletal, are more frequently seen at GP surgeries. It is essential to exclude cardiac disease. If there are items of Red Flags, uncertainty or suspicion, *urgent referral is needed* (see 'Red Flags').
> - The principal management of non-organic cases of chest pain is reassurance. Those with musculoskeletal chest pain require analgesics and possibly a chest x-ray to exclude any pathology.
> - Opioids are the mainstay of treatment of acute SCD pain.

ITEMS REPRESENTING RED FLAGS IN "CHEST PAIN" REQUIRING REFERRAL

- Family history of sudden unexpected death, genetic disorders of a cardiac nature, cardiomyopathy and hypercoagulopathy.
- History of cardiac intervention.
- Sharp, retrosternal pain that often radiates to the left shoulder, is aggravated on supine or taking a deep breath and is relieved on bending forward (suggestive of pericarditis). Squeezing, tightening or pressurizing sensation may suggest ischaemic heart disease.
- Exertional chest pain or exertional syncope.
- Abnormal cardiac findings:
  - › Tachycardia, which may worsen on lying down.
  - › Distant heart sounds, gallop rhythm, arrhythmia or non-innocent murmur.
  - › Associated palpitations.
  - › Abnormal ECG.
  - › Tall stature suggestive of marfanoid appearance.

COUGHING UP BLOOD (HAEMOPTYSIS)

Core Messages

➤ Haemoptysis is defined as coughing or expectoration of blood or the presence of blood-tinged sputum from the respiratory tract below the larynx. In contrast to adults, haemoptysis in children is an uncommon presenting symptom due to the rarity of lung neoplasms (Box 9.16). A massive haemoptysis is associated with a mortality rate of 10–15%.

➤ In general, the source of the bleeding is either from the lungs, the bronchial system or due to congenital heart disease. The amount of bleeding from the lung tends to be small compared to the bleeding from the bronchi, which produce more blood.

➤ Haemoptysis must be differentiated from haematemesis (Table 9.4).

BOX 9.16 Causes of haemoptysis

Pulmonary

- Vigorous cough
- Infection (pneumonia, TB, lung abscess)
- FB (mostly in children <4 years of age)
- Bronchiectasis
- CF
- Pulmonary embolism
- Pulmonary tumours (adenoma, haemartoma)
- Goodpasture's syndrome
- Sarcoidosis
- Haemosiderosis
- Hydatid cyst

Cardiac

- Congenital heart disease

Systemic

- Coagulopathy, e.g., disseminated intravascular coagulation (DIC)
- Hereditary haemorrhagic telangiectasia
- Systemic lupus erythematosus

TABLE 9.4 Differentiating haemoptysis from haematemesis

Haemoptysis	Haematemesis
• Sputum frothy	• Sputum not frothy
• Bright red or pink	• Brown or black
• Vomiting and nausea	• Associated vomiting and nausea
• Alkaline pH	• Acidic pH
• Concurrent lung disease	• Concurrent GI disease

Investigations

➤ FBC: Low Hb may confirm anaemia if the bleeding was large; leukocytosis in infection such as pneumonia; low platelets in thrombocytopenia or coagulopathy.

➤ Coagulation study with international normalized ratio (INR), prothrombin time (PT) and partial thromboplastin time (PTT) in case of coagulopathy.

➤ Sputum cytology for suspected TB or tumour.

➤ Sweat test for suspected cases of CF.

➤ Chest x-ray.

➤ Bronchoscopy and high-resolution CT scan of the lung may be indicated in unclear cases of haemoptysis or tumour.

PRACTICE POINTS

- After a careful history and physical examination, a chest x-ray should be performed. *If the diagnosis is not clear, a referral to a chest specialist should be considered.*
- Haemoptysis with high fever is most likely caused by pneumonia.
- Haemoptysis may occur in CF; approximately 5% of all patients will develop this symptom, which may recur.
- Among the differential diagnosis of haemoptysis is left-sided ventricular heart failure or mitral stenosis causing pulmonary hypertension.
- Pulmonary embolism may cause haemoptysis. This diagnosis should be considered if there is evidence of deep venous thrombosis (DVT).

Referral

➤ All cases with haemoptysis should be referred except mild self-limiting cases caused by a vigorous cough where the child is well and the chest x-ray is normal.

➤ Paediatricians may manage children with haemoptysis if the diagnosis is clear, e.g., pneumonia. Unclear cases should be referred to the chest unit to establish the diagnosis and treatment.

CHAPTER 10

Cardiology

INTRODUCTION

➤ Congenital heart defects (CHDs) are the most common congenital malformation, accounting for approximately 25–28% of all congenital anomalies. The incidence of CHDs is 0.8–1% of live births. CHDs are defined as structural malformations of the heart and/or the great intrathoracic vessels. Currently, over 90% of CHD patients survive into adulthood.

➤ CHDs in children are caused by a combination of genetic (about 15–20% of cases) and environmental factors. If the mother has CHD, the incidence of CHD increases from 1% in the general population to 15%. If a sibling has CHD, the risk of a second child having CHDs is 2–3%.

➤ The genetic basis of CHDs is divided into two groups: Syndromic CHDs (with other congenital anomalies and/or dysmorphic features) and non-syndromic.

➤ Other risk factors for CHDs include maternal diabetes mellitus, systemic lupus erythematosus (SLE), obesity, alcohol intake, medications (e.g., antiepileptic drugs, amphetamine) and congenital infections (e.g., rubella).

➤ The cardiovascular system (CVS) should be examined at the 6-week check. It is important that this is thorough, and it must include more than simply auscultation for murmurs (Box 10.1). It is vital that heart diseases are identified as early as possible to decrease morbidity and mortality.

➤ The main causes of acquired heart disease in children nowadays are Kawasaki's disease, myocarditis and rheumatic heart diseases. The latter are prevalent in low-income countries but rare in high-income countries.

BOX 10.1 Approach to the examination of the cardiovascular system

- Growth measurements of the child and plot on the centile chart.
- Observation looking for any cyanosis, anaemia, dyspnoea, chest shape and any finger clubbing.
- Palpation: Pulse (rate, rhythm, character); absent femoral pulse; precordium for parasternal thrill or heave; hepatomegaly; capillary refill.
- Auscultation: Heart sounds; murmurs: systolic or diastolic, grade, site of maximum intensity, radiation.
- Blood pressure measurement (for older children).

DOI: 10.1201/9781032642888-10

Growth

➤ Children with CHDs are at risk for poor growth, which manifests as wasting, stunting and underweight, caused by increased metabolic demand, reduced calorie intake (feeding fatigue) and haemodynamic instability. However, there is often a trend toward overweight and obesity in teenager age, similar to the general population.

➤ The increased metabolic demand also causes hypoxia and increased myocardial oxygen consumption to 2: 0–30% instead of the normal consumption of 10%.

➤ Therefore, nutritional rehabilitation for weight gain includes high calorie formulas with high calorie intake of 175–180 kcal/kg/day, instead of the normal requirement of 130–150 kcal/kg/day.

➤ There is no difference in pubertal timing between children born with CHDs and children born without.

Observation

➤ **Cyanosis**: Is there central cyanosis (blue lips or tongue) suggestive of cardiac or respiratory disease? Peripheral cyanosis is often normal.

➤ **Pallor**: Anaemia can cause tachycardia, a heart murmur (haemic murmur) and congestive cardiac failure.

➤ **Respiratory distress**: Symptoms and signs of respiratory distress such tachypnoea and subcostal recession may occur in both pulmonary diseases and cardiac failure. Liver enlargement, the presence of a heart murmur and gallop rhythm are suggestive of a cardiac cause of the respiratory distress.

➤ **Fatigue and exercise intolerance**: Infants may tire easily and sweat during feeding as an early sign of congestive cardiac failure. As a result, the infant is unable to take the full feed, resulting in poor weight gain. Older children may not keep up with other children.

➤ **Finger clubbing**: This may be a sign of cyanotic CHD or cystic fibrosis (CF).

Palpation

1. **Pulse**: Brachial and femoral pulses are felt. A delayed or absent pulse indicates coarctation of the aorta. The femoral pulses can be difficult to palpate in overweight or obese children. The apex beat is normally in the mid-clavicular line in the fourth to fifth intercostal space.

2. **Cardiac**: For a parasternal heave, by placing the palm over the lower half of the sternum. A heaving sensation indicates right ventricular hypertrophy. A thrill is a loud murmur that can be felt as a vibration.

3. **Liver**: Hepatomegaly (>3 cm below the right subcostal margin) suggests heart failure.

4. **Capillary refill**: A normal capillary refill time is up to 3 seconds; if longer, it is suggestive of poor circulation or shock.

Auscultation

➤ The bell of the stethoscope is placed lightly on the chest for detecting low-pitched sounds, while diaphragm side should be pressed firmly on the chest to detect high-pitched sounds. The first and the second heart sounds are high pitched. It is better to begin with the diaphragm because most murmurs are in the medium- to high-pitched range.

➤ Heart sounds: The first heart sound is due to closure of the mitral and tricuspid valves, and the second sound is due to closure of the aortic and pulmonary valves. Breathing causes splitting of the second heart sound. In atrial septal defect, the second sound does not vary with respiration, causing a fixed second sound.

➤ Murmurs are caused by turbulence of blood flow and may be innocent or pathological (Boxes 10.2 and 10.3). It is essential to check the murmur intensity both in lying and sitting positions. Systolic murmur may be ejection or pansystolic. Radiation can be checked in the axilla and back and over the carotid arteries.

> ➤ Venous hum: This is best heard just below the right clavicle. It disappears when the child lies down or turns the head to the other side. Its significance is that it can be confused with patent ductus arteriosus (PDA).

BOX 10.2 Criteria for diagnosing innocent murmur

- Short systolic ejection type of murmur.
- No or insignificant radiation to the apex, base or back.
- Varies in intensity and is usually louder in the supine position, with exercise and with fever and diminishes in sitting or standing position.
- Murmur quality is vibratory or musical.
- It is grade I or II in intensity (Box 10.4), best heard along left lower or midsternal border.
- Absence of symptoms and signs of heart disease, including no pansystolic murmur, diastolic murmur or greater in intensity than grade II.

BOX 10.3 Features of pathological murmur

- Diastolic or late systolic murmur.
- Loud murmur >2/6 in intensity.
- Continuous murmur with the exception of venous hum.
- A murmur that sounds like a breath sound.
- A murmur at the pulmonary area with fixed splitting of the second sound.
- Associated with any symptom or sign of heart disease such as fatigue, shortness of breath, tachypnoea and hepatomegaly.

BOX 10.4 Intensity grades of a murmur

- **Grade 1** • Difficult to hear, softer than the heart sounds.
- **Grade 2** • Intensity equal to heart sounds.
- **Grade 3** • Louder than the heart sounds, no thrill.
- **Grade 4** • Loud murmur associated with thrill.
- **Grade 5** • Is heard with only the edge of the stethoscope.

Referral

Referral to paediatrician if there is:

➤ Doubt about the significance of the murmur.
➤ Any pathological murmur.
➤ A new murmur which was not heard before.

Blood Pressure

➤ Although measurement of blood pressure (BP) is time consuming and may be difficult in children, it is an essential part of a cardiological assessment. In addition, hypertension in children is not as uncommon as previously believed. Recent data indicate the prevalence of hypertension has been increasing from about 1–2% to 4.5% in obese children. Childhood high BP is known to track into adulthood.
➤ It is important to choose the right size of cuff, which should cover almost the full length of the upper arm, the hand being supinated and the arm elevated to the level of the heart for proper position of the radial artery and to eliminate 'auscultatory gap'. The diaphragm of the stethoscope should be used to obtain a better seal.
➤ Children with coarctation of the aorta often present with hypertension. BP in the arm and legs should be measured in any child with hypertension to exclude this possibility.
➤ Table 10.1 shows normal values of pulse, respiratory rate (RR) and BP.

TABLE 10.1 Normal pulse, RR, systolic and diastolic BP

Age	HR Average (Ranges)	RR	SBP	DBP
Newborn	125/minute (70–190)	30–40	75 (60–90)	45 (40–60)
1–12 months	120/minute (80–160)	25–40	90 (80–100)	60 (50–70)
5 years	100/minute (80–120)	15–25	95 (90–115)	60 (55–75)
12 years	85/minute (65–110)	15–20	110 (95–125)	65 (60–80)

Note: A simple calculation of normal BP is 90+ the age of the child.

CARDITIS

Myocarditis/Pericarditis

➤ Although paediatric cases of myocarditis/pericarditis are uncommon, they are serious inflammatory diseases which can be life threatening.

➤ Presenting complaints vary from asymptomatic cases to sudden death. Symptoms are often non-specific. Carditis is mostly an infectious process, and cardiotropic viruses are the most common causes.

➤ In recent years, cardiac biopsy rates have been declining because of increasing reliance on cardiac magnetic resonance (CMR) imaging in addition to establishing clinical and laboratory diagnostic features (Box 10.5). CMR is non-invasive and is the gold standard for the diagnosis of carditis and clinical follow-up of patients.

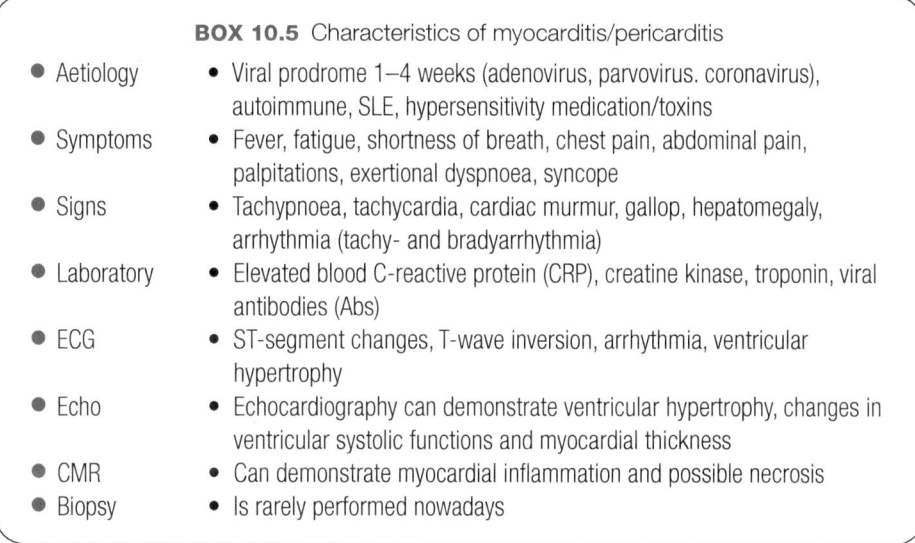

BOX 10.5 Characteristics of myocarditis/pericarditis

- Aetiology
  - Viral prodrome 1–4 weeks (adenovirus, parvovirus. coronavirus), autoimmune, SLE, hypersensitivity medication/toxins
- Symptoms
  - Fever, fatigue, shortness of breath, chest pain, abdominal pain, palpitations, exertional dyspnoea, syncope
- Signs
  - Tachypnoea, tachycardia, cardiac murmur, gallop, hepatomegaly, arrhythmia (tachy- and bradyarrhythmia)
- Laboratory
  - Elevated blood C-reactive protein (CRP), creatine kinase, troponin, viral antibodies (Abs)
- ECG
  - ST-segment changes, T-wave inversion, arrhythmia, ventricular hypertrophy
- Echo
  - Echocardiography can demonstrate ventricular hypertrophy, changes in ventricular systolic functions and myocardial thickness
- CMR
  - Can demonstrate myocardial inflammation and possible necrosis
- Biopsy
  - Is rarely performed nowadays

Infective Endocarditis

➤ Before the 1970s, infective endocarditis (IE) was often caused by rheumatic heart disease. In the past 50 years, the prevalence of rheumatic heart diseases has declined in high-income countries. CHDs have become the predominant underlying condition because more children with CHDs are undergoing corrective surgeries, which enable them to survive much longer than a few decades ago. At least 50% of children with IE cases had previous cardiac surgery.

➤ In addition to the complication of corrective surgery for CHDs, the prevalence of rheumatic heart diseases and carditis has remained a major risk factor in low-income countries. Other risk factors include indwelling central line catheters. Table 10.2 shows characteristic features of IE.

TABLE 10.2 Characteristic features of endocarditis

CHDs and bacterial aetiology	• VSD, aortic valvular diseases, Fallot's tetralogy, PDA and shunts are the most frequent CHD predisposing to IE after surgery. • Staphylococci are the most common cause of acute IE. • *Streptococcus viridans* is the most common cause of subacute IE. • Enterococci occur more often in patients undergoing lower bowel or genitourinary procedures. • *Pseudomonas* bacteria may cause IE among IV drug users.
Clinical features	• History of CHDs; central indwelling catheter; dental, intestinal, or genitourinary procedures. • Symptoms with fatigue, fever, rigor, night sweats, arthralgia, myalgia, weight loss. • Signs with tachycardia, new or changing murmur, embolic signs such as splinter haemorrhage of the nailbed, splenomegaly, heart failure, Osler's nodes, glomerulonephritis. • Diagnosis: Blood culture, echocardiography, CMR.
Oral prophylaxis	• Amoxicillin: 50 mg/kg 1 hour before the procedure. • Clindamycin (20 mg/kg), cephalexin (50 mg/kg) or azithromycin (15 mg/kg) for children with penicillin allergy.

CARDIOMYOPATHY

➤ Cardiomyopathy (CM) is a rare disease in children with an incidence of around 7 cases per 100,000 people/year. It is defined as a disease of the myocardium associated with myocardial dysfunction which is unexplained by CHDs.

➤ There are multiple modes of inheritance, but autosomal dominant transmission is the most common genetic form of CM. First-degree relatives of affected individuals have a high risk of developing the disease. Therefore, screening those relatives for CM is paramount.

➤ Hypertrophic CM (HCM) is the most common inherited CM due to mutations in numerous genes. Dilated CM (DCM) is typically characterized by dilatation and impaired function of one or both ventricles. Both HCM and DCM are either primary (idiopathic) or secondary, and both forms of CM are the most important cause of sudden death among athletes. Viruses (parvovirus B19, coxsackie and adenovirus) can cause myocarditis, leading to CM (Box 10.6).

BOX 10.6 Summary of CM characteristics

Aetiology

• CM is either primary due to direct cardiac disease such as post-viral myocarditis (in 35–40%) or DCM, or secondary due to a systemic disease such as hypertension or valvular disease.
• CM is mostly inherited as autosomal dominant. About 70% of HCM and 35% of DCM are caused by gene mutations.
• Syndromic CM can be associated with Pompe disease, Friedrich ataxia, Noonan syndrome.

Presentation

- Asymptomatic.
- Symptoms of heart failure: Dyspnoea, orthopnoea, chest pain.
- Signs: Congestive oedema, arrhythmia, syncope, tachycardia. Murmur may or may not be present.
- Sudden death.

Diagnosis

- HCM is characterized by ventricular hypertrophy, particularly left ventricle (wall thickness >15 mm).
- Echocardiography: Confirms the hypertrophy and dilation.
- ECG: May show prolonged PR, ventricular hypertrophy.
- Cardiac MRI can confirm the ventricular hypertrophy or dilation.

Prognosis

- 20% experience normalization of myocardial function within 2 years of presentation.
- Mortality may occur in 30% within 2 years of presentation, unless undergoing a heart transplantation.
- Risk factors for sudden death include family history of CM, recent episodes of syncope, SVT or ventricular tachycardia (VT), a young age at the first presentation (<30 years) and a ventricular septal thickness >3 cm.

RED FLAG

Once a case of CM has been identified, immediate testing of all family members is required.

ARRHYTHMIAS

➤ Primary care practitioners are in the frontline position in detect and treat many childhood arrhythmias. CHDs are the most common underlying causes of childhood arrhythmia and responsible for 25–33% of all arrhythmias.

➤ Arrhythmia is divided into tachyarrhythmia and bradyarrhythmia.

Tachyarrhythmia

➤ **Paroxysmal supraventricular tachycardia (SVT)** is a regular rhythm at a rate of >180–220 beats/minute (Table 10.3). SVT is caused by impulses from the atrioventricular (AV) node re-entering the atria occurring in otherwise healthy children.

> SVT is the most common form of tachycardia in children, with an estimated incidence between 1 in 250 and 1 in 1000 patients.

➤ Wolff–Parkinson–White syndrome (WPW) is a congenital cardiac abnormality with characteristic ECG findings (short PR intervals <0.12 seconds, delta wave and wide QRS complex >0.11 seconds) and occurs in 25% of SVT. It can cause cardiac arrest.

➤ **Premature ventricular complexes (PVCs):** These are some of the most common arrhythmias seen in the ECG caused by early depolarization of left or right cardiac ventricular cells. They are often regarded as benign with a good prognosis, and no treatment is required in asymptomatic children. Some children experience symptoms such as palpitations. Poor prognosis is associated with cardiac structural and coronary artery diseases. Beta-blockers or the antiarrhythmic drug flecainide is used.

TABLE 10.3 Some characteristic features of SVT

	Infants	Children
• Tachycardia • Symptoms/ Signs	• >220/minute Irritability, poor feeding, sweating, signs of heart failure, respiratory distress	• >180/minute Palpitation, dyspnoea, dizziness, nausea, chest pain, syncope
• ECG (both)	• Narrow complex (QRS <0.12 seconds) tachycardia, regular with no P waves, and signs of WPW syndrome	
• Treatment	• Ice packs on the face • Adenosine (rapid IV push) 0.15 mg/kg	• Vagal manoeuvres • Valsalva manoeuvres (blowing against closed glottis for 10–15 seconds) • Adenosine (rapid IV push) • Child >12 years: 3 mg IV

Bradyarrhythmia

➤ **Long QT syndrome (LQTS)** is either autosomal dominant inherited (Romano–Ward syndrome), autosomal recessive (Jervell–Lange–Nelson syndrome) or acquired (myocarditis or electrolyte disturbance). It is an important cause of loss of consciousness and may mimic epilepsy. Children may recover immediately after the episode or die during the event.

➤ LQTS has an estimated incidence of 1 in 5000 people and is identified by QT prolongation on ECG during clinical evaluation of an unexplained syncope, as part of a family study with a member who died because of sudden cardiac death or in the investigation of patients with congenital neural deafness.

➤ Clinical criteria of LQTS are shown in Box 10.7.

➤ **Congenital heart block (CHB)** is associated with a heart rate of about 50/minute. The congenital type of heart block is often caused by:

➤ An autoimmune disease, such as SLE, of a mother who is either symptomatic or, more often, asymptomatic. The block occurs through passive immune-mediated acquired transfer of autoantibodies.

➤ CHB may be associated with CHDs such as atrioventricular septal defect.

BOX 10.7 Clinical criteria of LQTS

Clinical

- Mostly asymptmatic
- Low heart rate for age
- Syncope, chest pain, palpitatuion
- Sudden cardiac death (SCD)

Family History

- Family members with LQTS
- Unexplained SCD

Diagnosis

- Family history of LQTS and positive genetic testing.
- ECG shows corrected QT (QTc) ≥480 ms. The presence of unexplained syncope and QTc ≥460 ms is also diagnostic. T-wave abnormalities included notched wave and T-wave alternans.

➤ **Brugada's syndrome** is an autosomal dominant inherited arrhythmia associated with sudden cardiac death in about 10–20% of cases. Its prevalence ranges from 1 to 2000–5000 people. Most patients are asymptomatic, and the diagnosis is based on ECG findings consisting of ST-segment elevation in the precordial leads V_1–V_3. Some patients present with syncope.

CHEST PAIN

➤ Chest pain is a common complaint affecting about 10% of school-age children. Chest pain is the second most frequent cause of referral to the paediatric cardiologists after cardiac murmur. Box 10.8 lists causes of chest pain.

➤ In the paediatric age group, most cases of chest pain are benign and non-cardiac, therefore, the term idiopathic, which is the most common cause of chest pain, occurring in 70–75% of cases. The condition is defined by an absence of a cause after thorough history taking, physical examination and laboratory testing.

➤ The important aspect of examining children with chest pain is to detect those uncommon cases with organic causes, including life-threatening pathologies.

➤ Children presenting with cardiac chest pain (4–5% of cases) have often other cardiac symptoms, including exertional chest pain, syncope, palpitation and dyspnoea. Physical examination may reveal a cardiac murmur and/or arrhythmia.

BOX 10.8 Main non-cardiac and cardiac causes of chest pain

Non-Cardiac (95–96%)
- Idiopathic
- Anxiety or stress
- Musculoskeletal, e.g., costochondritis
- Direct trauma to the chest
- Pulmonary (pneumonia, asthma, pleurisy)
- Sickle cell anaemia with acute chest syndrome
- Acid reflux

Cardiac (4–5%)
- Severe aortic stenosis/mitral valve prolapse
- Myocarditis/pericarditis
- Hypertrophic cardiomyopathy (HCM)
- Arrhythmia: Long Q-T syndrome, SVT
- Dissecting aortic aneurysm in Marfan's syndrome

PRACTICE POINTS

- Although most causes of chest pain in otherwise healthy children are benign and non-cardiac, it is important to do a thorough examination to ensure that cardiac causes are definitely not the underlying condition. It is also important to ask about any stressful events or signs of anxiety that could have triggered the chest pain.
- Musculoskeletal chest pain such as costochondritis (Tietze's syndrome) is frequently caused by a viral infection and is characterized by localized swelling of the costochondral, costosternal or sternoclavicular joints, mostly involving the second and third ribs. Chest movements or taking a deep breath may worsen the pain, and there is a tenderness on pressing the previously mentioned areas of the chest.
- Chronic (lasting >6 months) or recurrent episodes of chest pain without abnormal findings are likely to be psychogenic. This cause accounts for 5–10% of cases.
- Typical for non-cardiac cause of chest pain: Sharp quality, of short duration and unrelated to exercise. Chest pain of cardiac origin manifests as a deep heavy pressure, choking or squeezing sensation, and it is usually triggered by exercise. It is not sharp and is not affected by respiration.

SYNCOPE

➤ Syncope is caused by a variety of conditions (Box 10.9). Vasovagal syncope (VVS; fainting) is by far the most common cause (60–70%) and is defined as a transient loss of consciousness (TLC) associated with an inability to maintain postural tone caused by global cerebral hypoperfusion. It is characterized by a rapid onset, short duration, pallor and spontaneous complete recovery. VVS is a common paediatric complaint affecting approximately 30–40% of children below the age of 18 years.

➤ Postural orthostatic tachycardia syndrome (POTS) is another cause of TLC, typically diagnosed in adolescents. Episodes are characterized by dizziness, palpitation, headache, light headedness and fatigue. It causes a significant interference with learning and social activities. POTS has recently been linked with autoimmune diseases. Diagnostic criteria:
  ➤ Increase in heart rate of at least 30 beats per minute when rising from supine to standing during a 10-minute standing test.
  ➤ A drop of at least 20 mm Hg systolic or 10 mm Hg diastolic BP during standing position.
➤ Syncope requires special attention, as this can be cardiac in origin (around 6% of syncope cases). Cardiac causes of syncope are either structural heart diseases (e.g., aortic stenosis, CMs) or cardiac diseases associated with brady- or tachyarrhythmia (atrioventricular block or SVT). While the prognosis of VVS is excellent, the mortality of cardiac causes rises to 18–33%.
➤ The most common condition that can be confused with VVS is an epileptic syncope, which includes stiffness or brief tonic-clonic movements during the episode. Table 10.4 shows a differential diagnosis among VVS, cardiac and epileptic syncope.
➤ Psychogenic pseudosyncope (PPS) is another cause of an apparent TLC without cerebral hypoperfusion, accounting for about 4% of syncope. PPS is a conversion disorder characterized by a prolonged duration of TLC, eye closure during the episode, high frequency of recurrences and the episode usually occurs in the presence of an audience.

BOX 10.9 Main causes of syncope

- Vasovagal faint/Autonomic failure
- Cardiac syncope (e.g., structural CHDs and/or arrythmia)
- Seizures (e.g., atonic seizures)
- Trauma, head injury
- PPS (conversion symptoms)
- Cyanotic or pallid form of breath-holding spells
- Toxins/Poisoning/Medication

PRACTICE POINTS

- The differential diagnosis of syncope is diverse. It is vital to accurately identify patients with cardiac or epileptic syncope. Primary care physicians should differentiate between those patients in low-risk (VVS) and high-risk groups and decide if the patient is fit to be sent home or referred for investigation.
- Syncope without warning (a drop) is highly suggestive of a cardiac origin. A detailed history is imperative to make the diagnosis and avoid recurrence, which may be fatal. Other clinical presentations of CHDs include squatting,

hypoxic spells, angina and peripheral oedema. Bradycardia and low BP are often associated with cardiac syncope.
- Tilt-table test is used to clarify unexplained syncope and to confirm the diagnosis of VVS.
- *Referral should be considered for:*
  - All cases of syncope apart from infrequent vasovagal/autonomic failure. Occasional cases can be referred for tilt-table testing.
  - Unexplained cases of syncope should be referred to paediatric services. Cardiac syncope should be referred to paediatric cardiology services.
  - Frequent episodes of syncope irrespective of the aetiology, including vasovagal cases.

TABLE 10.4 Differential diagnosis among VVS, cardiac and epileptic syncope

	Vasovagal Syncope	Cardiac Syncope	Epileptic Syncope
Relevant history	• Previous episodes, healthy otherwise	• History of sudden death in the family; family or own history of CHD	• History of epilepsy
Sex	• Often in girls	• Boys or girls	• Boys and girls
Age	• Adolescents, uncommon before 10–12 years	• Any age; more often in teenagers	• Any age beyond infancy
May be preceded by	• Sweating, nausea, vomiting	• Palpitation or chest pain	• Unpredictable
Typical triggers	• Long standing in hot days, inadequate food or drinks, unpleasant smells, emotional stress	• During exercise (e.g., running or swimming), or no triggers or warning (a drop); attack may occur in supine position	• None
Diagnosis by	• Short duration, rapid recovery, examination, normal tilt-table testing	• Abnormal cardiac examination (presence of a murmur and/or arrythmia, abnormal ECG)	• Muscle contractions often with cyanosis, tongue biting, urine incontinence, slow recovery, confusion on awakening; EEG is often diagnostic

CHAPTER 11

Urogenital Diseases

URINARY TRACT INFECTION

➤ Urinary tract infection (UTI) is one of the most infectious diseases, affecting 2.8% of children annually, with recurrence rates ranging from 8% to 30%. Risk factors for UTI are shown in Box 11.1. It is a major cause of antibiotic prescriptions and hospitalization in children.

➤ Boys have a greater incidence of UTI in the neonatal period and early infancy, particularly in uncircumcised boys. Girls overtake boys in the incidence of UTI after the first year of life, and this persists into adulthood.

➤ Permanent renal scarring occurs in 15% after the first episode of UTI and in 40% after recurrence of UTI leading to hypertension, renal failure and proteinuria later in life. The important aim of childhood antibiotic therapy is to prevent renal scarring and further complications.

BOX 11.1 Risk factors for developing UTI

High Risk
- Vesicoureteral reflux (VUR)
- Congenital abnormalities of the urinary tract
- Ureteropelvic obstruction
- Urethral valve
- Neurogenic bladder

Low Risk
- Incomplete bladder emptying
- Constipation
- Gender
- Phimosis, uncircumcised boys
- Insufficient fluid intake

Definitions

➤ UTI is Urine infection caused by a single organism of >**100,000** colony-forming units per millilitre and a combination of clinical features presenting as an:
  ➤ Upper UTI (involving the ureter and kidney) is defined as UTI with a fever of 38°C or higher in association with non-specific symptoms and signs. Fever is the most common presenting sign of UTI in infancy and may be the only sign.

DOI: 10.1201/9781032642888-11

➤ Lower UTI (involving the bladder and urethra) is defined as a collection of well-recognized symptoms, and fever is often absent (see later).

➤ Recurrent UTI (up to 30% experience recurrences after the first episode of UTI):
  ➤ Two or more episodes of UTI with acute upper UTI.
  ➤ One acute upper UTI plus one or more episodes of lower UTI.
  ➤ Three or more episodes of lower UTI.

Urine Collection

Urine collection is crucial for the diagnosis of UTI. Children presenting with unexplained fever of ≥38°C should have their urine tested using the following collection methods:

➤ A clean catch urine sample is a valid method with low rates of contamination.

➤ If a clean catch urine sample is unobtainable, a urine sterile plastic bag or urine pads attached to the genitalia are commonly used in daily practice, but they have high rates of contamination. The culture result may be accurate if the bag is placed for less than 20 minutes.

Dipstick Results

➤ When nitrite and leukocyte esterase results are positive, the diagnosis of UTI is sufficiently likely to allow empirical antibiotic therapy. When both are absent, a UTI is unlikely.

➤ When only leukocyte esterase in dipstick testing is positive, the indication to commence antibiotic treatment depends on clinical suspicion.

➤ Urine culture should always be performed in cases of positive dipstick results in children.

Diagnosis

➤ Diagnosis of UTI is challenging due to its non-specific presentation. It should be considered in children presenting with fever (≥38°C) without an apparent source. Fever may be the only clinical sign in young children (Table 11.1). The presence of malodorous urine is not a helpful sign in the diagnosis of UTI.

➤ Blood tests (full blood count [FBC], C-reactive protein [CRP], renal function tests) are recommended for young febrile infants and those requiring hospitalization. Blood tests are not indicated in an older afebrile child with a lower UTI.

➤ Gram-negative organisms are the most common uropathogens in culture results, with *Escherichia coli* accounting for 70–80% of cases, followed by *Klebsiella* spp., *Enterobacter* spp., *Proteus* spp. and *Pseudomonas aeruginosa*, which is associated with severe UTI.

➤ Antibiotic treatment of asymptomatic bacteriuria (significant bacteriuria without clinical signs and symptoms of UTI) is not indicated.

TABLE 11.1 Symptoms and signs of UTI

Age Group	Symptoms/Signs
• <3 months	• Fever, lethargy, unwell, feeding difficulty, irritability, jaundice, vomiting, haematuria
• >3 months	
❯ Upper UTI	• Fever, abdominal pain, lethargy, haematuria, failure to thrive; loin pain and tenderness
❯ Lower UTI (usually >3 years, girls)	• Frequent and/or painful urination, urinary incontinence, nocturnal enuresis, abdominal and/or suprapubic pain, pruritic genitalia

Management of UTI

➤ **Infants <3 months with a possible UTI (high risk of serious illness)**
   ➣ Should be referred immediately to the care of a paediatric specialist for parenteral antibiotic therapy.
➤ **Children >3 months to <3 years (intermediate risk of serious illness)**
   ➣ A urine sample should always be collected for culture before antibiotic therapy.
   ➣ Empirical antibiotic therapy is indicated in all children present with fever >38.0°C and urine dipstick positive for nitrite and/or leukocytes.
   ➣ A combination of penicillin and beta-lactamase inhibitors or third-generation cephalosporins are suitable treatment. Aminoglycosides are an appropriate alternative in cases of allergy to beta-lactams. The empirical use of amoxicillin and trimethoprim–sulfamethoxazole should be avoided because of the worldwide emergence of a high rate of resistance.
   ➣ Antibiotic therapy should be continued for 7–10 days in patients with febrile uncomplicated UTI and for 10–14 days in patients with complicated UTI.
   ➣ If the child remains unwell and/or feverish after 24–48 hours, reassessing the case should be performed, another urine sample should be submitted for culture and an alternative diagnosis should be excluded.
   ➣ If oral antibiotics cannot be used (e.g., refusal or vomiting), children should be referred to a paediatric department where they are likely to receive an IV antibiotic agent for 1–2 days followed by oral antibiotics.
   ➣ Guidelines for investigation after UTI are shown in Box 11.2.
➤ **Children ≥3 years with cystitis/lower UTI (low risk of serious illness)**
   ➣ Urine sample for microscopy and culture or dipstick testing.
   ➣ In children with lower UTI, an antibiotic therapy, such as trimethoprim or nitrofurantoin, for 3–5 days is sufficient. Strict genital hygiene, increasing fluid intake, avoiding incomplete bladder emptying and voiding bladder dysfunction will add to the treatment success.

➤ Long-term management
➤ Antibiotic prophylaxis should not be routinely recommended following first-time UTI for children with uncomplicated UTI.
➤ There is insufficient evidence on the effectiveness of cranberry juice and probiotics in preventing recurrences of UTI.

Investigation after an Acute UTI

BOX 11.2 Imaging for infants <6 months with UTI

● **Renal ultrasound**	● Indicated for all children at least 2–4 weeks after a first febrile UTI. Recommended in all children <3 years with a first UTI and in cases of complicated or atypical UTI. In children of this age who respond well to antibiotic therapy, ultrasound may not be needed.
● **Fluoroscopic contrast voiding cystourethrography (VCUG)**	● The gold standard to diagnose vesicoureteral reflux is indicated if the ultrasound reveals abnormalities suggestive of urological malformation.
● **Dimercaptosuccinic acid (DMSA)**	● A radioisotope scan which is recommended in all children with VUR grades IV and V at least 6 months after the first UTI to detect renal scarring.
● **Mercaptoacetyltriglycine (MAG3) scintigraphy**	● To assess renal clearance and function.

URINARY STONES (NEPHROLITHIASIS)

Core Messages

➤ In contrast to adults who have a 10–20% lifetime risk of developing renal calculus, the prevalence of paediatric nephrolithiasis is uncommon and estimated to be around 1%. However, this prevalence has increased significantly in the past two decades.

➤ *The four main types of stones are*: 70–80% calcium oxalate, 10–15% struvite, 10% calcium phosphate and around 5% uric acid.

➤ Children with renal calculi are at risk of developing chronic renal disease such as renal failure, low bone mineral density and fractures. Hypercalciuria and a negative calcium balance contribute to low bone mineral density and increased fracture risks. Box 11.3 shows risk factors for developing renal stones.

➤ Conservative management of renal calculi is a priority in children. There is a high chance of spontaneous passages for small stones with sizes <3 to <5 mm. The decision for surgical intervention should be made on an individual basis. Stone recurrence is estimated to be 50% within 3 years after surgical intervention.

BOX 11.3 Risk factors for developing renal stones

- Family history of renal calculus
- Genetic, e.g., cystinuria (autosomal recessive)
- Recurrent UTI
- Obesity
- Neurogenic bladder
- Hyperlipidaemia
- Immobility, lack of exercise
- Prematurity
- Medications such as loop diuretics (furosemide) and antiepileptic drugs (AEDs)

Diagnosis

➤ Patients usually present with:
  - UTI
  - Renal colic with abdominal or flank pain
  - Following an episode of gross haematuria, dysuria, urgency and frequency of urination
➤ Midstream urine (MSU) typically shows haematuria without significant proteinuria or casts.
➤ Renal ultrasound scan is the investigation of choice.
➤ The presence of hypercalciuria (the most common biochemical abnormality associated with stones), hyperoxaluria or cystinuria to identify causes of stones.

Management

➤ All patients with suspected renal colic should be seen at the primary care clinic for assessment and management. Acute cases are likely to be referred. *Consider referral urgently if there is:*
  - Persistent pain
  - Associated fever
  - Signs of obstruction
➤ *For asymptomatic and non-obstructive renal calculi:*
  - Analgesics: NSAID such as diclofenac orally.
  - Renal ultrasound scan: Within 24 hours whenever possible. There should be a plan for periodic ultrasonography and regular follow-up at the GP surgery.
  - Urine should be sent for microscopy and culture. A UTI with splitting organisms such as *Proteus* can increase ammonia phosphate (struvite) and stone formation.
  - Increase fluid intake (low urine output increases solute concentration and the risk for stone formation). Children should drink enough fluid to produce at least 30 mL/kg/day to prevent renal calculi. Pupils should be allowed to have water bottles in the classroom and be encouraged to attend the toilet for urination.

➤ Preventing stone recurrence can be achieved by diet modifications, which should include avoidance of excessive protein consumption to decrease uric acid, hypercalciuria and hyperoxaluria. Sodium intake should be <2000 mg/day. Calcium intake should not be restricted, as this can increase the risk of stones.

➤ Blood tests should include FBC, plasma electrolytes, urea, creatinine, bicarbonate, calcium, phosphate and uric acid. Urine should be tested for hypercalciuria.

➤ Medical expulsive therapy in the form of alpha-blockers (e.g., tamsulosin or doxazosin) may occasionally be indicated to dilate the ureter and vesicoureteral junction, and this should be initiated following consultation with the urologists.

➤ The stone should always be sent for chemical analysis.

There are surgical options for managing renal stones including:

➤ Extracorporeal shock wave lithotripsy (ESWL), which can shatter most renal stones; often more than one treatment may be needed.

➤ Percutaneous nephrolithotomy (PCNL)

➤ Ureteroscopy

➤ Open surgery

NOCTURNAL ENURESIS

Core Message

➤ Nocturnal enuresis (NE) is defined as an involuntary voiding of urine at night into the bed or clothes at least twice a week for at least 3 successive months after the age of 5 years in the absence of organic diseases. It affects the child's self-esteem and social, emotional and psychological wellbeing. Definitions of terms related to this subject are shown in Box 11.4.

BOX 11.4 Definition of terms

- **Primary nocturnal enuresis** (PNE) refers to children who have never achieved urinary continence at night. It accounts for about 80% of all cases, and it is often associated with a family history of NE.
- **Secondary** is NE in a child who has previously been dry for at least 6 months. This form is often associated with stress and psychological trauma.
- **Monosymptomatic** is NE without daytime incontinence or urological symptoms such as UTI, dysuria or frequent urination.
- **Non-monosymptomatic** is NE with other lower urinary tract symptoms such as daytime incontinence or urgency.
- **Nocturnal polyuria** is the amount of urine produced at night that exceeds the maximum bladder capacity (MBC).
  - ❯ MBC is calculated by the following formula: age of the child $\times$ 30 + 30. A 7year old should have 240 mL MBC.
- **Overactive bladder** (formerly detrusor instability) is uninhibited bladder capacity which results in decreased MBC.

Risk Factors

➤ **Genetic:** The risk of NE is 15% if neither parent was affected, 40% if one parent was affected and 75% if both had the condition. Research has identified a genetic link to chromosomes 13q, 12q, 8q and 22q.

➤ **Smaller bladder capacity:** In children, the bladder capacity is calculated according to the following formula: The age in years $\times$ 30 + 30. Bedwetting is thought to occur when the volume of urine produced exceeds the functional bladder capacity. In enuretic children, bladder capacity is often smaller compared to non-enuretic children.

➤ **Nocturnal polyuria:** Normally, there is a decrease in overnight urine production as a result of an increase in plasma levels of the antidiuretic hormone arginine vasopressin (AVP). Urine output falls by approximately 50% at night in children who don't wet the bed, whereas 75% of children who wet the bed produce large volumes of urine at night (nocturnal polyuria). The overproduction of urine at night appears to be a direct result of a nocturnal AVP deficiency.

Investigations

➤ Urinalysis and culture should be performed for every child with enuresis, particularly if there is an associated symptom of diurnal incontinence.

➤ Renal ultrasonography should be performed on all enuretic patients with:
  ➢ Non-monosymptomatic EN such as daytime urinary incontinence to detect any renal or bladder abnormalities such as bladder wall thickness and to measure pre- and postvoid bladder capacity.
  ➢ Neurological abnormalities or cutaneous signs on the spine

Management

General

➤ Children and parents should be informed that their bedwetting is not their fault and that there is overwhelming evidence that children will be dry eventually. Punitive measures should not be used. Parents and children should be reassured about the high spontaneous cure rate.

➤ Reasonable rewards and star charts can help many children with NE.

➤ Adequate fluid intake and healthy diet should be encouraged, but caffeine-based drinks should be avoided.

➤ The child is encouraged to empty their bladder before bedtime, every 2 hours during daytime and promptly so in case of an urge to urinate.

➤ Constipation should be excluded and, if present, treated.

Specific Treatment

➤ Treatment is divided between an enuresis alarm and desmopressin or both (Table 11.2).

➤ Desmopressin is a synthetic analogue of AVP administered orally in a dose of 200–400 micrograms once at bedtime. It is also available as a fast-melting sublingual

TABLE 11.2 Comparison features between enuresis alarm and desmopressin

	Enuresis Alarm	Desmopressin
• Age to use	• >7 years	• >5 years
• Motivation	• Required	• No
• Deep sleep	• Less suitable	• Suitable
• Easy to use?	• No, labour intensive	• Yes
• Effect starts?	• Few weeks	• Rapid onset
• Success rate	• High, first-line therapy	• High relapse rate after discontinuation

dose 120–240 micrograms at bedtime. Fluid should be limited 1 hour before to 8 hours after its administration. Recommended duration of treatment is 3 months. The medication is suitable for short-term need, and it is associated with high relapse rates after discontinuation.

➤ Enuresis body-worn alarms are effective for children with monosymptomatic enuresis and should be the first line of treatment. It teaches children to hold their urine during sleep and awakens them for urination.

Referral Criteria

Children with monosymptomatic NE can be managed effectively by the primary care providers. *Referral may be required for*:

➤ Children with refractory NE with no response to alarm and/or desmopressin.
➤ Non-monosymptomatic NE.
➤ Any associated physical or neurological problems such as developmental attention or learning difficulties, behavioural or family problems.

GENITALIA

Penile Swelling

Core Messages
➤ Swelling of the penis, often with inflammation and pain, may occur in association with nappy rash or forceful attempt to retract the foreskin. Other common causes are balanitis (inflammation of the glans) and posthitis (inflammation of the pre-puce). Balano-posthitis refers to inflammation of both sites. Priapism, a non-erotic, unwanted persistent erection, is a relatively frequent complication in children with sickle cell anaemia (SCA). Trauma is another important cause of priapism, which may be high-flow due an arteriovenous shunt or low-flow when there is obstruction to the venous outflow.
➤ The oedema of nephrotic syndrome (NS) or Henöch-Schönlein-Purpura (HSP) accumulates in dependent sites and often causes penile swelling. It is easy to

differentiate balanitis from oedema; the latter lacks redness and other inflammatory signs.

➤ Practically all cases of penile swelling require immediate medical attention, and most require referral. Causes are shown in Box 11.5.

BOX 11.5 Common causes of penile swelling

- Penile causes
  - ❯ Balanitis
  - ❯ Trauma
  - ❯ Paraphimosis
  - ❯ Penile torsion
  - ❯ Tumour (including carcinoma)
  - ❯ Epidermal inclusion cyst
  - ❯ Condom-induced allergy (latex allergy)
- Systemic causes
  - ❯ Priapism
  - ❯ Generalized oedema (e.g., NS, HSP)
  - ❯ Congenital lymphoedema
  - ❯ Drugs (cocaine, serotonin reuptake inhibitors)

PRACTICE POINTS

- The foreskin is normally non-retractile and attached to the glans in neonates. It becomes retractile in about 40% aged 1 year, 90% aged 4 years and 99% aged 15 years.
- Balanitis, the most common cause of penile inflammation, may result from allergy, seborrhoeic dermatitis, insect bites or any erosion of the skin allowing bacteria (usually staphylococci) to invade. Sexually transmitted infection (STI) should be considered in sexually active adolescents.
- Attempts to forcefully retract the foreskin (e.g., for cleansing) are dangerous; this can lead to balanitis or paraphimosis.
- Cases of paraphimosis (a retracted foreskin behind the corona glandis which can't be repositioned) require immediate attention if ischaemia of the glans is to be prevented. Firm manual compression, with EMLA cream and gauze, will usually reduce the constriction.
- Although SCA is the most common and well-known cause of priapism, penile neoplasms, leukaemia (particularly chronic granulocytic leukaemia), cocaine abuse and scorpion bite are other rarer causes.
- Parents of children with SCA should be informed of priapism as a possible complication and advised to seek immediate medical assistance if it occurs.
- Immediate management of children with priapism includes ice packs, bed rest, emptying the bladder, oral or IV hydration and analgesics. Morphine may be required.

- Priapism requires immediate medical assistance, as it can lead to ischaemia, erectile dysfunction and impotence if not treated.
- The oedema in NS is initially subtle, appearing around the eyes and in the lower legs, but the penile swelling is more recognizable and may be the first initial sign of the disease.

Scrotal Swelling

Core Messages

➤ Scrotal swelling is common in children and may be acute or chronic, painful or painless (Box 11.6).

➤ The two most common painless causes are hydrocele and inguinal hernia. Hydrocele is caused by drainage of peritoneal fluid through a narrow patent processus vaginalis, while inguinal hernia is due to a wide patent processus vaginalis that allows omentum or bowel to pass into the scrotum. Inguinal hernia is frequently associated with undescended testis, prematurity and connective tissue diseases such as Marfan's syndrome.

BOX 11.6 Common causes of scrotal swelling

Painless	Painful
● Idiopathic scrotal oedema (ISO)	● Testicular torsion
● Inguinal hernia	● Torsion of testicular appendage
● Hydrocele	● Epididymitis/orchitis
● Generalized oedema (NS)	● Torsion of the spermatic cord
● Testicular tumour (e.g., hamartoma)	● Incarceration inguinal hernia
● Varicocele	● Trauma (scrotal haematoma)

PRACTICE POINTS

- In a mobile child with hydrocele, the size characteristically increases during the daytime and decreases overnight. Abrupt onset of painful scrotal swelling is usually caused by incarcerated hernia or testicular torsion. The onset of pain in torsion of the testicular appendix is usually gradual.
- Epididymitis is the most common cause of scrotal swelling in sexually active young adolescents. This is an ascending infection from the urethra.
- Epididymitis/orchitis may mimic testicular torsion; the inflammation, however, is commonly secondary to viral infection (e.g., mumps) or STI. In addition, the pain is more gradual in epididymitis/orchitis; nausea and vomiting is uncommon; and it is often associated with fever, dysuria and pyuria.

- ISO, usually caused by allergy, may mimic torsion. The scrotum is swollen and red in ISO, there are no symptoms, and the testis characteristically feels normal and not tender. ISO often extends to the groin and perineum. Parents can be reassured that the swelling will disappear in a few days (without treatment), leaving some purpuric discolouration.
- Varicocele occurs in about 5% of all adolescent boys and is a common cause of subfertility.

Vaginal Discharge (Vulvovaginitis)

Core Messages
➤ Physiologically, vaginal discharge (VD) is a common finding in neonate girls who often experience vaginal discharge (pseudo-menstruation) as a result of withdrawal of the maternal oestrogen hormone. A rise of oestrogen at the onset of puberty causes another physiological discharge (leukorrhoea).
➤ Prepubertal VD is the most common gynaecological problem in children and the most frequent reason for referral to paediatric and adolescent gynaecological services. While the most common isolates in prepubertal girls with VD are opportunistic bacteria of faecal origin, girls' VDs in puberty usually grow bacterial vaginosis and *Candida albicans*, which are rarely isolated in prepubertal girls.
➤ Non-specific vulvovaginitis is the most common cause of VD, affecting 25–75% of prepubertal girls and accounting for up to 70% of all cases (Box 11.7). It is usually caused by poor perineal hygiene, especially at an age when girls start to attend the toilet independently. Young girls often touch the nose and mouth and the genitalia, thereby spreading the pathogens to the genital area. In addition, the tendency of the labia minora to open on squatting and the proximity of the anal orifice to the vagina allow transfer of faecal bacteria to the vagina. Other contributory factors include wearing tight-fitting clothes and the use of irritants such as detergents and bubble baths.
➤ Sexual abuse is a serious problem, and a high index of suspicion is required to make the diagnosis (see 'Practice Points').

BOX 11.7 Summary of features of VD and vulvovaginitis

Presentation
- Vulvar itching, burning and soreness, frequent urination, dysuria, sleep disturbance

Signs
- Red vulva, vaginal introitus and labia minora, often associated with dried secretion of desquamated cells (known as smegma) and whitish/yellowish vaginal discharge in the interlabial area

Main Causes

- Physiological
- Non-specific vulvovaginitis (70–80% of all cases)
- Specific vulvovaginitis (due to specific pathogens such as group A streptococci, chlamydia or gonococci)
- Foreign body
- Child abuse
- Dermatosis (lichen sclerosis, atopic dermatitis)

Predisposing Factors

- Female anatomy (as noted earlier)
- Poor genital hygiene
- Tight underclothing, particularly if made of synthetic fibre
- Physiological low oestrogen deficiency
- Obesity
- Threadworms

Management: See Box 11.8

PRACTICE POINTS

- UTI is common in association with VD. Unless the UTI and/or threadworms are treated, treatment for VD is inadequate and VD will recur. Threadworm infection typically causes recurrent vulvovaginitis and manifests as nocturnal scratching due to female worms depositing eggs on the perineum.
- While VD of prepubertal girls characteristically grows no pathogens, culture of the vaginal discharge is an important test to identify pathogens implicated in vulvovaginal infection.
- *Child sexual abuse (CSA)* refers to the use of children in sexual activities (including fondling, masturbation and penetration) of any kind which they do not understand and give consent to. Data from European countries indicate that CSA affects 10–40% of girls and 5–10% of boys. Most perpetrators of child abuse are close relatives or family friends.
  - › Most children suspected of CSA do not yield abnormal findings. This does not exclude child abuse. Common presenting symptoms are rarely related to genitalia and include sleep disturbance, non-specific sudden behaviour changes, phobias, anorexia, poor school performance and social withdrawal. Other uncommon complaints are anogenital pain, dysuria and itching.

> The interview of the child suspected of being sexually abused is the most valuable component of medical evaluation, using the child's words for body parts, drawings and age-appropriate questions.

- Foreign body should always be considered when the discharge has a foul odour. Common objects include clumped toilet tissue or small parts of toys. Examination under general anaesthesia may be indicated.
- Lichen sclerosus is an autoimmune chronic inflammatory disease which is characterized by a sharply demarcated area of hypopigmentation around the vulva and the perianal area. It is associated with intense itching and bleeds easily with normal toilet activities, e.g., genital wiping. The mean age of disease onset is 5 years.

BOX 11.8 Summary of management of vulvovaginitis

- Eliminate predisposing factors such as threadworms.
- Discontinue all external irritants such as bath additives, washing lotions and wet wipes.
- Genital hygiene by rinsing and washing with water instead of soap, proper bladder emptying and stool wiping front to back. Keep the area as dry as possible.
- Loose, cotton knickers are recommended; no tight underclothing.
- Sitz bath with sodium chloride for 10 minutes, rinsing with water and then thoroughly drying.
- Local application of a neutral lipid-containing cream
- Urine specimen and vaginal swab (in the presence of VD) for culture.

RECTAL PROLAPSE

Core Messages

➤ Rectal prolapse (RP) refers to a protrusion of the rectal mucosa through the anus, termed partial or mucosal RP, and usually is <2 cm. Protrusion that includes the entire rectal wall is termed procidentia. It usually presents as a painless, red mass at the anal verge.

➤ Most cases of RP occur during the first few years of life, with a peak incidence of 1–3 years of age. The condition is uncommon in children older than 4 years of age, who are more likely to require surgical intervention.

➤ RP should be viewed as a symptom rather than a specific disease and should always be considered a presenting sign of an underlying condition (Box 11.9).

➤ Most cases of RP respond well to conservative management. RP rarely becomes chronic; if so, complications, such as ulceration, bleeding and inflammation (proctitis) are likely consequences.

➤ RP is more common in tropical and developing countries due to the high prevalence of diarrhoea, malnutrition and parasitic infestation. One of the most important causes of RP in high-income countries is cystic fibrosis (CF), which accounts for 20% of cases. RP may be the first manifestation of CF.

BOX 11.9 Causes of RP

Idiopathic (about 15–20%)

Secondary

- CF (about 20%)
- Chronic constipation (25–30%)
- Chronic diarrhoea (e.g., coeliac, ulcerative colitis; 20%)
- Connective tissue diseases
- Malnutrition
- Intestinal parasites
- Chronic cough (e.g., pertussis)
- Repair of imperforate anus
- Meningomyelocele

PRACTICE POINTS

- The diagnosis of RP is often based on history, as the physical examination is usually normal because prolapse cannot be evoked in the clinical setting. Parents should be encouraged to take photos or video to establish the diagnosis. Management of RP is shown in Box 11.10.
- In contrast to adults, the incidence and recurrence of RP decrease as children grow older, and conservative management is usually successful and indicated. Approximately 90% respond to conservative management with resolution of the RP. Spontaneous resolution is less likely after the age of 4 years.
- CF is one of the most common causes of RP, occurring in about 20% of cases. The diagnosis should always be considered if there is a history of meconium ileus, persistent cough and/or failure to gain weight adequately.
- RP should be differentiated from rarer causes of prolapse resembling RP such as prolapsed intussusception, haemorrhoids and prolapsed polyp. The latter appears as a dark, plum-coloured, red mass (in contrast to the lighter red mucosa appearance of the RP), and they do not have a hole in the middle. Intussusception is associated with intermittent severe abdominal pain.

BOX 11.10 Management of RP

- RP should be promptly and gently reduced manually. Parents and the child should be taught how to reduce the prolapse as soon as it appears outside the anus and to seek medical assistance if this is not achieved.
- A sweat test is indicated in all children with RP who present without a known underlying cause.
- Treatment of the underlying cause is important. Children with constipation should be treated with laxatives and diet including high-fibre diet, adequate fluid intake and advice to avoid prolonged straining. Prolonged sitting on a child's potty and straining predisposes for RP, and this should be avoided.
- Surgical options are recommended for children with persistent RP, particularly for those children with frequent episodes of rectal prolapses or if the RP is associated with symptoms such as discomfort or difficulty to reduce the prolapse.
- Sclerotherapy with ethyl alcohol and circumferential sutures or the use of hypertonic saline are common procedures.

CHAPTER 12

Throat, Ear and Nose

UPPER RESPIRATORY TRACT INFECTIONS

Introduction

➤ Upper respiratory tract infections (URTIs) are the most common cause of fever, reasons for doctor consultations, health service utilizations and antibiotic use in children. The infections have a significant impact on the child and family life and carry a considerable economic burden. Common and rare causes of URTI are shown in Box 12.1.

➤ The majority of URTIs are self-limiting viral illnesses that are not accompanied by secondary bacterial infections. The infections are uncommon in children younger than 1 year of age and peak at the age of 2–4 years. An infection rate of six to eight infections a year is considered normal. A higher incidence occurs in those who attend nursery and whose siblings attend nursery or school. Daycare attendance is an established risk factor for URTI.

BOX 12.1 Main causes of URTI/sore throat

Common

- Viral URTI (including tonsillopharyngitis)
- Bacterial tonsillitis
- Acute otitis media (AOM)
- Otitis media with effusion (OME)
- Sinusitis
- Laryngitis/stridor
- Herpetic gingivostomatitis

Rare

- Herpangina
- Scarlet fever
- Retropharyngeal or peritonsillar abscess
- Oropharyngeal thrush
- Aphthous ulceration

DOI: 10.1201/9781032642888-12

➤ The most common cause of bacterial tonsillitis is group A *Streptococcus* (GAS). Symptoms and signs of viral URTI and bacterial GAS tonsillitis may overlap. Therefore, GAS infection needs to be excluded by clinical criteria and throat culture or rapid antigen detection test.

➤ Cough subsequent to URTI occurs commonly in >50% of cases and may persist for 2–3 weeks. Another common complication includes acute otitis media, particularly affecting children under the age of 2 years.

➤ Judicious antibiotic prescribing practices for URTI are recommended, as antibiotic prescription for URTI remains a common practice.

Management of URTI

Relief of Fever

➤ The main effect of antipyretics is to relieve the child's discomfort and thereby the parents' anxiety. Paracetamol is the most commonly used antipyretic and analgesic drug. A therapeutic dose is 10–15 mg/kg every 4–6 hours.

➤ Ibuprofen suspension is available for children who are at least 6 months old. Its anti-inflammatory and analgesic properties provide additional therapeutic advantages over paracetamol. Ibuprofen is used as an antipyretic in a dose of 5 mg/kg three times daily. A dose of 10 mg/kg is more potent and has longer-lasting fever suppression than paracetamol.

➤ Paracetamol is frequently used in an alternating manner with ibuprofen. The practice is common but has no scientific basis.

➤ Saline nasal spray may be beneficial and it can reduce the nasal symptoms.

➤ Physical measures (fan, tepid sponging) for fever are unnecessary and unpleasant for the child; their use is discouraged. Offering extra fluids, keeping the room cool and dressing the child lightly are beneficial.

Relief of Cough

➤ Medications for treating cough (over-the-counter and prescription medications), including cough suppressants, mucolytics, sedatives and antihistamine drugs, have failed to provide efficacy, lacking scientific evidence, and are associated with significant side effects.

➤ Honey has been recommended, including by the World Health Organization (WHO), as a potentially valuable demulcent for treating URTI with cough. It has anti-inflammatory, antibacterial and antioxidant effects. It increases saliva production and improves swallowing by coating the inflammatory areas and has effects on sensory receptors that send irritative signals to the brain cortex resulting in reduction of cough.

Antibiotic Prescription

➤ The majority of URTIs are viral infections (around 90%) that are not complicated by bacterial infection. Antibiotic use for acute URTI is usually not indicated. The common practice of prescribing antibiotics for URTIs will contribute to the global threat of antimicrobial resistance.

➤ Promoting non-use of antibiotics in URTI can be achieved by education of healthcare providers and parents, use of clinical-decision algorithms and the use of rapid diagnostic testing to reduce uncertainty in the diagnosis.

TABLE 12.1 Summary of managing bacterial throat infections

	Signs/Symptoms	Tests	Treatment
Tonsillitis	• Fever >38.5 • Odynophagia • Purulent tonsils • Lymphadenopathy • Absence of runny nose/cough	• FBC, CRP • U&E • Monospot test	• IV/oral antibiotics • Dexamethasone
Peritonsillar abscess	• As above+: ❯ Trismus ❯ Unilateral peritonsillar swelling, bulging of soft palate, contralateral uvula deviation		• As above+: Incision & drainage

ACUTE TONSILLITIS

➤ Tonsillitis is an infection confined tom the tonsillar parenchyma in association with odynophagia, fever, purulent exudate, lymphadenopathy and absence of nasal signs such as runny nose.

➤ The incidence of acute tonsillitis and deep neck space infections has increased significantly in the past 25 years, while the number of tonsillectomies has decreased.

➤ There is variation in antibiotic prescribing practices for recurrent sore throats among GPs; most discourage their use. Signs and symptoms are not powerful enough to differentiate bacterial tonsillitis from other types of sore throats, particularly viral URTI. Diagnosis and management are shown in Table 12.1.

➤ Primary care physicians are advised to use a diagnostic scoring system based on Centor (Box 12.2) to determine the likelihood of bacterial cause of tonsillitis. A positive score of 3 should trigger a pharyngeal rapid swab testing or culture to detect haemolytic streptococci. On the other hand, antibiotics are unlikely to be indicated with Centor score 0, 1 or 2.

➤ A frequent cause of fever with tonsillitis is glandular fever and periodic fever, including aphthous stomatitis, pharyngitis and adenitis (PFAPA). There is no diagnostic test for PFAPA but the condition responds well to steroid therapy.

➤ The Centor criteria (Box 12.2) can be used for diagnosis and treatment.

BOX 12.2 Centor diagnostic criteria and treatment

	No	Yes
• Age 3–14 years	0	+1
• Exudate or swelling on tonsils	0	+1
• Tender/swollen anterior cervical area	0	+1
• Temperature	0	+1
• Cough	+1	0

• Patients with a score of:

❼ Zero to 1 are at low risk from streptococcal pharyngitis, and no further diagnostic testing is needed.

❼ 2 or 3 should be tested using rapid a streptococcal test or throat swab.

❼ ≥ 4 should be considered for empirical antibiotics.

Tonsillectomy

➤ Tonsillectomy is one of the most frequently performed surgical procedures, particularly in children. There were **37,000** paediatric tonsillectomies performed in England in 2016–2017. The main complication is post-tonsillectomy haemorrhage, occurring in 1–2%.

➤ Studies have not been conclusive in finding a clear clinical benefit of tonsillectomy in children. A Cochrane review showed only modest benefit of tonsillectomy/adenotonsillectomy in the treatment of recurrent tonsillitis. Some benefits may not persist over time.

➤ Enlargement of the tonsils and adenoids can cause obstruction of the upper airway, leading to oxygen desaturation and obstructive sleep apnoea (OSA). An overnight sleep study by a polysomnography is performed to diagnose OSA. This condition is associated with poor quality of life and low cognitive skills if it becomes chronic. Tonsillectomy is the primary treatment for children with OSA. Other indications for tonsillectomy are shown in Box 12.3.

➤ OSA is common in children with Down's syndrome (DS) due to craniofacial anatomy, macroglossia, hypotonia and increased prevalence of obesity. It is recommended that these children undergo a universal screening with polysomnography to exclude OSA.

BOX 12.3 Indications for tonsillectomy

● Watchful waiting is more appropriate than tonsillectomy for children with mild and recurrent sore throats.
● Sore throats due to acute tonsillitis and that warrant consideration that are:
  ❯ Debilitating and prevent normal functioning.
  ❯ Seven or more documented and adequately treated episodes of tonsillitis in the preceding year, or five or more such episodes in each of the preceding 2 years or three or more such episodes in each of the preceding 3 years.
● Peritonsillar abscess.
● OSA, e.g., in children with obesity or DS.
● Periodic fever, aphthous stomatitis, and cervical adenitis (PFAPA).

OBSTRUCTIVE SLEEP APNOEA (OSA)

Assessment and Management

➤ **General**
  ➢ OSA is a common paediatric sleep disorder characterized by recurrent partial or complete obstruction of the upper airway resulting in oxygen desaturation and/or arousal from sleep gasping for air.
  ➢ The prevalence is 2–4% and is increasing, which is coinciding with the rising levels of children's overweight and obesity. Predisposing conditions are listed in Box 12.4.

➤ **Symptoms**
  ➢ Snoring, apnoea and chronic mouth breathing observed by the parents. Sleep disturbance characterized by labour respiration, restlessness and waking at night; unusual sleep positions to maintain a patent upper airway.
  ➢ Daytime somnolence, impaired daytime and school performance.
  ➢ In severe cases: Right-sided heart failure, arrhythmia and developmental delay.

➤ **Assessment**
  ➢ Physical examination during wakefulness may be entirely normal.
  ➢ Confirming the enlarged tonsils and adenoids as the most common cause.
  ➢ Diagnosis is confirmed by overnight polysomnography. Continuous pulse oximetry (when polysomnography is not available) may show intermittent oxygen desaturation overnight.
  ➢ MRI is the best device to evaluate the upper airway for suspected obstruction.
➤ **Treatment**
  ➢ Medications (e.g., nasal decongestants) have limited value.
  ➢ Weight reduction (if obese), intranasal corticosteroids and watchful waiting are appropriate for mild cases. Moderate/severe cases should be referred to an ENT specialist. Cardiological evaluation may be indicated in these cases.
  ➢ First-line treatment is tonsillectomy with or without adenoidectomy.

BOX 12.4 Conditions predisposing to OSA

● Adenotonsillar hyperplasia
● DS
● Congenital craniofacial abnormalities
  ❯ Small nasopharynx
  ❯ Micrognathia
  ❯ Macroglossia
● Obesity
● Persistent nasal obstruction
● Neuromuscular diseases

SINUSITIS

➤ Acute bacterial sinusitis is defined as inflammation of the mucosal lining of one or more paranasal sinuses, usually preceded by a viral URTI, which promotes the obstruction of the sinus ostia. The viruses of URTI can induce proliferation of pathogenic bacteria. Persistence or worsening symptoms of URTI suggest the diagnosis of sinusitis.
➤ The diagnosis of acute sinusitis is made on clinical criteria and imaging (Box 12.5).
➤ Of the many viruses causing URTI, respiratory syncytial virus (RSV) and rhinovirus are the main pathogens. *Haemophilus influenza* (non-typeable), *Streptococcus pneumonia* and *Moraxella* bacteria are the major pathogens that cause bacterial sinusitis.

BOX 12.5 Diagnostic criteria for acute bacterial sinusitis

● Persistent symptoms of nasal discharge and daytime cough lasting 10 days with no improvement.
● A worsening course of nasal discharge, daytime cough or fever after initial improvement.
● Severe onset of symptoms with fever of >39.0°C and purulent nasal discharge for at least 3 consecutive days.
● Uncommon symptoms include decreased sense of smell, facial pain and tenderness (more common in adults).
● A contrast-enhanced CT scan can confirm the diagnosis.

PRACTICE POINTS

- High annual rates of URTI and the severity of the initial URTI are associated with a high risk of developing bacterial sinusitis.
- Amoxicillin with or without clavulanate is the treatment of choice in a dose of 50–90 mg/kg/day, depending on the severity of symptoms at presentation, for 2–3 weeks.
- Clinicians should reassess the initial symptoms and signs of patients with sinusitis within 48–72 hours of the initial consultation.
- *Referral is indicated for* persistent or worsening symptoms despite the antibiotic therapy.
  - *Urgent referral* in case of severe facial pain or ocular symptoms.

LARYNGITIS AND STRIDOR (SEE ALSO CHAPTER 9)

Core Messages

➤ Croup (or laryngotracheobronchitis) is characterized by a viral URTI affecting the subglottic area, followed by an abrupt nocturnal onset of barking cough, inspiratory stridor, hoarseness and varying degrees of respiratory distress. Symptoms are usually mild and transient, typically affecting those in the 6 months to 3 years age group, with usually excellent prognosis. Only about 1–2% of children with viral croup have severe symptoms requiring intensive care. Microorganism causes (Table 12.6):
  - ❯ Croup is mostly caused by viruses including parainfluenza type B (causing 50% of cases as the major pathogens), RSV, adenoviruses and influenza A and B viruses.
  - ❯ Bacterial causes are rare and include *Mycoplasma pneumoniae, Staphylococcal aureus* and *H. influenzae.*

BOX 12.6 Causes of croup

Acute

- Laryngotracheobronchitis (viral croup)
- Spasmodic croup
- Infectious mononucleosis
- Aspiration of foreign body
- Epiglottis
- Bacterial tracheitis (staphylococcal infection)
- Hypocalcaemic tetany

Persistent

- Laryngomalacia
- Tumour: Papilloma, haemangioma, laryngeal web
- Vascular ring
- Chiari's malformation

➤ In neonates, laryngeal injury may occur subsequent to birth trauma and results in unilateral vocal cord paralysis (usually left side), producing hoarseness with mild stridor. Bilateral paralysis of the vocal cord causes dyspnoea as well. The prognosis of post-ventilation aphonia/hoarseness is good, and recovery is expected.

➤ Persistent stridor commencing in the first few weeks of life is mostly caused by laryngomalacia because of collapse of the supraglottic structure during inspiration. A child with laryngomalacia has a normal cry without hoarseness.

Investigations for Persistent Stridor

➤ Thyroid function test (TFT) to exclude hypothyroidism.

➤ Serum calcium to confirm hypocalcaemia.

➤ Chest x-ray may diagnose vascular ring or aspiration.

➤ Direct laryngoscopy to diagnose laryngeal node (post-ventilation), haemangiomas and unilateral or bilateral paralysis of the vocal cord.

➤ CT scan or MRI of the head to diagnose Chiari's malformation.

PRACTICE POINTS

- In neonates, laryngeal injury may occur after a birth trauma and results in unilateral vocal cord paralysis (usually left side) producing hoarseness with mild stridor. The prognosis is good, and recovery is expected over the next few weeks.
- Nocturnal onset of acute stridor with barking cough and hoarse voice is almost certainly croup, viral or spasmodic. Their prognosis is excellent. Only about 1–2% of children with viral croup have severe symptoms requiring intensive care and intubation.
- A child with croup who rapidly becomes unwell with high fever has developed extension of the infection into the respiratory tract, has bacterial tracheitis as a complication of the viral croup or has bacterial epiglottis.
- The most important aspect of acute stridor is to differentiate between a life-threatening and benign conditions.

Management

➤ Most children with croup have a mild and short-lived illness and are managed in the primary care setting (Box 12.7). Children should be made comfortable, which is best achieved in the lap of a parent or caregiver.

➤ Monitoring the patient is important, particularly respiratory and pulse rates. Their increase may be the first signs of hypoxia. Assessing croup severity using various severity score systems (Table 12.2 and Box 12.8) are useful for research studies, but they do not enhance routine clinical care.

BOX 12.7 Summary of pharmacological management of croup

- Corticosteroids reduce inflammatory oedema and are given as:
- Dexamethasone 0.15 mg/kg by mouth with a single dose.
- Higher doses of corticosteroids of 0.6 mg/kg are also recommended.
- Same dose to be given before transfer to hospital for severe croup.
- Oral prednisolone 1 mg/kg is an alternative drug to dexamethasone.
- Nebulized adrenaline is recommended for moderate-to-severe croup which can improve the symptoms of respiratory distress within 10–30 minutes.

TABLE 12.2 Assessment of severity of croup

	Mild Croup (Can Be Managed at Home)	Severe Croup (for Referral)
• Mental status	• Normal	• Agitated or exhausted
• Severity of stridor	• Mild	• Severe
• Ability to talk	• Yes	• Difficult
• RR, pulse rate	• Normal	• Increased
• Fever	• Absent or low grade	• >39.0°C
• Accessory muscle use	• No	• Yes
• Air entry	• Normal	• Decreased
• Level of consciousness	• Normal	• Drowsy

➤ Although humidified air has not shown to influence croup severity in clinical trials, the use of steam from a shower in a closed bathroom or steam from a vaporizer seems helpful and may terminate the laryngeal spasm within a few minutes.

➤ Children with respiratory distress and/or low oxygen saturation should receive oxygen treatment, which can be given (to avoid agitating the child) via a plastic tube with the opening held within a few centimetres of the child's nose and mouth.

➤ Antibiotics, decongestants and short-acting beta-2 agonists have not been shown to be beneficial in croup management. However, the use of analgesics/antipyretics is reasonable to reduce the child's discomfort.

➤ Systemic corticosteroids are the main treatment for croup, with a single dose of dexamethasone. The oral or IM route of corticosteroids is either equivalent or superior to budesonide inhalations. Adding inhaled budesonide to oral dexamethasone does not provide extra benefit.

➤ In comparison to oral prednisolone, dexamethasone is superior in reducing rates of returning to hospitals but not in reducing croup scores.

BOX 12.8 Westly croup severity score

Level of Consciousness
- Normal   (0 point)
- Disorientation   (5 points)

Cyanosis
- None   (0 point)
- With agitation   (4 points)
- At rest   (5 points)

Stridor
- None   (0 point)
- With agitation   (1 point)
- At rest   (2 points)

Air Entry
- Normal   (0 points)
- Decreased   (1 point)
- Markly decreased   (2 points)

Retraction
- None   (0 point)
- Mild   (1 point)
- Moderate   (2 points)
- Severe   (3 points)

Total Score:

Score interpretation: 0–2 = mild; 3–7 = moderate; 8–11 = severe; 12–17 = impending respiratory failure.

SWALLOWING DIFFICULTY (DYSPHAGIA)

Core Messages

➤ Swallowing is a complex mechanism involving approximately 50 muscle pairs (agonists and antagonists) to bring swallowed material to the stomach. Swallowing is developed as early as 20 weeks of gestation and is established at 33–34 weeks of gestation.

➤ Dysphagia is defined as a difficulty in swallowing due to impaired transfer of fluids or food from the oral cavity to the oesophagus (pre-oesophageal) and from the oesophagus to stomach (oesophageal dysphagia) (Box 12.9).

➤ Dysphagia may include discomfort or pain during swallowing (odynophagia), food sticking in the throat, feeling of a lump in the throat, chest pain or regurgitation through the mouth or nose. In infants, dysphagia may manifest as low interest in food, body stiffness or vomiting during feeding, unusual lengthy feeding and coughing or gagging during feeding.

BOX 12.9 Causes of dysphagia

Pre-Oesophageal

- Upper airway obstruction (tonsillitis, tonsillar abscess, epiglottitis)
- Neuromuscular (e.g., myasthenia gravis, bulbar palsy)
- Plummer–Vinson syndrome (iron deficiency)
- Globus hystericus

Oesophageal

- Oesophagitis (GO reflux)
- Vascular ring
- Achalasia
- Lower oesophageal ring (Schatzki's ring)
- Drugs (potassium chloride, quinidine)

LYMPHADENOPATHY AND NECK MASS

Core Messages

➤ Lumps in the neck are common and have multiple causes (Box 12.10). Cervical lymphadenopathy is the most common finding, which is usually benign and reactive to viral infections resulting in small, non-tender mobile lymph nodes, measuring <1 cm for cervical and axillary lymph nodes and <1.5 cm for inguinal lymph nodes. Generalized lymphadenopathy indicates the presence of lymph nodes in more than two node regions.

➤ About one-third of neonates have palpable lymph nodes <1 cm in diameter. They are commonly present in the inguinal area (due to the prevalence of infection of the nappy area) but may also be palpable in the cervical or axillary region.

➤ Pathological lymphadenopathy is suggested by either abnormally large lymph nodes (>1–1.5 cm in diameter), tenderness on palpation, matted together, fixed to the skin or underlying structures or if they are localized in the supraclavicular area.

BOX 12.10 Causes of lymphadenopathy and neck mass

Lymph Nodes

- Infections
  - › Reactive lymphadenitis due to local infection
  - › TB lymphadenitis
  - › Mononucleosis
  - › Kawasaki's disease
- Autoimmune diseases
  - › Rheumatoid arthritis
  - › Systemic lupus erythematosus (SLE)
- Malignancy (e.g., lymphoma)
- Lymphangioma (cystic hygroma)

Neck Cyst

- Dermoid cyst
- Thyroglossal cyst
- Branchial cyst

Others

- Sternomastoid tumour
- Goitre
- Pharyngeal pouch

Investigations

➤ Chest x-ray is first-line investigation in suspected cases of TB or lymphoma.
➤ Full blood count (FBC): Leukocytosis suggests bacterial infection; atypical lymphocytes for mononucleosis; leukopenia for SLE; anaemia for chronic infection or lymphoma.
➤ Liver function tests (LFTs).
➤ Monospot test or IgG/IgM for mononucleosis.
➤ Tuberculin skin test for suspected TB adenitis.

PRACTICE POINTS

- Reactive lymphadenopathy is the most common lump in the neck. Parents usually fear the possibility of cancer and need to be reassured, including that the lymphadenopathy may last months and years and may enlarge again in response to another viral infection.
- *A neck mass greater than 1 cm in diameter, which is matted or fixed to the underlying structures, requires urgent referral to exclude lymphoma.*
- Generalized lymphadenopathy suggests either systemic infection (e.g., viral infections such as mononucleosis or toxoplasmosis), autoimmune disease (e.g., rheumatoid arthritis) or malignancy (e.g., leukaemia).

- Cervical lymphadenopathy should be differentiated from tuberculous lymphadenitis. The latter is suspected if the lymphadenopathy is associated with persistent or unexplained fever, night sweats, anorexia or does not undergo spontaneous regression of its size within 6–8 weeks. Biopsy carries a small risk of causing fistula.
- A thyroglossal cyst, which develops from a remnant thyroglossal duct, is painless and localized in the midline but becomes enlarged and tender if infected. A pathognomonic sign is its vertical movement on swallowing and tongue protrusion. The cyst should not be excised unless the presence of thyroid tissue is excluded.
- The usual branchial cyst looks like an insignificant papule on the side of the neck (in contrast to a thyroglossal cyst). *A referral to ENT is recommended.*
- The most common acquired goitre in children is Hashimoto's thyroiditis, with normal TFT or one suggestive of hypothyroidism.

EAR

Earaches (Otalgia)

➤ Otalgia is a common reason for seeking medical attention. Its causes are shown in Box 12.11. Acute otitis media (AOM) is the most common reason for otalgia and is mostly caused by viruses, e.g., adenovirus, RSV and influenza. Otitis externa (OE) is the second most common cause of otalgia and is mostly caused by *Pseudomonas* and staphylococci.

➤ In contrast to adults, referred pain from outside the ears (extrinsic causes) is common in paediatrics, occurring via five main sources: Trigeminal nerve (sensory distribution of the face, teeth and gums); facial nerve (temporomandibular joint or Bell's palsy); glossopharyngeal nerve (tonsils, pharynx); vagus nerve (laryngopharynx or oesophagus) or via the second to third cervical vertebrae (cervical spine). In all of these cases patients have a normal otological examination.

➤ Ramsay Hunt syndrome (auditory herpes zoster) usually presents with severe ear pain. Clues for this syndrome are vesicles on the pinna and in the external auditory canal in the distribution of the sensory branch of the facial nerve.

BOX 12.11 Causes of otalgia

- Infective AOM
- Infective OE
- Referred pain (toothache, tonsillopharyngitis)
- Foreign body (FB)
- Infected eczematous dermatitis
- Mastoiditis
- Temporomandibular arthritis
- Ramsay Hunt syndrome (herpes zoster oticus)

OTITIS MEDIA

➤ OM is a spectrum of diseases, which include several disorders (Table 12.3).
➤ Viruses of a URTI can ascend through the eustachian tube to the middle ear, paving the way for bacterial OM.
➤ The incidence of OM has decreased since the 1990s due to the introduction of strict diagnostic criteria that recommend judicious antibiotic use and the introduction of pneumococcal conjugate vaccination.

TABLE 12.3 Umbrella term of OM

Term	Definition
• OM	• General term comprising AOM, OM with effusion and chronic OM.
• AOM	• Moderate-severe bulging of TM, mild bulging TM and recent (within 24 hours) onset of earache, or pain or intense redness of TM or acute ear discharge.
• OM with effusion (OME)	• See next under "OM with effusion."
• Chronic OME	• Persisting signs of OME ≥3 months from the time of diagnosis.

AOM = acute OM; TM = tympanic membrane.

Management (Box 12.12)

BOX 12.12 Management of AOM

● Oral analgesics with paracetamol or ibuprofen.
● Antibiotics for AOM are particularly indicated if the child is:
  ❯ Ill-looking.
  ❯ <2 years of age, with bilateral OM.
  ❯ Immunocompromised.
  ❯ Has craniofacial malformation.
● Choices of antibiotics include:
  ❯ Amoxicillin or (as a second choice) co-amoxiclav* 5–7 days.
    ❯ Macrolides, e.g., azithromycin.
    ❯ Cephalosporine.
● Decongestant, antihistamines and steroids are of no value.
● Ventilation tubes are not helpful for recurrent AOM.

* These are first-line drugs to treat OM.

➤ Prevention of viral URTI and OM can be achieved by influenza vaccines, which are recommended at >6 months of age in the United States and >2 years in the UK.
➤ Pneumococcal vaccination is associated with significant reduction of OM incidence by reducing or eliminating nasopharyngeal colonization of S. *pneumoniae*, non-typeable H. influenza and *Morella catarrhalis*.

PRACTICE POINTS

- The TM of a crying baby is often red on inspection, and so OM should not be misdiagnosed.
- The presence of otalgia in the absence of otologic findings indicates the need for a thorough workup to determine the source of referred pain.
- Bloody discharge may follow a direct trauma or be subsequent to an FB insertion in the ear. Cancer is a rare cause that should be considered.
- A child with suppuration in the middle ear or mastoid is at risk of developing subdural or extradural abscess, meningitis and brain abscess. Persistent fever with little or no response to antibiotic therapy, severe otalgia and persistent headache, vomiting, lethargy or irritability and a tender mastoid area on pressing are alarming features.
- Children with recurrent OM should undergo baseline immune evaluation, which includes IgG subclass checking (e.g., FBC and immunoglobulins).
- In Ramsay Hunt syndrome, the associated hearing loss and the facial palsy may be permanent (in about 50%).

Referral should be considered for the following:

➤ Concerns about hearing/speech following OM.
➤ Recurrent OM, e.g., >6 episodes with 12 months.
➤ Persistent otorrhoea.
➤ Concern about OM complication, e.g., mastoiditis, meningitis.

Otitis Media with Effusion (OME)

➤ **Characteristics**
  ➣ Defined as fluid in the middle ear without signs of inflammation or infection.
  ➣ TM is usually retracted, has impaired mobility, is opaque appearing and is not red.
  ➣ Usually associated with a transient, mild degree of hearing loss (20–30 dB).
  ➣ Risk factor: Following suppurative OM, effusion will be present:
    - 80% of cases at 2 weeks.
    - 40% at 1 month.
    - 20% at 2 months.
    - 10% at 3 months.
➤ **Initial management**
  ➣ Watchful waiting is indicated if the effusion has persisted for <3 months and the child is not significantly symptomatic.
  ➣ Review after 3 months.
  ➣ Ventilation tube insertion may be indicated with documented hearing loss.
  ➣ Antibiotics, antihistamines or decongestants are generally ineffective.

➤ **When to refer**
  ➤ Hearing impairment persistent for >3 months.
  ➤ Any hearing impairment that is causing speech delay.
  ➤ Hearing impairment and the child is symptomatic.
  ➤ Significant hearing loss after 3 months often entails myringotomy with insertion of tympanostomy tubes to improve middle ear ventilation.
  ➤ In cases of persistent OME despite tympanostomy tubes, adenoidectomy may be considered.

Ventilation Tubes (Grommets)

➤ AOM is one of the most frequent reasons for primary care visits. While most children have one AOM, some suffer from recurring AOM, defined as 3 episodes of infection in 6 months or ≥4 within 1 year.
➤ Grommets facilitate middle ear ventilation and drainage of middle ear fluid to prevent OM effusion and AOM.
➤ Although surgery (insertion of grommets, adenoidectomy or both) results in short-term reduction of AOM and hearing gain (about 12 dB improvement in hearing), evidence for its long-term benefits is lacking. Box 12.13 shows some practice points for children with grommets.

BOX 12.13 Practice points for children with grommets

● After insertion of grommets, many children (reported incidence 26–75%) develop episodes of otorrhoea through the tube while the tube is properly placed and patent. These episodes may be accompanied by foul odour, pain and fever. Otorrhoea persists in 5% at 1 year.
● Grommets should fall out in 6–9 months, and the perforation heals concurrently.
● Persistent perforation occurs in <1% of cases, and surgery may be required later.
● While surface swimming is allowed without earplugs, in case of diving or using water chutes, well-fitting silicone rubber earplugs should be worn. Beware that bath water is much worse than swimming pool water because of the germs from the rest of the body and irritant soap.

OTITIS EXTERNA

➤ **Characteristics**
  ➤ OE is defined as an infection of cutis/subcutis of the external auditory canal, with possible involvement of the TM and the pinna.
  ➤ More than 90% of OE cases are caused by bacteria, mainly *Pseudomonas* or *S. aureus*.

> OE is usually due to trauma (e.g., manipulation to remove cerumen), water in the ear canal (following swimming, soap and shampoo) or due to dermatitis of the external canal.
> Severe pain is a predominant symptom, which typically worsens with pressure on the tragus and pinna. There is otorrhoea, itching, erythema and swelling inside the ear canal. The surrounding lymph nodes are tender.

> **Initial management**
>> Tuning fork or audiogram examination to assess conductive hearing.
>> Swab from the ear discharge.
>> Cleansing the ear canal, topical antiseptic. Topical antibiotic preparations containing neomycin, polymyxin or colistin in the absence of systemic manifestations such as fever.
>> Oral antibiotic treatment is indicated only if the infection has spread beyond the ear canal causing systemic symptoms.

> *When to refer*
>> Severe ear pain not relieved by analgesics.
>> Cellulitis beyond the ear canal (child usually requires IV antibiotics).

PRACTICE POINTS

- OE, also called swimmer's ear, tends to recur in children who often swim. Instillation of 2% acetic acid (Earcalm spray) immediately after swimming is the most effective prevention.
- During and after an acute OE, children should not swim and the ears should be protected from water during bathing.
- Some topical otic preparations (neomycin, colistin, polymyxin) used to treat OE can cause contact dermatitis, which manifests as erythema, vesiculation and oedema.

REMOVAL OF CERUMEN AND SYRINGING

Core Messages

> Cerumen provides a protective film on the ear canal and needs to be removed only if there are symptoms of pain or discomfort, hearing impairment or interference with a proper view of the TM.
> Elderly people, young children, cognitively impaired children (e.g., DS), those wearing hearing aids and those with an anatomically deformed ear canal are at high risk for cerumen impaction.
> Irrigation of the ear canal gently with warm water (see next) is effective, provided the eardrum is intact and there is no history of OE, previous ear surgery or unilateral deafness.

➤ Cerumenolytic agents include sterile saline solution, olive oil, almond oil or sodium bicarbonate ear drops. There are no significant differences between them.
➤ The child should lie down with the affected ear up for 5–10 minutes after the ear drops have been instilled.
➤ If the cerumen is impacted, ear drops may be used twice daily for a few days before syringing or cleansing with micro-suction.

Syringing

EQUIPMENT REQUIRED

➤ Auroscope
➤ Tissue
➤ Towel
➤ Propulse ear syringe
➤ Noots tank

PROCEDURE

➤ Explain the procedure to the child and parent. Ask the child to indicate any discomfort.
➤ Ensure that a softening agent, olive oil, has been used for 2–3 days prior to the procedure and that the cerumen is soft.
➤ Use the largest speculum on the auroscope that will fit into the ear.
➤ Gently pull the pinna upwards and backwards to straighten the canal.
➤ Protect the child with a towel.
➤ Ask the child (if old enough) or parent to support the Noots tank.
➤ After the cerumen is removed, ensure it has been completely removed by doing a final check.
➤ Discuss prevention by not using cotton buds, and indicate the natural cleaning procedure.

HEARING (See Also Chapter 1)

It is estimated that 1–2 newborns/1000 live births have varying degrees of bilateral sensorineural hearing loss (Table 12.4). Box 12.14 lists the main risk factors for hearing impairment.

TABLE 12.4 Degrees of hearing loss

• <25 dB	Normal hearing
• 25–35 dB	Mild hearing loss
• 40–60 dB	Moderate hearing loss
• 60–90 dB	Severe hearing loss
• >90 dB	Profound hearing loss

BOX 12.14 High risks for hearing loss in children

- Parental concern.
- Delayed speech.
- Family history of deafness.
- Low birthweight, particularly <1500 g.
- Use of ototoxic drugs, e.g., gentamicin.
- Craniofacial malformations.
- The presence of preauricular pit or tag.
- Severe perinatal asphyxia.
- Severe jaundice >400 µmol/L.
- Congenital infections, e.g., toxoplasmosis, rubella.
- History of CNS infection, e.g., meningitis.
- Recurrent or persistent OME >3 months.
- Trauma associated with loss of consciousness.

Detection of Hearing Impairment

➤ This should begin as early as possible. Parental concerns usually precede medical detection and diagnosis of hearing impairment. Primary care physicians are in a unique position to respond to these concerns and to show knowledge about normal speech development (Table 12.5), which suggests normal hearing.

➤ In the high-risk category for hearing loss or if children are significantly slow in achieving the previously mentioned developmental milestones or if the screening hearing test was inconclusive or abnormal, hearing tests should be considered (Table 12.6). Figure 12.1 shows the summary diagnostic steps for children suspected of hearing loss.

TABLE 12.5 Speech development with normal hearing

Age (Months)	Normal Developmental Milestones
0–1	• Startles, blinks or quiets briefly to loud sounds (bell)
2–4	• Coos, increases vocalization when spoken to, quiets to mother's voice, laughs, turns the head toward the sounds
5–6	• Shows excitement to voices, localizes the sounds presented in a horizontal plane, vocalizing 'ah-goo'
7–12	• Imitates sounds, responds to name when called, can say 'mama or dada' • One word with meaning (10 months)
15	• Four or five words
18	• Should follow simple spoken direction
21	• 20–50 words, combines two words
24	• At least 50 words, 3-word sentence

TABLE 12.6 Available hearing tests

Age	Test	Comments
Birth	• Otoacoustic emission (OAE)	• Quick, simple and sensitive test; can detect low hearing loss.
	• Brainstem-evoked potential (BSEP)	• Too time consuming for universal screening.
6–9 months	• Distraction testing	• Low sensitivity of the test and many cases with hearing impairment can be missed. Careful techniques such as quiet conditions and adequate sound level are required.
>3 years	• Pure tone audiometry	• Best diagnostic test at all ages once cooperation is possible. Children are referred to ENT specialist if thresholds are worse than 25 dB.

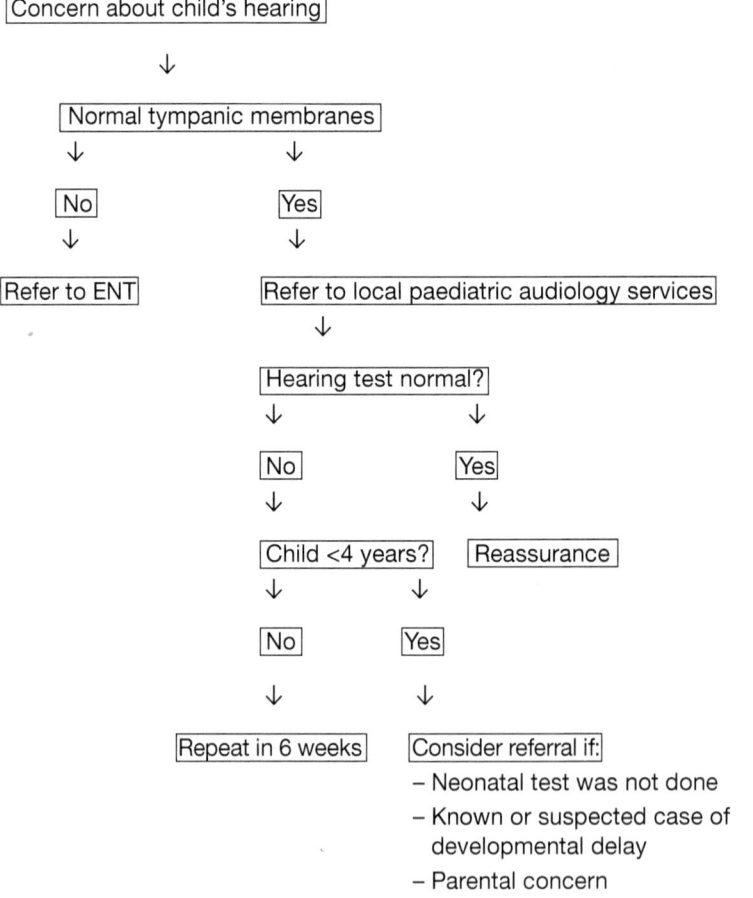

FIGURE 12.1 Summary steps for management of hearing impairment.

NOSE

Nasal Discharge/Blocked Nose

Core Messages
➤ By far the most common causes of persistent nasal discharge or blockage are viral infectious rhinitis, allergic rhinitis (AR) and adenoid hypertrophy.
➤ In neonates and young infants, blocked nose (snuffles) is common due to the presence of mucus in a narrowed nasal passage. It is loud during feeding and sleep and disappears aged 4–5 months; reassurance is the best medicine. Nasal malformations such as congenital narrowing of the nasal passage, choanal atresia and stenosis have to be considered in the differential diagnosis, particularly if the symptoms are persistent.
➤ Although most causes of nasal discharge/blocked nose are benign and self-limiting, serious conditions may occur (Table 12.7).
➤ It is easy for the clinician to diagnose polyps clinically: In contrast to the highly vascularized pink turbinate tissue, polyps are grey, shiny, grape-looking masses present between the nasal turbinates and the septum.

Acute Nose Bleeding (Epistaxis)

➤ Nosebleed is very common, and about 60% of the population experience a nosebleed at least once in their life.

TABLE 12.7 Causes of persistent nasal discharge/blockage

Cause	Diagnosis	Comments
Congenital	• Baby snuffles	• Caused by mucus in a narrowed nasal passage. Inspiratory noises become loud during feeding and quiet at sleep, disappears aged 4–5 months. Snuffles is an important sign of congenital syphilis.
	• Ciliary dyskinesia	• Persistent nasal congestion, sinusitis, recurrent infections of ear and lungs.
Infection	• Viral rhinitis (VR)	• Very common, first watery, may become viscous and green in colour, nasal congestion. Itching or sneezing usually absent. Symptoms last 7–10 days, usually self-limited. Rhinovirus occurs in 50%.
	• Chronic rhinitis	• Symptoms last for at least 12 weeks; sinusitis and adenoiditis are usually present.
	• Bacterial rhinitis	• About 10% of viral rhinitis cases can be complicated by bacteria (*S. pneumonia, H. influenza, Moraxella*).
Allergy	• Seasonal/Perennial	• In addition to watery rhinorrhoea/nasal obstruction, itching and sneezing are present. Symptoms are triggered by exposure to allergens in a usually atopic patient (see Allergic Rhinitis, Chapter 5).
Obstruction	• Adenoid hypertrophy	• Nasal obstruction, snoring, open mouth at night.
	• Foreign body	• Persistent purulent nasal discharge. No VR signs.
	• Nasal polyposis	• Nasal obstruction, runny nose, decreased sense of smell. Cystic fibrosis should be excluded.

➤ In 90–95% of cases the source of the bleed is in the area of the anterior part of the nasal septum: Kiesselbach's area. The remaining 5–10% occur in the posterior area.

➤ There are many causes of nosebleed (Table 12.8). Trauma due to digital manipulation (nose picking) is the most frequent cause. Management is shown in Box 12.15.

TABLE 12.8 Main causes of nosebleed

• Trauma	• Digital manipulation, foreign body
• Haematological	• Thrombocytopenia, von Willebrand syndrome, haemophilia
• Inflammatory	• Viral and allergic rhinitis
• Drugs	• Anticoagulants, steroid nasal spray
• Tumour	• Juvenile nasopharyngeal angiofibroma
• Syndromes	• Osler–Weber–Rendu (hereditary haemorrhagic telangiectasia)

BOX 12.15 First aid measures for nosebleed

- Patient in upright position.
- Patient leans forward to avoid blood trickling into pharynx.
- Pinch the lower part of the nose gently for about 5 minutes; repeat the procedure if re-bleed. Ice application to the neck.
- If these measures fail, local application of antiseptic cream; a solution of oxymetazoline, xylometazoline or ephedrine drops may help.
- If the bleeding stops, patient is kept for 30 minutes' observation.
- If the bleeding persists: *Emergency referral to otorhinolaryngology; if the source of bleeding is not visible, an anterior nasal pack needs to be inserted.* If the source of bleeding is visible: Electrocautery or silver nitrate cautery.
- Blood pressure measurement.

CHAPTER 13

Ophthalmology

ACUTE RED EYES

Core Messages

➤ Acute red eye is common and caused by a variety of conditions (Table 13.1), including eye diseases of the conjunctiva (conjunctivitis), cornea (keratitis), iris, ciliary body and choroid (uveitis), and the sclera (scleritis).

➤ Neonatal conjunctivitis (ophthalmia neonatorum) is a potentially blinding disease if not treated in time. Neonates present aged 5–15 days after birth with redness and an initial watery discharge. It is mostly caused nowadays by *Chlamydia trachomatis* and rarely by gonococcal infection. The infection rapidly produces profuse purulent discharge. The cornea is often affected.

TABLE 13.1 Main causes of acute red eyes

Cause	Presentation	Treatment
Infectious		
• Viral	Acute burning or gritty feeling, watery discharge, abrupt onset in one eye and infect the other eye within 24–48 hours, other signs of viral URTI, e.g., cough, runny nose.	• Self-limited, symptomatic with cool compress. • Povidone iodine 5% eye drops.
• Bacterial	Pain, discomfort, mucopurulent discharge, with redness maximal at the inferior conjunctive, mattered and adhered in the morning.	• Topical antibiotic. • Erythromycin ointment.
Non-Infectious		
• Allergic	Bilateral involvement, swelling with watery discharge, chemosis and crusts on lid margins in the morning; itching is prominent and characteristic.	• Avoiding allergen exposure topical and/or oral antihistamine (e.g. azelastine).
• Foreign body (FB)	Acute unilateral eye pain with an FB sensation and sensitivity to light.	• Removal of FB.

DOI: 10.1201/9781032642888-13

➤ Beyond the neonatal period, most causes of acute red eye are as follows:
   ➤ **Viral conjunctivitis** shows abrupt onset of redness of almost the whole conjunctiva with watery discharge and a follicular appearance of the tarsal conjunctive (Figure 13.1A). The infection is usually caused by adenovirus in association with a viral upper respiratory tract infection (URTI). Herpes simplex virus (HSV) has a similar presentation, often with a characteristic vesicular eruption on the face.
   ➤ **Bacterial conjunctivitis**, usually caused by *Haemophilus influenza* (non-typable), *Moraxella catarrhalis* or staphylococci. Discharge should be cultured.
   ➤ **Allergic conjunctivitis** is usually seasonal and caused by airborne allergens such as pollen, dander or dust. Family history of atopy is often positive. It is a type 1 hypersensitivity, IgE-mediated.
   ➤ **Keratitis** (Figure 13.1B), with redness surrounding the cornea (circumcorneal). An associated impaired vision differentiates keratitis from conjunctivitis.
   ➤ **Uveitis** present with pain, lacrimation, photophobia and eye hyperaemia. It is often associated with pauci-articular form of rheumatoid arthritis.

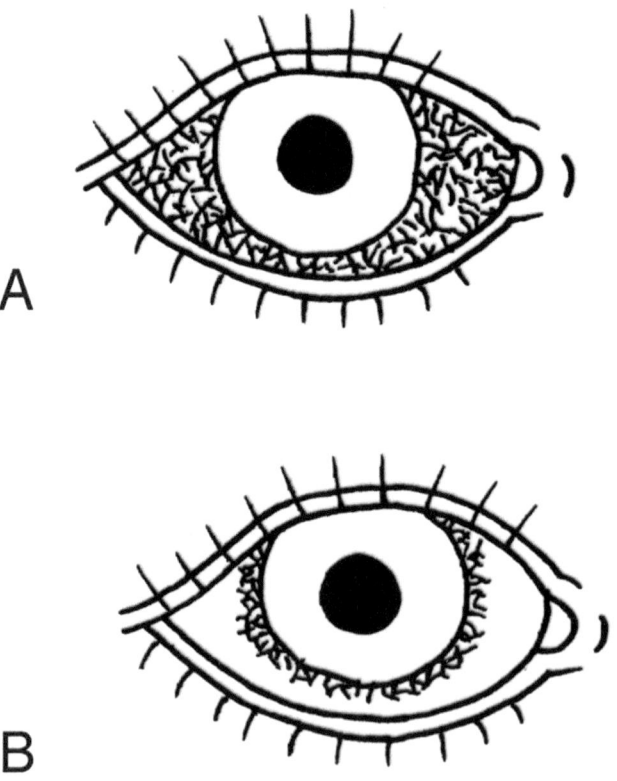

A

B

FIGURE 13.1 A: Diffuse redness of the conjunctiva seen in viral conjunctivitis. B: Circumcorneal redness seen in anterior uveitis and corneal ulcer.

PRACTICE POINTS

- Physical examination of the eyes should always include vision assessment by testing each eye separately using Snellen charts (see 'Strabismus'). For children too young to use Snellen charts, vision can be broadly assessed by seeing if the child can focus on a book or colour pictures.
- Episcleral and retinal haemorrhages in neonates are common during vaginal delivery. Although these are alarming to parents and clinicians, they are harmless and disappear within 2 weeks.
- At birth, the nasolacrimal duct is often blocked, causing watering eyes (epiphora), sticky eyes and recurrent conjunctivitis. Diagnosis is made by the history and by refluxing discharge with a pressure over the lacrimal sac. The blockage resolves spontaneously in over 95% over the next few months, rarely until the age of 1 year, and very rarely needs surgery.
- Steroids should never be prescribed unless herpes infection is excluded. If the diagnosis is not clear, *referral to an ophthalmologist is indicated.*
- Orbital cellulitis presents as red and swollen eye. *Urgent referral is indicated for possible intravenous antibiotic treatment.*

Referral

Referral to an ophthalmologist is indicated whenever the diagnosis is unclear; cases with severe conjunctivitis; or suspected uveitis, keratitis or scleritis. Most cases with lacrimal or nasolacrimal duct obstruction and viral, bacterial or allergic conjunctivitis can be treated by primary care clinicians.

STRABISMUS (SQUINTS)

Core Messages

➤ **Strabismus** – misalignment of the eyes – is a common ophthalmic problem, affecting 4–5% of children younger than 6 years of age. Strabismus may be either congenital (or better termed infantile, as this allows inclusion of cases of strabismus developed within the first few months of life) or acquired, transient or constant, manifest or latent. Of the most important and serious causes of acquired type of strabismus is retinoblastoma (Box 13.1).

  ➤ Risk factors for having strabismus include prematurity, family history of strabismus, craniofacial anomalies, maternal smoking and associated cataract.

  ➤ Because of different causes and treatments, strabismus is divided into non-paralytic and paralytic. Non-paralytic strabismus includes inward deviation (esophorias; commonly known as convergent, inward or crossed eyes), outward deviation (known as exophorias or divergent strabismus), hyperdeviation (upward) and hypodeviation (downward). Paralytic strabismus involves palsy of the third, fourth, or sixth cranial nerve.

➤ In a child with any ocular disorder, including strabismus, assessment of the visual acuity is essential. Untreated amblyopia (reduced visual acuity) results in permanent vision impairment. Paradoxically, amblyopia can cause strabismus.

BOX 13.1 Main causes of strabismus

Primary

- Pseudo-strabismus
- Congenital (infantile) strabismus
- Idiopathic

Secondary

- Paralytic strabismus (cranial nerve III, IV, VI)
- Intracranial lesion (infection, mass)
- Retinoblastoma
- Amblyopia
- Migraine ophthalmoplegia
- Thyroid disease
- Möbius syndrome

How to Examine for Squints

➤ **Eye movements**: The child is asked to (or attracted to) look at an object/toy, which is moved in different directions at one-third of a metre distance from the face. Paralytic squint can easily be detected.

➤ **Corneal light**: Useful for children who are not cooperative (below the age of 3 years). A light source is held between the examiner and the child at 50–75 cm. The light reflection in normal ocular alignment will generate an identical light reflection in each child's pupil in healthy eyes and in children with pseudo-strabismus. In strabismus, there is a deviation of 30 dioptres if the light reflex is at the edge of pupil, 45 dioptres if between the pupil and limbus and 60 dioptres if at the edge of the limbus.

➤ **Red reflex**: Holding an ophthalmoscope at a distance of 0.5 m in front of a child, an identical red reflex in both eyes is produced. Unequal sizes, shape or colour is abnormal.

➤ **Cover test**: This is a suitable test for children who are cooperative with reasonably good vision in each eye. The child's attention is directed to a target, and the examiner covers one eye and watches for movement of the uncovered eye. If no movement occurs, there is no squint.

➤ **Uncover test**: This is followed by rapidly covering and uncovering each eye. If there is any malalignment, the eye rapidly moves as the cover moves to the other eye.

PRACTICE POINTS

- Pseudo-strabismus is a common cause of referral to ophthalmologists. It is usually caused by epicanthic folds or a broad, flat nasal bridge. The normal alignment can by shown by the normal corneal light reflexes and cover test.
- Up to the age of 6 months, intermittent strabismus is a normal developmental milestone, occurring particularly as outward deviation in about two-thirds of neonates. After the age of 6 months, any degree of strabismus needs to be evaluated. Strabismus should never be ignored; it is never outgrown.
- Accommodative strabismus usually manifests aged 2–4 years and is a convergent strabismus occurring during accommodation (focusing) caused mainly by hyperopia (farsightedness).

- Cases with red flag signs (see Red Flags) should be referred urgently. Retinoblastoma, with an incidence of 1 in 20,000 births, is the most important cause of acquired strabismus. The tumour presents with a unilateral or bilateral leukocoria (a white pupil) or a red eye. Retinoblastoma is the most curable if diagnosed early; high mortality is inevitable if untreated.
- Recent onset of paretic ocular muscle usually presents with double vision that increases in one direction and an increase in the eye deviation when fixating with the paretic eye. Brain tumour could be the underlying cause.
- A fourth ocular nerve palsy causes a contralateral head tilt, i.e., a head tilt to the right caused by left-sided nerve palsy and vice versa. Conversely, sixth nerve palsy causes an ipsilateral head tilting. The reason for the tilt is to avoid diplopia.
- Möbius syndrome is rare and characterized by paretic facial muscles (expressionless face, impaired sucking and smiling), inability to move eyes from side to side and associated limb and chest wall defects.

WARNING SIGNS (RED FLAGS) IN CHILDREN WITH STRABISMUS

- Acute onset
- Abnormal red reflex
- Diplopia
- Headache
- Nystagmus
- Limited abduction
- Associated with neurological signs

Referral

➤ All cases with strabismus after the age of 6 months require timely referral to an ophthalmologist.

➤ Any patient with red flags on history or examination should be referred urgently.

➤ A diagnosis of pseudo-squint should be established (observation and corneal light reflex) to avoid unnecessary referral.

➤ The first episode of ophthalmoplegic migraine may also require referral to establish the diagnosis, but recurrent episodes may not need a referral.

VISION IMPAIRMENT AND SCREENING

Core Messages

➤ Visual acuity develops rapidly after birth and reaches full development around the age of 8 years. Early vision impairment can lead to psychomotor and cognitive impairment as well as increased risk of mortality.

➤ Vision impairment is defined as mild with a visual acuity worse than 6/12, moderate if worse than 6/18 and severe if worse than 6/60 Snellen metres. The leading cause of severe vision impairment globally is cataracts. In high-income countries, uncorrected refractive errors (defined as the inability to bring parallel rays into focus on the retina) are the leading causes.

➤ Amblyopia is a decreased visual acuity in a structurally normal eye or, less frequently, in an eye with structural abnormality. Conditions causing vision impairment, including sudden visual loss, are collectively uncommon in high-income countries and are either due to abnormalities within the eyes or systemic causes listed in Box 13.2.

➤ Intraocular causes are easy to detect, e.g., corneal opacity, cataract or optic atrophy, while the eyes remain structurally normal in systemic causes of vision impairment.

➤ Most causes of cortical visual loss occur in children with neurodisability, which may follow asphyxia at birth with or without seizures, and development of spasticity or hypotonia. Rarely, cortical visual loss occurs as an isolated neurological phenomenon.

➤ Age-appropriate vision screening, including an eye check, in the 6- to 8-week baby check is shown in Box 13.3.

BOX 13.2 Main causes of vision impairment/loss

Orbital

- Refractive errors (myopia, hyperopia, astigmatism)
- Strabismus
- Retinopathy of prematurity (ROP)
- Infection/inflammation, e.g., trachoma, keratitis, uveitis
- Congenital glaucoma
- Corneal scarring
- Retinal detachment
- Optic neuritis

Systemic

- Migraine
- Amaurosis fugax
- Occipital lobe seizures
- Medications (e.g., corticosteroids).
- Raised intracranial pressure (ICP; optic glioma, posterior fossa tumour)
- Congenital varicella
- Conversion symptom (hysteria)
- Cortical blindness
- Familial transient visual loss

In Low-Income Countries

- Cataract, eye infection, vitamin A deficiency

BOX 13.3 Age-appropriate eye screening

• External inspection	• To detect any structural abnormality, e.g., ptosis or (all ages) nystagmus, or one cornea is larger than the other, which suggests congenital glaucoma.
• Red reflex test	• By directing the ophthalmoscope light toward both eyes (all ages) from 50 to 75 cm. A normal symmetric red reflex should be observed from both eyes, while an absence of red reflex may suggest congenital cataract.
• Fix and follow	• This is assessed by drawing the child's (from 3 months of age) attention to a handheld light or toy and slowly moving the target to different directions.
• Pupillary testing	• Checking for any irregular shape, unequal size, poor or (all ages) unequal reaction to light.
• Visual acuity	• Testing involves identification of optotypes that consist of letters, numbers (for older children) or symbols for young children. Optotypes for older children include Sloan letters or Snellen charts.
• Corneal light reflex	• To compare the position of the corneal light reflection (aged >1–2 months) from 30 cm: Normal light reflex shows symmetric reflexes centred on the pupils. If the eyes are non-aligned, the light reflex will not be symmetric.
• Cover test	• While the patient is fixing on a distant target, the examiner occludes one eye while observing the other eye for any refixation movement (for older children). No eye movement of either eye indicates normal eye alignment.

Recommended Investigations

➤ Electrophysiological testing with electroretinography (ERG) for retinal causes of visual impairment.
➤ MRI of the eyes and head for suspected tumour.
➤ EEG for cases with seizures.
➤ TORCH screening test (IgM for cytomegalovirus [CMV], herpes simplex, rubella), urine for rubella virus isolation, as indicated clinically.
➤ HIV DNA detected by polymerase chain reaction (PCR), if clinically indicated.

PRACTICE POINTS

• GPs should be able to diagnose most eye abnormalities. Observation is the most important technique to detect these abnormalities including visual defects. Visual acuity is tested during the first few months of life by the child's ability to fixate and follow an object (bright-coloured toy). Older children are tested using the Snellen chart. Examination of the visual fields (looking for the wiggly fingers) can also be carried out if indicated. Fundoscopy is usually not necessary.

- Detection of visually impaired children is essential because of possible treatment including cataracts, ROP, glaucoma and retinoblastoma. Many of these conditions have genetic implications.
- The most common cause for transient visual loss in children is due to a visual aura in classic migraine. Aura is defined by the International Headache Society as a recurrent disorder that develops over 5–29 minutes and lasts for <1 hour (see also Chapter 14).
- Transient monocular visual loss lasting 1–5 minutes is usually referred to as amaurosis fugax resulting from cerebral ischemia. While migraine aura may present with flashes of light (photopsia), amaurosis fugax presents as complete blackout of vision or a curtain across the vision.
- Occipital seizures (such as benign partial epilepsy with occipital paroxysm) are not rare; visual symptoms are prominent and include amaurosis, multicoloured illusions or hallucinations and eye deviation, followed by hemi-clonic seizures or automatisms. EEG is usually diagnostic.
- A child with leukocoria, a white pupil, has a major clinical implication: The likely cause is either retinoblastoma or a cataract.
- Some systemically administered medications, e.g., steroids, may cause cataract. Steroids can also cause glaucoma.

Referral

All children with acute loss of vision should be referred to an ophthalmologist except infants with intermittent squints and in children with recurrent ophthalmoplegic migraine.

PROPTOSIS (EXOPHTHALMOS)

➤ Proptosis, exophthalmos or protrusion of the eyes, is a forward displacement of the eye, which has a variety of underlying causes (Box 13.4).
➤ The condition usually has serious underlying causes, and so all cases of proptosis should be referred.

BOX 13.4 Main causes of proptosis

Local (Orbital)
- Orbital capillary haemangioma
- Shallow orbit (e.g., Crouzon's syndrome)
- Optic nerve glioma
- Trauma (orbital haemorrhage)

Systemic
- Metastatic neuroblastoma
- Plexiform neurofibroma
- Graves' disease (thyroid orbitopathy)
- Meningioma (involving sphenoid wing)
- Histiocytosis X
- Sarcoidosis
- Deep dermoid cyst

PRACTICE POINTS

- Clinicians dealing with a child with proptosis should do a full ophthalmic examination, including assessment of visual acuity, ocular muscle movement, measuring of proptosis, pupillary size and reaction to light, fundi and a systemic examination.
- A proptotic eye not adequately protected by the lids is at risk of keratopathy, strabismus, diplopia, optic nerve atrophy and decreased visual acuity.
- Orbital capillary haemangioma is the most common orbital tumour in children, often affecting the upper lid. The tumour has a rapid growth during the first 6 months of life and regresses spontaneously at 4–6 years of age.
- Optic gliomas are usually benign and often asymptomatic and commonly present with visual disturbance. Unilateral glioma typically presents with afferent pupillary defect: A light source on the affected eye produces pupil dilatation (instead of constriction), while the unaffected eye produces bilateral pupil constriction.
- Proptosis caused by Graves' disease may occur in older, more often female, children. Optic neuropathy, corneal problems and extraocular muscular involvement are significantly less common in children than in adults.
- Neuroblastoma, the most common solid tumour of childhood, metastasizes frequently into the orbit. It arises either from the adrenals, cervical sympathetic chain or mediastinum.

DIPLOPIA (DOUBLE VISION)

Core Messages

➤ Diplopia, simultaneous perception of two images of a single object, is less common in children than in adults mainly because of the lower incidence of strokes and other intracranial lesions.

➤ Diplopia is either binocular (true diplopia) or monocular (Box 13.5). Diplopia is usually binocular, and the most common cause of diplopia in children is misalignment of the visual axes (strabismus). Monocular is caused by abnormality in the cornea (e.g., severe astigmatism), in the lens (e.g., cataract, dislocated lens) or in the vitreous humour (e.g., vitreous cysts). A detailed history and examination will make it clear which muscles and ocular nerves are affected and what is the likely cause.

➤ Diplopia is often the first manifestation of many systemic muscular or neurologic disorders. Some are of a serious nature such as disorders affecting the cranial nerves (third, fourth and sixth), which innervate the six ocular muscles.

➤ *Some cases of diplopia are red flags and need an urgent referral* (see 'Red Flags').

BOX 13.5 Causes of diplopia

Binocular

- Physiological
- Strabismus
- Myasthenia gravis (in association with ptosis)
- Cranial nerve palsies (III, IV and VI)
- Increased ICP
- Ophthalmoplegic migraine

- Thyroid ophthalmopathy
- Drugs (e.g., antiepileptics)

Monocular

- Intraocular diseases (e.g., dislocated lens)
- Cataract
- Corneal scarring
- Trauma

RED FLAGS IN DIPLOPIA

- Acute onset
- A dilated pupil
- Associated headache, vomiting
- Cranial nerve palsies
- Any case following exclusion of strabismus

Recommended Investigations

➤ Blood pressure measurement
➤ Blood glucose
➤ Thyroid function tests for suspected cases of hyperthyroidism
➤ MRI of the head may show tumour or area of infarction.
➤ Anti-acetylcholine antibodies in plasma and electromyography (EMG) for suspected myasthenia

How to Examine a Child with Diplopia

➤ Take a detailed history.
➤ Assess ocular mobility: Does the patient follow a moving torchlight in all directions?
➤ Does the object double vertically (one on top of the other) or horizontally (side by side)? Are the two images of the same intensity, or is there one as a faint image?
➤ Does the double vision disappear after closing one eye (binocular) or persist (monocular)?
➤ Corneal reflex test is done from about 33 cm to detect any strabismus and the extent of deviation: 30 dioptres if the reflex appears at the edge of pupil, 45 dioptres if between the pupil and limbus and 60 dioptres if at the edge of the limbus.

PRACTICE POINTS

- Differentiating monocular from binocular diplopia is simple: Covering each eye will correct diplopia in binocular, while diplopia persists in the monocular of the affected eye.
- Common causes of diplopia are strabismus, cranial nerve palsies and brain tumour. The brain of a young child often learns how to suppress the image of the weaker, misaligned eye. Therefore, head tilting (and not diplopia) may be the presenting symptom.
- In third nerve palsy, the eye will deviate in a down-and-out position. In fourth nerve palsy, the affected eye is deviated high in the eye. In sixth nerve palsy, the affected eye deviates inward. Young children with fourth nerve palsy typically present with head tilting opposite to the affected eye, while in sixth nerve palsy, the head tilting is toward the palsied nerve.
- Migraine may present as a third nerve palsy on the side of the headache during the attack (ophthalmoplegic migraine). A typical basilar artery migraine (e.g., diplopia, vertigo, ataxia and headache) should be differentiated from intracranial tumour.
- When a child presents with diplopia and ptosis, myasthenia gravis, third nerve palsy or Horner's syndrome should be considered. Small pupil and reduced sweating on the affected side suggest the latter possibility.
- Diplopia may be the first compliant in children with a dislocated lens, including those with Marfan's syndrome or homocystinuria (malar flush, neurodisability, thromboembolic events).
- Although adolescents with hysteria may present with diplopia, the diagnosis of hysteria should be one of exclusion.

Referral

Although diagnosing which ocular muscles are affected is fairly easy, a final diagnosis is unlikely to be reached in a primary setting. Referral to an ophthalmologist is usually required for all pathological causes of diplopia.

DISORDERS OF THE EYELID

➤ Eyelid disorders are common in children and range from benign, self-resolving to serious malignant processes (Box 13.6). Therefore, a complete ophthalmic and systemic examination is required.

➤ Epicanthic folds are semilunar skin folds across the inner corner of the eyes (canthus), usually originating from the upper eyelid and causing pseudo-strabismus (see 'Strabismus [Squints]' earlier). They are present in most infants and become less apparent with peaking of the nasal bridge by the end of the first year of life. Persistent epicanthic folds beyond infancy occur mostly in Asian populations.

➤ Congenital ptosis (droopy eye) refers to an abnormally low-lying upper eyelid resulting in narrowing of the palpebral fissure. It is a common and often overlooked sign and present either at birth or in the first year of life. Congenital ptosis is usually due to dysgenesis of the levator muscle, often associated with strabismus (in about 30%), astigmatism and amblyopia (Box 13.7). The upper eyelid is innervated by the third cranial nerve (oculomotor) and cervical sympathetic system.

➤ Congenital myasthenia syndrome is rare and caused by genetic defective signal transmission at the neuromuscular junction due to mutations in >30 genes. It is mostly inherited as autosomal dominant or recessive. The diagnosis is suspected if there is easy fatigability, facial weakness (ptosis) and respiratory difficulty.

BOX 13.6 Main abnormalities of the eyelid

Congenital

- Epicanthic folds
- Coloboma (may be associated with Goldenhar's syndrome)
- Congenital and acquired ptosis

Acquired

- Tumour (haemangioma, dermoid cyst)
- Eyelid retraction (a vertically larger-than-normal opening of the eyelid, often associated with autoimmune thyroid diseases)
- Acute blepharitis
- Chalazion (inflammation of the meibomian cyst)

Eyebrow Abnormality

- Sparse or absent eyebrows (ectodermal dysplasia, alopecia)

BOX 13.7 Causes of ptosis

Congenital (90%)

- Dysgenesis of superior levator muscle (usual cause)
- Marcus–Gunn jaw-winking phenomenon and Möbius syndrome
- Congenital myasthenia

Acquired (Manifests > Age of 1 Year)

- Bell's palsy
- Ophthalmoplegic migraine
- Muscular dystrophy, e.g., myotonic dystrophy, muscular dystrophy
- Hornor's syndrome (ptosis, miosis and anhidrosis)
- Botulism (caused by an exotoxin produced by *Clostridium botulism*)

Investigations

➤ A chest x-ray and CT scan in cases of myasthenia gravis for evidence of an enlarged thymus and thymoma, in addition to EMG, autoantibodies (particularly anti-acetyl antibodies) and genetic testing.

➤ CPK in blood for muscular diseases.

➤ ECG for cases of muscular dystrophy and myopathies.

➤ EMG may be diagnostic in cases of myasthenia gravis and myotonic dystrophy.

PRACTICE POINTS

- Although most eyelid disorders are dealt with by ophthalmologists, these conditions are important to clinicians because they are associated with systemic diseases such as myasthenia gravis, myotonic dystrophy or botulism.
- Meibomian glands are situated under the inner surface of the eyelid and secrete meibum to lubricate the eye surface. Chalazion (meibomian cyst) is a sterile, chronic inflammatory granuloma caused by blockage of the meibomian glands. The resulting lump is painless and is found typically in the middle of the upper eyelid. In contrast to chalazion, a stye is a painful red lump that grows from the base of the eyelashes. It is usually caused by bacterial infection (such as Staphylococcus) of the hair follicle and is self-resolving in most cases.
- Ptosis (blepharoptosis) is defined as the distance between the centre of the pupillary light reflex and the upper eyelid margin of <2 mm (normal distance 4–4.5 mm). It can cause cosmetic, functional and psychosocial problems.
- Children with ptosis often present with abnormal postures such as backward tilt of the head with chin lifting in an attempt to maintain binocular vision.
- In Marcus–Gunn jaw winking (5% of all cases with ptosis), the upper lid rises as the jaw opens (e.g., during sucking, eating or chewing). This synkinesis (simultaneous movement) occurs as a result of an anomalous connection between the third and fifth cranial nerves.
- Children with ptosis should be referred for ophthalmic opinion and surgery, particularly if they have cosmetically unacceptable abnormal head posture, amblyopia (lazy eyes) and abnormal visual field.
- Entropion (inward turning of the lid margin and lashes) can cause corneal damage. Infants commonly present with irritability. Larsen's syndrome (multiple joint dislocations, cleft palate and neurodisability) has to be excluded. Urgent consultation with an ophthalmologist is required.
- Patients with ectropion (outward turning of the lid margin) are at risk of exposure keratopathy, overflow of tears and conjunctivitis. This may occur in association with facial palsy resulting from weakness of the orbicularis muscle. Again, urgent ophthalmic consultation is required
- Eyebrow abnormalities include sparse or absent eyebrows (e.g., alopecia, ectodermal dysplasia) and eyebrows joining together medially (Waardenburg's syndrome, Cornelia de Lang's syndrome).

Referral is required for all cases with eyelid disorders except clear and benign cases of, for example, epicanthic folds or chalazion and stye.

CHAPTER 14

Neurology

CONGENITAL ANOMALIES OF THE CNS

Anencephaly

➤ This anomaly occurs when the cephalic (head) end of the neural tube fails to close, usually between the 23rd and 26th days of pregnancy, resulting in the absence of a major portion of the brain, skull and scalp.
➤ Affected infants are either stillborn or die within a few days of birth.
➤ Incidence is approximately 1:1000 live births; risk of recurrence is 4%.

Macrocephaly and Megalencephaly

➤ Measurement of head circumference (HC) is an essential component of the physical examination in paediatric practice.
➤ Macrocephaly and megalencephaly are defined as an abnormal HC, which is greater than 2 standard deviations (greater than 98% centile on growth chart) above average for the age and sex. While macrocephaly is an increase of HC due to bone skull structure, megalencephaly refers to an increase of the brain parenchyma (oversized brain).

BOX 14.1 Diagnostic criteria of familial macrocephaly

- Dominant-inherited condition (familial macrocephaly).
- The abnormal large HC remains unchanged later in life.
- Child is asymptomatic with no evidence of a syndrome or increased intracranial pressure (ICP).
- A parent or sibling with macrocephaly.
- Normal imaging such as head ultrasound scan (if fontanelle is patent) or MRI (imaging is usually unnecessary).

➤ The condition is common, affecting up to 5% of the paediatric population. It is mostly benign and familial (Box 14.1), and parents can be reassured, providing that signs of red flags are absent (see Red Flags). If one or more than one important red flags are present, pathological conditions can be the underlying causes of large HC such as hydrocephalus (Box 14.2). *An urgent referral is needed.*

 DOI: 10.1201/9781032642888-14

RED FLAGS IF A LARGE HC IS ASSOCIATED WITH

- Developmental delay
- Neurological impairment
- Tense/bulging fontanelle, squint, gait abnormality, vomiting
- Unexplained irritability
- Suspected child abuse
- Cutaneous vascular marks
- Poor weight gain

BOX 14.2 Pathological conditions causing an abnormal large HC

- Hydrocephalus with progressively enlarged HC
- ASD* (15% of ASD cases have abnormal HC)
- Sotos syndrome
- Achondroplasia
- Increased ICP
- Fragile X syndrome
- Lysosomal storage disease
- Café-au-lait (neurofibromatosis type 1)
- Organic acid disorders

* ASD = autism spectrum disorder.

Microcephaly

➤ The measurement of HC between 0 and 24 months (the period of the greatest postnatal brain growth) is an important anthropometric indicator of brain growth.

➤ Microcephaly is defined as a small head circumference >2 standard deviations (SD) below the mean for age and sex. Most children develop normally, while those with >3 SD often have comorbidities including epilepsy and developmental delay. A simple classification is shown in Box 14.3.

BOX 14.3 Classification of microcephaly

- **Congenital (Primary) Microcephaly**
  - ❼ Genetic (e.g., autosomal recessive)
  - ❼ Intrauterine infection (e.g., cytomegalovirus [CMV], toxoplasmosis)
  - ❼ Zika viral infection
  - ❼ Alcohol consumption during pregnancy
  - ❼ Drugs taken during pregnancy
- **Secondary Microcephaly (Postnatal)**
  - ❼ Genetic
  - ❼ Infection, e.g., meningitis
  - ❼ Trauma (head injury)
- **Syndromic Microcephaly** (e.g., Down's syndrome)

➤ Microcephaly is a neurodevelopmental condition caused by defects in the formation of the cortical cells resulting in a thinner cortex and reduced brain size.

➤ Comorbidities include developmental delay, microphthalmia, skeletal malformation and cortical/subcortical calcification on brain MRI scan.

Hydrocephalus

➤ Hydrocephalus develops from an imbalance between cerebrospinal fluid (CSF) production and absorption, resulting in abnormal CSF volume, progressive dilatation of the brain ventricles and increased ICP. Subsequently, HC increases and crosses the centile lines upward in infancy. The incidence in the paediatric population is about 0.1–0.6% of live births. Causes of hydrocephalus are shown in Box 14.4.

BOX 14.4 Main causes of hydrocephalus

Primary (Congenital)
- Congenital structural malformation
- X-linked hydrocephalus
- Stenosis of the aqueduct of Sylvius
- Chiari malformation

Secondary (Postnatal)
- Post-intraventricular haemorrhage of prematurity
- Infection (e.g., meningitis)
- Trauma

Syndromic Hydrocephalus
- Crouzon's and Pheiffer's syndromes
- Neurofibromatosis

➤ Hydrocephalus occurs predominately in infants who have a different presentation than older children:
- ❼ **In infants:** Tense, full or bulging fontanelle; sutures widely separated with prominent skull veins and downward gaze of the eyes; irritability; poor feeding; vomiting; and high-pitched cry.
- ❼ **Older children:** Headache; vomiting; changes in vision, personality and behaviour; slow cognitive deterioration; gait abnormalities; cognitive and developmental changes.

➤ Hydrocephalus needs to be differentiated from macrocephaly, which is a much more common cause of head enlargement. Current treatment is almost exclusively surgical by placement of a shunt.

➤ Treatment of hydrocephalus includes surgical interventions such as intermittent CSF drainage and continuous CSF diversion by placing a shunt (current treatment of choice). Non-surgical treatment includes acetazolamide or hyperosmolar therapy with mannitol, gene therapy, and implantation of mesenchymal stem cells.

Prognosis and Complications of Hydrocephalus

➤ Hydrocephalus is a serious and lethal condition if left untreated. Death may occur due to medical comorbidities (e.g., respiratory failure) rather than the hydrocephalus itself. The second cause of death is shunt complications, including shunt failure, obstruction or infection.

➤ Although most hydrocephalic children after treatment can enjoy independence, attend normal school and are capable of learning, problems vary significantly according to the aetiology of hydrocephalus. Children with posthaemorrhagic hydrocephalus have a high rate of learning difficulty and cognitive skills (around 40%) compared to those without cerebral haemorrhage.

➤ In addition, hydrocephalic children have high rates of epilepsy (up to 30% of children), hearing difficulties, psychological impairment, mobility disorders and urination and defecation problems.

➤ Close follow-up of these children, with rehabilitation and referral to various specialties, plays a key role in improving their outcomes.

Plagiocephaly

➤ This common condition is usually caused by a continuous external pressure such as a preferential sleeping position. It is characterized by a flattening of one side (rarely affecting both sides of the occiput). The greatest deformity usually occurs in the first 3 months. Diagnostic features are shown in Box 14.5.

BOX 14.5 Diagnostic features of positional plagiocephaly

● The usual finding is asymmetric unilateral flattening of one side of the skull occurring during the first 3 months of life.
● Normal patent skull sutures with normal HC.
● Characteristic signs (detected when standing behind the infant and looking from above): The head flattening is associated with compensatory ipsilateral protrusion or bulge of the forehead with an ipsilateral anteriorly positioned ear (In the case of lambdoid synostosis, the forehead bulge is on the contralateral side with no ipsilateral anteriorly positioned ear).
● The diagnosis of plagiocephaly is clinical. A skull x-ray to confirm the patency of the skull sutures is sometimes required in cases of uncertainty or suspected craniosynostosis. A high-resolution ultrasound scan can identify the normal patent suture and exclude lambdoid synostosis.

➤ The incidence has increased dramatically due to the 'Back to Sleep' campaign in 1992, which was designed to reduce cases of sudden infant death syndrome (SIDS). Consequently, the incidence of SIDS decreased significantly while the incidence of positional plagiocephaly increased by more than 600% because children are being put to sleep on the back.

➤ The simplest way to assess the severity of plagiocephaly is to use a diagonal calibre (during physical examination), which measures the difference between the diagonal lengths of each side of the head. A mild plagiocephaly is 0.9–1.2 cm, severe is >1.2 cm.

➤ The condition is more common in premature infants, infants with hypotonicity and in those with developmental delay. In case of congenital muscular torticollis, the intense neck muscles lead to the infant holding their head in one position. Its importance is usually cosmetic, and the shape of the head is likely to correct itself over time, usually by 12–18 months.

➤ While most scholars have viewed plagiocephaly as a minor and cosmetic issue, a few studies suggest an association between plagiocephaly and developmental delay involving motor and language development but not cognitive and social development.

Management

➤ When the diagnosis of positional plagiocephaly is certain, parents need reassurance because they are often concerned with the cosmetic appearance of their child's head. The parents can be told that slow improvement will continue, and the deformity does not interfere with brain development.

➤ Early recognition is very important. The younger the child is when plagiocephaly is recognized (before 2–3 months), the better the chance of improvement.

➤ Daytime: The more time babies spend on their tummies when playing, the better and earlier the shape of the head will be corrected.

➤ Sleeping pattern: The baby's sleeping pattern is adjusted so that anything exciting (e.g., red toy) is positioned so that it encourages them to turn their head in that direction. A rolled-up towel under the mattress can help the child sleep with less pressure on the flattened part of the head.

➤ Physiotherapy can help if the deformity is more than mild, particularly for those babies who turn their head in one direction only.

➤ Helmet and bands. The use of these is controversial and generally not supported by evidence. Wearing a helmet for 23 hours/day for months is not a happy experience.

Craniosynostosis

➤ Cranial sutures are essential to allow skull growth and the expansion of the rapid brain growth in the first 2 years of life. Premature fusion of the cranial sutures impedes the growth of the skull, resulting in a characteristically abnormal head shape and a risk of increased ICP (Box 14.6).

BOX 14.6 The most common forms of suture synostosis

Non-Syndromic Suture Synostosis (in Order of Prevalence)

- Sagittal   Scaphocephaly
- Metopic suture   Trigonocephaly
- Unilateral coronal   Frontal plagiocephaly
- Unilateral lambdoid   Pachycephaly

Syndromic Suture Synostosis

- Apert's syndrome
- Muenke's syndrome
- Crouzon's syndrome

➤ Craniosynostosis is a congenital cranial malformation in which one or more cranial sutures are fused already in utero. The incidence ranges from 1 in 2100 to 2500 births/year.

➤ The most common form of non-syndromic synostosis (also termed isolated) is scaphocephaly caused by premature fusion of the sagittal suture. Frontal synostosis caused by fusion of the coronal sutures leads to unilateral flattening of the forehead. Unilateral lambdoid synostosis, due to premature fusion of one lambdoid suture, is an important deformity because of the flattening occiput and the possible difficulty in differentiating it from positional plagiocephaly (see earlier).

➤ Syndromic suture synostosis is differentiated from non-syndromic synostosis by associated dysmorphic features, birth defects and the presence of synostosis in more than one suture.

SPINA BIFIDA

➤ Spina bifida (SB) is a congenital spinal neural defect (SND) in which the spinal column is split (bifid) because of a failure to close the embryonic neural tube during the fourth week of postfertilization.

➤ The most common vertebral sites involved are either S1 alone or S1 and S2 together.

➤ Causes are heterogenous and include chromosomal abnormality, genetics and teratogenic exposure. Up to 70% of SB can be prevented by folic acid supplement.

➤ High antenatal levels of alpha-fetoprotein (AFP) may indicate an open neural tube defect, which can be confirmed by ultrasonography. SND identified early can be potentially repaired antenatally or within 48 hours postnatally.

Spina Bifida Occulta (SBO)

SBO is the most common (incidence is up to 22% of population) and the mildest type of SB anomaly, resulting from a midline defect of one or more vertebral bodies. The defect is usually covered by a layer of normal skin, but sometimes it is covered by patches of hair, a small dimple or vascular skin naevus. There is no neural tube defect. The condition is usually asymptomatic. In some cases, SBO has been linked with voiding problems, including nocturnal enuresis.

Meningocele

This is the modest type of SB, which is a midline defect in the posterior vertebral arches through which meninges with CSF protrude to form a sac. The protrusion is usually covered by normal skin and presents as a fluctuant midline mass. The spinal cord is usually normal, and there is little or no neurological damage.

Meningomyelocele

Spinal cord and nerves are exposed through opening of the spine, resulting in partial or complete paralysis of the parts of the body below the spinal opening. Other complications include hydrocephaly, urinary incontinence and constipation.

SUDDEN-ONSET HEADACHE

Core Messages

➤ Headaches are a common complaint, occurring in about 50% of children aged 7 years and 80% of children aged 15 years. Children with a history of infantile colic, regurgitation, abdominal migraine and cyclic vomiting are at risk of migraine.

➤ Although most causes of headaches in children are benign, it is essential to consider an underlying systemic disease: Worsening headache in the morning, increased by stooping or straining, can suggest increased ICP. Infants or toddlers with headache may present with irritability, unwillingness to play, crying while holding their head or vomiting.

➤ Trigeminal autonomic cephalalgias include cluster headache, paroxysmal hemicrania and unilateral neuralgiform headache with conjunctival injection.

➤ Neuroimaging is not indicated on a routine basis in children with recurrent headaches and normal physical examination. It is mainly indicated with an abnormal neurological examination, progressive headaches or coexisting seizure.

➤ The classification of headache disorders differentiates primary from secondary headaches (Box 14.7). Primary headaches are caused by independent pathology mechanisms and not by other disorders.

BOX 14.7 Primary and secondary causes of headaches

Primary
- Migraine
- Tension headaches
- Trigeminal autonomic cephalalgias
- Other primary headaches (e.g., primary stabbing, exercise, cough)

Secondary
- Viral upper respiratory infection (URTI)
- Head injury
- Acute sinusitis
- Substance or drug abuse
- Increased ICP, including benign ICP
- Hypertension

MIGRAINE AND TENSION HEADACHES

➤ Migraine is defined as a recurrent headache disorder manifesting as attacks lasting 2–72 hours, typically pulsatile. In children, migraine headaches are commonly bilateral (in adults, typically unilateral), frontal (in adults, temporal or ocular) and shorter (often <30 minutes in young children).

➤ Auras are defined as recurrent attacks of unilateral and fully reversable visual, sensory or other CNS symptoms that usually develop gradually, last a few minutes and usually precede the headache.

➤ Migraine without aura (common migraine) is the most common type of migraine with certain diagnostic criteria (Box 14.8). Criteria for diagnosing migraine with aura (classical migraine) are shown in Box 14.9.

BOX 14.8 Criteria for diagnosing migraine without aura

- Five or more attacks fulfilling the following criteria:
  - ❼ Headache lasting 0.5–48 hours
- Headache has at least two of the following four criteria:
  - ❼ Bilateral or unilateral location
  - ❼ Pulsating quality
  - ❼ Moderate to severe
  - ❼ Aggravated by physical activities.
- At least one of the following accompanies headache:
  - ❼ Nausea and/or vomiting
  - ❼ Photophobia and phonophobia

BOX 14.9 Criteria for diagnosing migraine with aura

- At least two attacks fulfilling the following criteria.
- At least three of the following four characteristics:
  - ❼ One or more reversible aura symptoms
  - ❼ At least one aura develops gradually >4 minutes
  - ❼ No aura symptoms lasting >1 hour
  - ❼ Headache follows aura with a free interval of <1 hour but may begin before or simultaneously with aura

➤ Establishing a diagnosis of migraine in primary care and referring the patient to a headache outpatient clinic has been shown to decrease further GP visits for migraine crisis.

➤ Alternating hemiplegia may be the first sign of later migraine. Beware that frequent vasoconstriction causing the hemiplegia causes ischaemia, which may lead to cerebral injury and developmental delay later.

Management of Migraine

➤ As children will often seek out a dark space at the onset of migraine, this should be encouraged as well as sleeping, as this can terminate the episode. Children are also encouraged to take frequent small sips of water to remain hydrated.

➤ Management guidelines for treatment of migraine are shown in Table 14.1.

TABLE 14.1 Management guidelines for migraine

Medication	Dose (mg)	Frequency
• Paracetamol	• 15 mg/kg	• 4–6 hourly
• Ibuprofen	• 10 mg/kg	• 8 hourly
• Naproxen	• 5–7 mg/kg	• 8–12 hourly
• Sumatriptan		
• Nasal	• 10–20 mg	• Single dose, repeat at least 2 hours later
• Oral	• 25–50 mg	• As noted earlier
• Subcutaneous	• 6 mg	• Single dose, repeat at least 1 hour later (indicated for acute cluster headache)
• Zolmitriptan		
• Nasal	• 5 mg	• Single dose, repeat at least 2 hours later PRN
• Oral	• 2.5 mg	• As noted earlier

➤ Although evidence-based treatment or prophylaxis is lacking, analgesics such as paracetamol, ibuprofen and sumatriptan are effective first-line treatment.

➤ Excessive use of analgesics may cause analgesic-induced headache with a rebound effect.

➤ Migraine prophylaxis should be considered if the child is missing >3 days of school in a month and/or has more than one to two attacks per week that interfere with daily activities. Propranolol (first choice) and pizotifen are frequently used as prophylaxis.

➤ *Tension headache* is the second most common type of headache. Diagnostic criteria and therapeutic guidelines for therapy are provided in Boxes 14.10 and 14.11, respectively.

➤ *Tension headache* is divided into infrequent (one or fewer episode/month), frequent (1–14 episodes/month for >3 months) and chronic (>15 episodes/month for >3 months).

➤ It is simple to differentiate between the two most common causes of headaches: Migraine disrupts the child's activity; tension headache does not.

BOX 14.10 Diagnostic criteria for tension-type headaches

- Previous episodes of headache fulfilling the following:
  - ❼ Headache lasting a few minutes to 7 days
- At least two of the following pain characteristics:
  - ❼ Pressing or tightening (not pulsating)
  - ❼ Mild or moderate intensity (children continue to play despite their headache)
  - ❼ Bilateral location
  - ❼ Not aggravated by physical activities
  - ❼ No nausea or vomiting
  - ❼ No photophobia or phonophobia
  - ❼ No evidence of structural or metabolic disease

BOX 14.11 Therapeutic guidelines for tension headache

- Avoiding or minimizing causes or triggers.
- A trial with analgesics is indicated.
- Cutting down frequent and excessive analgesics, as these can make headache worse.
- Infrequent/chronic headache, medications such as tricyclic antidepressants (amitriptyline), muscle relaxants, anticonvulsants (topiramate or gabapentin) and serotonin reuptake inhibitors (paroxetine or fluoxetine) have been used.
- Tranquilizers such as diazepam should not be used because of their side effects.
- Relaxation training or biofeedback.

Warning Signs of Headaches (Red Flags)

➤ Sudden-onset headaches can be the main symptom of a life-threatening neurological condition. Warning features of serious underlying causes are listed in Table 14.2.

TABLE 14.2 Warning headache features requiring immediate referral (Red Flags)

Symptoms	Signs
• Pain that wakens the child from sleep or worse when waking up	• Drowsiness
• Recent head trauma	• Cranial nerve palsy
• Associated with severe vomiting, particularly in the morning	• Blurred vision, diplopia
• Occipital	• Abnormal gait
• Drowsiness	• Abnormal neurological signs
• Recent changes in mood or personality	• High BP with bradycardia
• Pain worsened by coughing or Valsalva manoeuvre	
• <5 years	

➤ Benign ICP is characterized by increased ICP (e.g., headaches, vomiting and papilloedema) with normal CSF and ventricular size (as evident by CT scan or MRI). Focal neurological signs are absent. *An urgent same-day referral to the hospital is required to exclude a brain tumour.*

➤ Basilar migraine (presenting with vertigo, diplopia, blurred vision and ataxia) should be differentiated from posterior fossa tumour.

MIGRAINE VARIANTS

In families with a history of migraine, migraine variants are common and include items shown in Table 14.3.

TABLE 14.3 Clinical presentation of migraine variants

Abdominal migraine	• Episodic abdominal pain, moderate to severe, typically periumbilical, often in the absence of headache • Accompanied by nausea with or without vomiting, pallor • Usually lasts a few hours, range 1–72 hours; is terminated by sleep • Typical age 4–8 years, very rarely before 2 years • Strong family history of migraine
Cyclic vomiting	• Bouts of vomiting which may lead to dehydration • Headache may or may not be felt • Infants are typically affected
Ophthalmic migraine	• Unilateral eye pain and third nerve palsy with ptosis, papillary dilatation and external eye deviation
Basilar artery migraine	• Ataxia, vertigo, dysarthria, weakness, syncope, scotoma or transient blindness
Acute confusional state	• Change in orientation, personality or behaviour (restless, hyperactive) • Confusion may last minutes to hours • It may occur after minor head trauma
Benign paroxysmal Vertigo of childhood	• Sudden unsteadiness with nystagmus and vomiting occurring typically in toddlers (median age 18 months) • The spell lasts minutes and often occurs in clusters over several days, then subsides for weeks or months • Normal neurological examination and vestibular function • Typically there is a family history of migraine and the children will develop typical migraines in the future
Paroxysmal torticollis of infancy	• Recurrent episodes of head tilt associated with pallor, agitation and vomiting • Typically occur in infancy; spontaneous remission occurs aged 2–3 years • If the episode persists, abnormalities in the cervical vertebrae (e.g., dislocation) or posterior fossa tumour should be excluded

TREMOR

➤ Tremor is an involuntary and rhythmic movement. It is rare in the paediatric population but affects up to 4% of the adult population.

➤ Jitteriness, a rhythmic tremor, of equal amplitude, is common in healthy neonates, particularly premature infants and when babies are crying.

➤ Most tremors are action tremors, which occur with voluntary muscle contraction (Box 14.12). Essential tremor (ET) is the most frequent abnormal movement (around 1% of population), defined as an isolated tremor manifesting as an action tremor of bilateral upper extremities for a minimum of 3 years that occurs in the absence of other neurological signs. No neurological cause is found.

BOX 14.12 Classification of tremors

Rest Tremor (Limb Relaxed and Supported against Gravity)

- Juvenile Parkinson's disease
- Drug-induced (lithium, antiepileptics)
- Wilson's disease

Action Tremor (Limb Is Held in Position)

- Physiological (enhanced physiological tremor)
- Essential tremor (can occasionally be unilateral)
- Medications (beta-2 agonists for asthma)

Intention (Target-Directed Limb Movements)

- Cerebellar lesion (spinocerebellar degeneration, tumour)
- Multiple sclerosis
- Drug induced

PRACTICE POINTS FOR DIAGNOSING TREMOR

➤ Jitteriness in neonates needs to be differentiated from seizure caused by, for example, hypoglycaemia or hypocalcaemia. Normal jitteriness has no abnormal gaze or eye movement, bradycardia or tachycardia, with no cyanosis and can be stopped when a limb is held by an examiner or a parent.

➤ Drug addiction (e.g., cocaine, heroin, amphetamine) among pregnant women has increased steadily over the years. The result is an increased incidence of neonatal withdrawal syndrome with irritability, jitteriness and occasionally seizures.

➤ Physiological tremor is an action tremor and occurs in most individuals when the arms are extended. The tremor involves both hands and fingers. This is enhanced by anxiety, stress or caffeine. More subtle tremor can be demonstrated by holding a piece of paper on the outstretched hands.

➤ Childhood-onset ET often remains undiagnosed until later in life and misdiagnosed as physiological tremor. Children with ET have less functional impairment than adults.

➤ Asthma medications such as beta-2 agonists and theophylline, anticonvulsants such as valproate and tricyclic antidepressants are capable of inducing tremor. Although tremor caused by salbutamol is benign, parents should be made aware of it at the time the drug is prescribed to avoid parental anxiety.

➤ Tremor needs to be differentiated from tics, which are actually jerks, are non-rhythmic and can affect any muscles. Chorea is usually symmetric, is more rapid than tremor, is jerky and affects predominately the face.

➤ In any child with progressive or acute tremor, serious conditions such as Wilson's disease, hyperthyroidism, hypoglycaemia, hypocalcaemia, neuroblastoma and pheochromocytoma have to be excluded.

Investigations

➤ Blood glucose, calcium
➤ Thyroid function tests (TFTs) for suspected hyperthyroidism
➤ Urine for copper and serum ceruloplasmin for cases with Wilson's disease
➤ Imaging of the brain for cerebral or cerebellar causes

Referral

➤ A neonate or infant with tremor occurring in an awake and alert state
➤ The tremor is acute, rapidly progressive or may have an underlying cause such as hypoglycaemia or hypocalcaemia
➤ It is causing difficulty in children with writing or activities in daily life
➤ Aetiologically obscure
➤ There is excessive parental concern

OTHER MOVEMENT DISORDERS (SEE TABLE 14.4)

TABLE 14.4 The main non-tremor movement disorders

Ataxia	• Acute cerebellar ataxia, often follows a viral illness
	• Drugs such as phenytoin
	• Genetic, e.g., ataxia telangiectasia, Friedrich's ataxia
	• Metabolic, e.g., abetalipoproteinaemia
Chorea	• Sydenham's chorea as a manifestation of rheumatic fever
	• Systemic lupus erythematosus (SLE)
	• Drugs such as phenothiazines and haloperidol (tardive dyskinesia)
	• Huntington's chorea
Dystonia	• Genetic, e.g., dystonia musculorum deformans
	• Cerebral palsy
	• Drug-induced, e.g., phenothiazines, haloperidol
Tics	• Transient tics, lasting weeks and months
	• Tourette syndrome, associated with vocalization (obscene words), compulsive behaviour and ADHD
Myoclonia	• Myoclonic jerks, commonly occurring at sleep onset
	• Myoclonic epilepsy

SEIZURES

Core Messages

➤ Seizures are common in children, occurring in 5–7%. A new classification of seizures is shown in Box 14.13. Seizures are now divided into groups depending on where seizure onset starts in the brain and whether or not a person's awareness and movements are affected.

BOX 14.13 New classification of seizures

- **Focal Seizures** (seizure onset in an area on one side of the brain)
- **Aware seizures**
  - ❼ Motor onset (e.g., automatism, tonic, clonic, atonic)
  - ❼ Non-motor onset (e.g., autonomic, cognitive, sensory)
- **Impaired awareness**
  - ❼ Motor onset (as noted earlier)
  - ❼ Non-motor onset (as noted earlier)
- **Generalized Seizures** (seizure onset on both sides of the brain)
  - ❼ Motor onset (with visible physical movement)
  - ❼ Non-motor onset (e.g., absence, without physical movement)
- **Focal to Bilateral Seizures** (onset of seizure on one side of the brain and spreading to both sides)
- **Unknown-Onset Seizures**
  - ❼ Motor onset (e.g., tonic-clonic)
  - ❼ Non-motor onset (e.g., tonic-clonic)

➤ In children, febrile seizures (FSs) are the most common cause of seizures, occurring in 3–4% (Box 14.14), followed by epileptic seizures with an incidence of 1%. Children with seizures are more likely to experience comorbidities such as intellectual and learning disability, language development delay, depression and anxiety.

BOX 14.14 Criteria for diagnosing simple FS

- Healthy child with no neurological abnormality
- Age 6 months to 6 years
- No focal or prolonged (<10 minutes) seizures
- Presence of fever >38.0°C
- No subsequent paralysis
- Family and/or own history of FS (not always present)

➤ Epilepsy should not be diagnosed unless seizures recur and they are unprovoked (e.g., by fever, low calcium).

➤ Any seizure should be differentiated from pseudo-seizure occurring with conversion symptoms.

Management of Seizures in Primary Care

Prehospital Treatment (Figure 14.1)

> Airway
> Breathing
> Circulation
> Check blood glucose
> ↓
> Buccal: Midazolam 0.3 mg/kg (2.5–10 mg), to repeat after
> 10 minutes if needed
> Rectal: Diazepam 0.5 mg/kg (5–10 mg)
> IV: Lorazepam 0.1 mg/kg (max. 4 mg)
> IV: Diazepam 0.3/kg (max. 10 mg)

FIGURE 14.1 Prehospital treatment of seizure.

➤ Prompt seizure termination is the central aim of epilepsy treatment.
➤ Rapid administration of rescue medication of benzodiazepine (as the first-line treatment) is associated with a shorter duration of a generalized convulsive status epilepticus and a lower probability of recurrent seizures in the A&E department.
➤ After seizure termination, the child and family should be given information about:
  ➢ How to recognize further seizures.
  ➢ First aid and initial safety guidance in case of a further seizure.
  ➢ How to reduce the risk of further seizure.
  ➢ How to proceed to the nearest A&E urgently in case of further seizures.
  ➢ Epilepsy itself, including:
    • Safety issues of activities that should be adapted or avoided, e.g., showering rather than having baths, supervised swimming and water sports.
    • The importance of adherence to medication in addition to information on the side effects of the antiepileptic drugs (AEDs).
➤ Information and support should be provided at routine appointments with the GP, and children and young people should have access to a specialist nurse.
➤ Children presenting with a first afebrile seizure and those after complicated FS are at risk of further afebrile seizures, especially within 6–12 months.

Indications to Refer Children with Seizures

➤ Although primary care clinicians can provide excellent services for children with epilepsy, there is a limit to how much these services can offer, including lack of expertise and time. *Therefore, there is a need for referral to a paediatric outpatient clinic or epilepsy clinic.*
➤ Children should be referred urgently for an appointment within 2 weeks:
  ➢ For an assessment after a first suspected afebrile seizure
  ➢ For recurrent seizures (epilepsy)
  ➢ If children develop seizure recurrence after a period of remission

➤ *Referral of children with suspected or confirmed epilepsy to tertiary paediatric service if:*
  ➢ They are <3 years of age.
  ➢ They are <4 years and have myoclonic seizures.
  ➢ They have a unilateral structural lesion of the brain.
  ➢ They show deterioration in their behaviour, speech or learning difficulty.

Management of Epilepsy with AEDs (Table 14.5)

TABLE 14.5 Common anticonvulsants with first and second choices in treatment of epilepsy

Seizure Type	First-Line Drug	Second-Line Drug
• Generalized (e.g., tonic-clonic)	• Sodium valproate • Lamotrigine	• Carbamazepine
• Myoclonic	• Sodium valproate	• Lamotrigine, clobazam
• Absence seizure	• Sodium valproate	• Lamotrigine, clobazam
• Focal	• Carbamazepine, lamotrigine, levetiracetam	• Gabapentin, topiramate
• Infantile spasms	• Vigabatrin	• Prednisolone, valproate

➤ AEDs should be commenced once:
  ➢ The diagnosis of epilepsy has been established beyond doubt.
  ➢ The child and the parents should receive full information about the effects of the drugs and their side effects.
  ➢ The child's wish to take the AED should be taken into consideration.
➤ Most clinicians agree not to commence an AED after a single seizure. However, AED should be considered after a first unprovoked seizure if:
  ➢ There are signs of neurological deficit.
  ➢ If the patient or their family do not accept the risk of further seizure.
  ➢ EEG shows unequivocal epileptic activity.
  ➢ Brain imaging shows a structural abnormality.

Investigation of Epilepsy (Table 14.6)

➤ Diagnosis of epilepsy, aetiology and classification can often be made on detailed history alone (Table 14.7). Once the diagnosis is established and AEDs initiated, these children should be best followed up by primary care clinicians or community paediatricians. Occasionally, children initially seen in the primary care setting with clear and mild epilepsy who may not need or wish a referral can undergo some investigations.
➤ The objective of seizure treatment is to achieve complete or near-complete seizure control. Approximately 70% of people with epilepsy will became seizure free with optimal treatment of monotherapy with AED.

TABLE 14.6 Guidelines on investigation in children with epilepsy

Urine	With Clinitest for reducible substances if clinically indicated. Aminoaciduria is sometimes requested.
Blood	• First-line tests (can be performed at GP surgery): Electrolytes and urea, glucose, calcium, phosphorus and alkaline phosphatase, magnesium, acid–base status (as clinically indicated). • Second-line tests: Ammonia, lactate, metabolic screens, chromosomal analysis if there is evidence of dysmorphic features.
EEG	It will help establish whether the seizures are epileptic or non-epileptic. Interictal EEG has a range of diagnostic sensitivity between 25% and 55%. However, it can: • Confirm the diagnosis of epilepsy such as focal epilepsy or 3-second spikes and waves in the absence of seizures or hypsarrhythmia pattern in West's syndrome. • It helps with the AED choices.
Imaging	• Cranial ultrasound, performed when the anterior fontanel is open (it closes between 9 and 18 months). • Neuroimaging (CT scan and MRI) is particularly indicated in cases of focal epileptic seizures.
Radioisotope scanning	Single photon emission tomography (SPECT) and positron emission tomography (PET) are used in selected cases prior to surgery.

Prognosis

➤ The prognosis of children with epilepsy is generally good.
➤ In children with FS, deaths or persistent motor deficits occurring as sequalae of simple seizures are unusual. FSs are associated with increased intellectual deficits only among children with:
  ➤ Pre-existing neurological or developmental abnormalities.
  ➤ Subsequent afebrile seizures.
➤ In children whose anticonvulsant therapy has been withdrawn after prolonged control, nearly 30% may experience recurrence of seizures, and 85% of them relapse within 5 years of drug withdrawal.
➤ Factors associated with increased risk of relapse are:
  ➤ Long duration of epilepsy before control
  ➤ Pre-existing neurological deficits
  ➤ Abnormal EEG before anticonvulsants were discontinued
  ➤ If the seizures began early <2 years of age

Mortality

Mortality due to epilepsy is two to four times that of the population without epilepsy. Death in a child with epilepsy may be due to the following:

➤ Underlying cause, such as neurodegenerative disorder
➤ Accident during epileptic seizure (trauma, drowning, aspiration, suffocation)
➤ Status epilepticus
➤ Suicide

➤ Sudden death in epilepsy (SUDEP), defined as sudden, unexpected, non-traumatic and non-drowning death in an individual with epilepsy in which autopsy does not reveal an anatomical or toxicological cause for the death. SUDEP causes about 500 deaths each year in the UK. Criteria for SUDEP are:
- ➣ Patient has epilepsy, i.e., recurrent and unprovoked seizures.
- ➣ Patient died unexpectedly while in reasonable health.
- ➣ Death occurred suddenly within minutes.
- ➣ Death occurred under benign and normal circumstances.
- ➣ Death was not due to direct result of seizure or status epilepticus.
- ➣ An obvious medical cause could not be determined at autopsy.

➤ Certain factors known to be associated with an increased risk of mortality include:
- ➣ Symptomatic epilepsy (e.g., cerebral malformation, developmental delay)
- ➣ Uncontrolled generalized tonic-clonic seizures
- ➣ Patients with sleep seizures
- ➣ Poor compliance with AEDs, particularly omitting to take AEDs
- ➣ Sudden and frequent changes to AEDs
- ➣ Lack of sleep or food, presence of stress, excess alcohol intake
- ➣ Seizure occurrence when living alone

➤ Minimizing the risk of mortality:
- ➣ Identifying those with poorly controlled epilepsy and ensuring they have access to specialized centres. A referral to epilepsy specialists for regular review is important.
- ➣ Offering continued education/information about epilepsy. AEDs should always be taken as prescribed, and the patient should never run out of medications. The patient is to be advised to take the AEDs immediately once they remember they forgot to take them. Encourage patients to keep seizure diaries.
- ➣ Referring patient to practice nurse (e.g., for counselling, education).
- ➣ Recommending lifestyle restrictions, which may include:
  - Using shower instead of bath.
  - Swimming should be supervised.
  - Keeping regular sleep schedule and avoiding fatigue.
  - Avoiding recreational drugs, excess use of alcohol.

TABLE 14.7 Conditions mimicking seizures

Syncope (vasovagal syncope)	Condition is rare before 10 years of age. Episode typically is precipitated by prolonged periods of standing without moving in a warm environment. It manifests as sudden loss of tonus, falling with pallor and bradycardia. It may be rarely associated with brief tonic contraction, abnormal movements, upward deviation of the eyes and even urinary incontinence.
Breath-holding spells (BHSs)	Diagnosis of BHS is easy from the history: Both types (cyanotic and pallid) are triggered by an upsetting or painful event, followed by crying, breath holding and cyanosis, which precedes a rare seizure movement. Cyanosis in epileptic seizure occurs usually after the tonic seizure. Typical BHS occurs aged 6 months to 5 years and may occur a few times a day or every few months, and frequency decreases with age. In the pallid form of BHS, the child screams briefly followed by a loss of consciousness, hypotonicity and pallor. Recovery follows shortly.

(Continued)

TABLE 14.7 Conditions mimicking seizures (Continued)

Benign paroxysmal vertigo	Occurs typically aged 1–2 years (after the child learns to walk) and may last up to the age of 6 years. While standing and fully awake, the child suddenly becomes panicked, frightened and does not want to move until the event ends. The frequency decreases with age.
Benign sleep myoclonus (BSM)	BSM is characterized by repetitive, high-frequency myoclonic jerks in the arms, occasionally in the legs, which lasts for few seconds while falling asleep. The most important feature differentiating BSM is that it does not occur outside sleep.
Night terror	Occurs in the non-REM phase of sleep, typically 1.5–2 hours after falling asleep. Episode is characterized by screaming, sweating and hallucinations (see 'Sleep Disorders').
Pseudoseizure	Diagnosis is based on: • Occurs typically at 10–18 years of age, more often in females • Bizarre, unusual muscle contracture • Absence of cyanosis, tongue biting or injury • Normal EEG often showing excess of muscle artifacts • Normal serum prolactin (raised in true epilepsy)

HYPOTONIA (FLOPPY BABY SYNDROME)

Core Messages

➤ Hypotonia is defined as a diminished resistance of muscle to stretching. It poses a challenge for clinicians because hypotonia may be the presenting sign of both benign and serious conditions.

➤ Hypotonia is caused by disorders that affect any level of the CNS (Box 14.15). Central hypotonia can be caused by benign conditions such as benign congenital hypotonia (infants present early with floppiness but later develop normal muscle tone) or by cerebral injury such as hypoxic-ischaemic encephalopathy.

BOX 14.15 Causes of hypotonia

Central (Upper Motor Neurone, without Severe Weakness): >75% of Cases
● Benign congenital hypotonia
● Chromosomal abnormality (Down's syndrome, Prader–Willi syndrome)
● Hypoxic-ischaemic encephalopathy

Anterior Horn Cells (Lower Motor Neurone, Associated with Weakness)
● Spinal muscular atrophy (SMA)

Peripheral Nerves
- Congenital demyelinating neuropathy
- Familial dysautonomia

Neuromuscular Junction
- Congenital/transient myasthenia

Muscles
- Myotonic dystrophy

➤ A key distinction is to determine whether a child with hypotonia is with or without muscle weakness. While children with a central hypotonia present typically with floppiness but without weakness (have antigravity power, normal or brisk tendon reflexes), those with peripheral hypotonia often present with weakness, which is a decreased ability to voluntarily and actively move muscles against resistance. They usually have normal intellect, markedly reduced muscle power, reduced muscle tone and reflexes and fasciculation (present with anterior horn cell disease).

Diagnosis of Hypotonia

➤ Physical examination should differentiate between floppiness due to weakness and floppiness due to insignificant or no weakness. Delayed of motor development with normal social and language development makes CNS lesion unlikely. Brisk tendon reflexes indicate CNS lesion, while diminished or absent reflexes point strongly to lower motor lesion.
➤ Examination of a child with hypotonia should always begin with observation, including the head (shape and size), face (for dysmorphism) and eyes (for strabismus) (Box 14.16).

BOX 14.16 Characteristic signs of hypotonia

- Supine — Paucity of spontaneous movements, muscles feel floppy on palpation, significant head lag on pulling to sitting position (normally no head lag >4–5 months of age).
- Vertical suspension — A healthy baby infant should maintain the head upright after the age of 3 months (it tests the truncal/nuchal muscle tone).
- Standing — Inability or reduced ability for age to bear its own weight.
- Prone — Inability or reduced ability to lift the head above the ground (achieved aged 6 weeks to 3 months) and lifting the head with upper chest (4–6 months in healthy infants). Frog-legged: Hips abducted and knees flexed.

NECK PAIN AND STIFFNESS

Core Messages

➤ Neck pain and stiffness (NPS) is a common musculoskeletal problem in paediatrics and a common presenting complaint to both emergency and primary care clinicians. The symptom is extremely important because of the possibility of serious underlying conditions. Box 14.17 lists the main causes of NPS.

BOX 14.17 Localized and systemic causes of NPS

Localized (To the Neck)

- Viral URTI with cervical lymphadenitis
- Benign paroxysmal torticollis (BPT)
- Muscular torticollis (sternomastoid tumour)
- Text neck syndrome
- Cervical spine infection
- Trauma (neck injury)
- Chiari's malformation

Systemic (Outside the Neck)

- Migraine
- Meningism, meningitis, pneumonia (upper lobe pneumonia)
- Juvenile fibromyalgia
- Sandifer's syndrome (GO reflux)
- Dystonic drug reaction
- Rheumatoid arthritis
- Spasmus nutans

➤ In infants, mild head tilting may be caused by shortening of the sternomastoid muscle, a so-called sternomastoid tumour. In older children, an important cause is torticollis (wry neck), which is characterized by holding the neck tilted to one side with the chin rotated in the opposite direction.
➤ In contrast to torticollis and lymphadenitis, a child with meningism is usually ill-looking with fever.
➤ Meningism is an important subset and always requires emergency evaluation. It is characterized by the presence of signs of neck stiffness in addition to fever and ill-looking appearance.

PRACTICE POINTS

- Torticollis resulting from sternomastoid tumour is asymptomatic in the first few days of life. At 10–20 days, a mass is frequently felt in the muscle. The mass gradually disappears and the fibrous tissue contracts, causing limited head motion and mild tilting of the head (torticollis).
- BPT is characterized by a head tilt associated with vomiting, irritability and/or ataxia. BPT is associated with migraine. About 50% of children have a history of infantile colic.
- Children with torticollis and dystonic drug reaction look remarkably well despite the stiff neck, in contrast to those with CNS infection.
- Text neck syndrome (a 21st-century syndrome) is being increasingly recognized in older children and adolescents who for hours a day (average 5–7 hours) have frequent forward head flexion while looking at the screens of mobile devices and/or texting for a long period of time. The condition has caused cervical spinal degeneration.
- Although headache is a cardinal symptom in migraine and tension headache, neck pain with stiffness is a frequent associated finding in about 7% of cases. Neck pain can also be a trigger of migraine attacks.
- Drug history is of paramount importance to confirm a rare case of dystonic drug reaction (oculogyric crisis, especially with metoclopramide).
- Juvenile-onset fibromyalgia is characterized by widespread musculoskeletal pain with fatigue, sleep disturbance, anxiety and depression lasting >3 months. It affects mostly adolescent girls.
- Any child with meningism should be considered a case of meningitis until proved otherwise. Even if pneumonia is diagnosed, a child with meningism requires a lumbar puncture (LP) to confirm or exclude meningitis. The skin of a child with meningism should be carefully searched for any rash or petechiae if suspected meningococcal disease. Meningitis, particularly meningococcal disease (MCD), may initially mimic a virus-like illness. Within a few hours, the disease can rapidly progress to septic shock, hypotension, disseminated intravascular coagulation (DIC) and death.

ACUTE CONFUSIONAL STATE

➤ Acute confusional state (ACS) is characterized by sudden alteration of the mental state leading to an inappropriate interaction with people and the environment. It has an acute and dramatic onset of disorientation, impaired concentration and subtle motor signs such as tremor. In older children, disorientation for time is striking.
➤ In the absence of a relevant medical history (such as sickle cell anaemia or medication), the differential diagnosis can be quite difficult and challenging to clinicians. Box 14.18 lists causes of ACS.
➤ A child presenting with ACS should be regarded as a medical emergency. *Referral to hospital is urgently required.*

BOX 14.18 Main causes of ACS

Cerebral

- Migraine
- Encephalitis/encephalopathy
- Brain tumour
- Head injury
- Non-convulsive status epilepticus (NCSE)
- Psychosis

Non-Cerebral

- Side effect of medication (e.g., antihistamine, illicit drugs [cocaine, amphetamine and ecstasy drugs])
- Hypoglycaemia

PRACTICE POINTS

- The diagnosis of the first episode of acute confusional migraine is often difficult; drug abuse such as amphetamine, cocaine and ecstasy; encephalitis; and NCSE need to be considered.
- Family history of migraine and severe headache with visual symptoms prior to the confusion may suggest the diagnosis of migraine. A confusional state of migraine often lasts several minutes to hours. It may be the first presentation before being replaced by typical migraine attacks.
- Minor trauma can occasionally trigger a major ACS grossly disproportionate to the degree of trauma.
- Although patients with psychosis usually present with delusion, hallucination, and paranoid ideation, ACS can be the main presenting symptom.
- Psychiatric manifestations in patients with SLE include personality changes, depression and psychosis, which can be the presenting features in SLE.

SLEEP DISORDERS

Core Messages

➤ Children vary in their requirement for sufficient sleep. Sleep duration is age dependent. Young infants need on average 14 hours of sleep per 24 hours, which is almost evenly distributed during the day and night. Children aged 6–12 years require about 10–11 hours, and teens about 9 hours. An insufficient night's sleep is likely to affect the child's mood and behaviour during the day, leading to school problems such as reduced attention span, aggressiveness and poor performance.

➤ Sleep disorders (Box 14.19) include chronic insomnia with difficulty in initiating sleep, maintaining sleep and early awakening with inability to return to sleep, occurring at least 3 nights/week and is present for at least 3 months.

➤ Between 50 and 80% of children with ASD have insomnia, which adversely affects their mental and physical health.

➤ Parasomnia, which is disruptive sleep-related disorders occurring during non-rapid eye movement (NREM), includes sleepwalking, sleep talking, sleep terrors and confusional arousal.

➤ Kleine–Levin syndrome is rare and is characterized by long and recurrent hypersomnia, hyperphagia and sometimes hypersexuality.

BOX 14.19 Main sleep disorders and management of insomnia

- Insomnia for intercurrent illness, pain or itching
- Chronic insomnia as defined above.
- Persistent insomnia (with initiation and maintaining sleep)
- Parasomnia, such as sleep terrors (Box 14.20)
- OAS
- Hypersomnia (e.g., narcolepsy)
- Sleep-related epilepsies
- Kleine–Levin syndrome

Management of Chronic Insomnia

- Promoting daytime physical exercises but not too close to bedtime
- No electronics/screens at least 1–2 hours before bedtime (digital curfew)
- Adaptive bedtime routines including story reading, bathing
- Cognitive behavioural therapy (CBT) for insomnia
- Melatonin may be used for a short time: 0.5–1 mg, 30–60 minutes before bedtime for children with sleep-onset insomnia. Melatonin use should be avoided in children below the age of 2 years

---

BOX 14.20 Characteristics of sleep terrors

- Types
  - ❼ NREM: Sleepwalking, sleep terrors, confusional arousal
  - ❼ REM: Nightmares (occurring in the second part of the night)
- Sleep terrors are defined as a sudden arousal accompanied by autonomic signs (sweating, tachycardia, mydriasis). There is often a piercing scream, and the child looks flushed, frightened and agitated and is not easily aroused. The child can't recall the event the next morning. Common causes of sleep terrors include gastro-oesophageal reflux, medications and sleep deprivation.
- Nightmares are differentiated from sleep terrors by vivid and terrifying, well-remembered dreams; nightmares are not as intense as sleep terrors.
- Management includes reassurance that the condition will resolve spontaneously, often at adolescence age. It is important to search for a cause of the parasomnia and eliminate it before initiating medication. In case that the episodes are severe, violent and/or harmful, benzodiazepines may be used at night.

Narcolepsy is a rare neurological disorder characterized by excessive daytime sleepiness (Box 14.21). Narcolepsy (with cataplexy) is caused by loss of hypocretin-producing neurones which are responsible for the sleep–wake cycle.

BOX 14.21 Narcolepsy

Diagnostic Criteria
- Excessive daytime sleepiness
- Sleep-related hallucinations (hypnagogic)
- Cataplexy (sudden loss of muscle power, e.g., after laughter)
- Sleep paralysis
- Disruptive sleep
- Low CSF hypocretin

Management
- Patient and family should be informed that there is no cure
- Psychosocial support, lifestyle changes
- Regular physical activity
- Short, regular naps at times when patient feels sleepiest
- Swimming should be supervised
- Avoidance of emotional situations
- Effective medications include methylphenidate, amphetamine, tricyclic antidepressants and selective serotonin reuptake inhibitors (SSRIs)
  - ❼ Sodium oxybate is effective for the treatment of cataplexy

---

Obstructive Sleep Apnoea (OSA)

➤ An important cause of insomnia is OAS, which is characterized by snoring and apnoea due to partial or complete upper airway collapse or obstruction, which disrupts normal sleep patterns and ventilation.

➤ OAS is primarily due to hypertrophy of the tonsils and adenoid, which is commonly associated with Down's syndrome, obesity and neuromuscular diseases.

➤ Small infants often have transient apnoea episodes at night, which are harmless. Referral to hospital is not required if these episodes are not associated with cyanosis or bradycardia.

➤ Nocturnal polysomnography is the gold standard to diagnose OSA and its severity. Adenotonsillectomy in cases of hypertrophy and reduction of obesity are the treatment approaches.

Sleep-Associated Epilepsy

➤ Several sleep-related epileptic seizures are shown in Box 14.22. Autonomic symptoms and secondary generalization may occur in these sleep-related epilepsies and may mimic 'sleep disturbance'.

➤ Sleep generally has a significant seizure-promoting effect during NREM and an inhibitory effect on the REM phase.

BOX 14.22 Non-epileptic and epileptic seizures related to sleep

Non-Epileptic Seizures

- Benign sleep myoclonus — Face is never involved, facial colour normal. Cessation aged 3–6 months. EEG is normal.

- Juvenile myoclonic — Bilateral single or multiple myoclonic jerks, predominately the arms, occurring when drowsy or shortly after awakening. EEG is normal.

Epileptic Seizures

- Benign partial epilepsy — Unilateral parasthesias followed by tonic and/or centrotemporal clonic seizure involving the tongue, lips, cheek, spikes (rolandic) pharynx and occasionally the arm, occurring during sleep or awakening. EEG usually diagnostic.

- Benign occipital epilepsy — Partial epilepsy with onset (mainly nocturnal) of vomiting, pallor, sweating, tonic eye deviations and visual hallucinations.

- Nocturnal frontal lobe epilepsy — Presents with motor features (kicking, hitting, thrashing, epilepsycycling and scissoring of the legs) and vocalization (shouting, grunting, screaming and coughing). Seizures are usually brief and multiple, in contrast to night terrors which usually are longer and occur only once at night.

CHAPTER 15

Endocrinology and Transgender

DIABETES MELLITUS

Polyuria

➤ Polyuria is defined as a urine output >2 $L/m^2/24$ hours.
➤ Although polyuria has numerous causes (Box 15.1), the main causes are diabetes mellitus (DM), diabetes insipidus (DI), primary polydipsia (compulsive water drinking) and defects of renal tubular transport ability (renal tubular acidosis [RTA]). DM usually has a short history and is easily diagnosed. The remaining three causes may have a more protracted course, and the diagnosis can be difficult.

BOX 15.1 Causes of polyuria

- Diabetes mellitus
- Congenital and acquired nephrogenic DI
- Psychogenic polydipsia (compulsive fluid drinking)
- Renal tubular acidosis
- Cranial or nephrogenic diabetes insipidus
- Metabolic polyuria (potassium deficiency, hypercalcaemia)
- Chronic renal failure
- Drugs (diuretics, lithium, chlortetracycline)
- Renal tubular acidosis (e.g., Fanconi's syndrome)
- Pituitary tumours (craniopharyngioma, histiocytosis X)
- Barter's syndrome

➤ DI is caused by a lack of production/release of the hypothalamic hormone arginine vasopressin (also called antidiuretic hormone [ADH]).
➤ The fourth most frequent cause of polyuria (after DM, primary polydipsia and DI) is RTA. Children with RTA present with signs of dehydration, failure to thrive, anorexia and vomiting. Investigation reveals glycosuria, low serum bicarbonate and potassium and hyperchloraemia.
➤ It is essential to determine whether the child has frequent small urination or polyuria. Parents are usually good historians. Observation of the child's urination helps establish the diagnosis.

DOI: 10.1201/9781032642888-15

➤ All cases of polyuria should be referred to a paediatric setting for evaluation. An exception is possibly a child with clear symptoms of primary polydipsia who is well and thriving and whose polyuria ceases with fluid weaning.

➤ The diagnosis of a mild polyuria can be missed, and affected children may present with signs of dehydration including irritability, poor feeding, failure to gain weight, elevated body temperature (hyperthermia) and convulsion due to hypernatraemia.

➤ Long-standing polyuria may cause enlarged bladder, thickening of the bladder wall, mega-ureter and hydronephrosis.

TYPE 1 DIABETES MELLITUS

➤ Diabetes refers to a group of chronic metabolic disorders that result from an immune-mediated destruction of the pancreatic islet β-cells leading to hyperglycaemia. Environmental factors, the microbiome and the genome play major roles in developing diabetes. There is an annual increase in diabetes of 2–3% in the UK.

➤ Type 1 diabetes mellitus (T1DM) is characterized by a marked insulin deficiency in the presence of hyperglycaemia and positive autoantibody tests to glutamic acid decarboxylase, pancreatic islet β-cells and 1A-2b zinc transporter and/or insulin.

➤ Of the estimated 4.3 million people with diabetes in the UK, about 10% have T1DM and about 90% have type 2 diabetes (T2DM). Presentation and diagnostic criteria of T1DM are shown in Box 15.2. The incidence of T1DM in the UK is estimated to be 24.5 per 100,000 (0–14 years).

BOX 15.2 Presentation and diagnostic criteria of type 1 diabetes mellitus

- History is typically short (few days to 2–3 weeks), appearing at any age, with two noticeable peaks: 4–7 years old and 11–14 years old.
- Presentation
  - ❼ Cardinal symptoms of polyuria, polydipsia and polyphagia.
  - ❼ Other symptoms include tiredness, consciousness that ranges from alertness to drowsiness, obtunded or coma, dry mouth and reduced skin turgor.
  - ❼ Diabetic ketoacidosis (DKA), occurring in about a third of patients.
- Diagnostic criteria of DM
  - ❼ Fasting blood glucose level of >7.0 mmol/L (≥126 mg/dL)
  - ❼ Random blood glucose level >11.1 mmol/L (≥200 mg/dL)
  - ❼ Glycated Hb (HbA1c) of >48 mmol/mol (≥6.5%)
  - ❼ An abnormal result from an oral glucose tolerance test
- Diagnostic criteria of DKA
  - ❼ Blood glucose >11 mmol/L with venous pH <7.3 or bicarbonate <15 mEq/L

➤ T2DM can occur in children and young people, particularly if there is a family history of the condition, they are obese and they are from an Asian or Black family background, and they do not usually need insulin. Measurement of C-peptide and autoantibodies can distinguish between T1DM and T2DM.

➤ Non-T1DM and non-T2DM include monogenic diabetes, which accounts for 1–3% of all diabetes and is due to a single diabetic gene defect. It includes neonatal diabetes, maturity onset diabetes of the young (MODY) and syndromic diabetes (Box 15.3). Other rare types include insulin-resistance syndrome and mitochondrial diabetes. The diagnosis should be suspected if the diabetes occurs in the first year of life, patients never or rarely develop ketones during episodes of hyperglycaemia or have other associated features such as deafness or optic atrophy.

BOX 15.3 Monogenic diabetes

- Neonatal diabetes (NDM, congenital diabetes) is characterized by
  - ❼ Frequent genetic mutations (80%); the most common one is on the 6q24 locus.
  - ❼ Persistent hyperglycaemia diagnosed within the first 6 months due to reduction of the pancreatic islet β-cells. The condition is usually resolved by 18 months of age.
  - ❼ Clinically: Polyuria, dehydration, intrauterine growth restriction, failure to thrive, epilepsy, muscle weakness and developmental delay.
  - ❼ About 50% of NDM cases can be treated without insulin using oral hypoglycaemic medications such as sulfonylurea.
- MODY
  - ❼ Is usually autosomal dominant inherited diabetes.
  - ❼ Most patients with MODY are overweight or obese.
  - ❼ There is often a history of neonatal hypoglycaemia.
- Syndromic diabetes
  - ❼ Wolfram's syndrome is characterized by diabetes insipidus, optic atrophy and deafness, bleeding peptic ulcer and defective platelet aggregation.
  - ❼ Lipodystrophy due to complete/partial lack of hormones from adipose tissue.
  - ❼ Mitochondrial diabetes presenting with neurological signs such as seizures.

Management

A comprehensive management plan for children and young people with T1DM was published by National Institute for Health and Care Excellence (NICE) in August 2015 and last updated in May 2023, which is summarized in Box 15.4.

BOX 15.4 Summary of NICE guidelines on type 1 diabetes mellitus

Children and young people (CYP) with T1DM and their family, as appropriate, should be:

- Offered an integrated package of care by a multidisciplinary paediatric diabetes care team. In case of a new diagnosis of T1DM, *an immediate referral (same day) to the team or to the paediatric A&E should be carried out.* Oral hypoglycaemic agents should not be offered.
- Encouraged to attend clinic four times/year and explain that regular contacts with the diabetes team will help maintain optimal blood glucose levels (<7 mmol/litre fasting and pre-eating) and <9 mmol/litre after meals. HbA1c should be 48 mmol (6.5%) or lower.
- Informed to inject rapid-acting insulin before eating and that these injections help optimize blood glucose after meals. The dose of insulin may be adjusted after each blood glucose measurement.

- Offered information about management of insulin therapy, including rotating injection sites, blood glucose and HbA1c monitoring.
- Measured for height and weight, as well as their body mass index (BMI) calculated at each clinic visit.
- Informed about how diet, physical exercise and intercurrent illness affect blood glucose and how to check blood glucose and ketone bodies and possibly changing insulin doses in these situations.
- Encouraged to have regular dental checks.
- Offered access to mental health professionals, as psychological disturbance (e.g., anxiety, depression, behavioural problems) may interfere with the management and wellbeing.
- Offered screening testing for:
  - ❼ Coeliac disease and thyroid function at diagnosis and annually.
  - ❼ Retinopathy annually from the age of 12 years. Eye examination by an optician at least every 2 years.
  - ❼ Microalbuminuria annually from the age of 12 years.
  - ❼ Blood pressure measurements annually from the age of 12 years.
- Informed that they may experience a partial remission phase (honeymoon period) during which a low dosage of insulin (0.5 units/kg body weight) may be sufficient.
- Offered the types of insulin (Table 15.1) which suit their individual needs and with the aim of obtaining HbA1c <48 mmol (<6.5%) without disabling hypoglycaemia and with maximizing quality of life. Optimal glycaemic control requires multiple-dose rapid-acting insulin regimens that mimic physiological insulin release.
- Offered testing of their HbA1c levels four times per year. The optimal preprandial blood glucose level is 4–7 mmol/L and postprandial is <9 mmol/L.
- Encouraged to measure their blood glucose four or more times a day and more often if they have intercurrent illness.
- Offered information about the insulin pump if they experience severe hypoglycaemia, provided:
  - ❼ Multiple-dose insulin therapy has failed.
  - ❼ Those receiving it have the commitment and competence to use it effectively.
  - ❼ A specialist diabetic team has agreed to give the insulin pump.

TABLE 15.1 Available types of insulin regimens

Types of Insulin	Onset and Duration of Action
Rapid-acting	10–15 minutes; 2–5 hours
Short-acting	30–60 minutes; up to 8 hours
Intermediate-acting	1–2 hours; 12–18 hours
Long-acting	1–2 hours; 18–26 hours
Glargine*	1–2 hours; 24 hours

* Glargine is a synthetic version of human insulin with more consistent basal insulin levels throughout the day and fewer nocturnal hypoglycaemia compared to human insulin.

- Educated and trained, including their family and school nurse, in how to treat episodes of hypoglycaemia including the use of fast-acting glucose liquid carbohydrate (easier to swallow than solid) and IM glucagon for severe hypoglycaemia.
- Encouraged for annual immunization against influenza, starting when they are 6 months of age.
- Encouraged to wear or carry a badge to tell they have T1DM.
- Informed how to find out about government disability benefits and how to obtain the Public England Green.
- Informed that their total energy intake is approximately as follows:
  - ❼ Carbohydrate >50%
  - ❼ Protein 10–15%
  - ❼ Fat 30–35%
- Encouraged to have healthy eating habits, good knowledge of nutrition and eating foods with low glycaemic index such as fruits and vegetables, as well as regular exercise.

Other Treatments

➤ Pancreas transplants have been performed for over 50 years but have become mainly a standard treatment in individuals who develop end-stage renal failure and require simultaneous kidney and pancreas transplant.

➤ Islet transplantation has been carried out for years, but it has not achieved long-lasting insulin independence in the majority of cases.

➤ Ultra-rapid inhaled insulin has limited use so far due to its fixed dosing, issues with consistent delivery, cost and the need for pulmonary function testing.

➤ Immunotherapy is a new treatment that reprograms the immune system so that it no longer attacks and destroys pancreatic β-cells.

PRIMARY (PSYCHOGENIC) POLYDIPSIA

➤ Primary polydipsia (PP) in children is defined by water volume consumption exceeding 2 L/m²/day.

➤ PP is a clinical disorder characterized by excessive thirst and a pathological fluid intake leading to hypotonic polyuria and a decreased serum osmolality with dilutional hyponatraemia. The condition is not caused by production or release of ADH and is not associated with psychiatric comorbidity.

➤ PP is mostly seen in healthy young children when polydipsia becomes a habit after a period of increased thirst following, for example, fever or hot weather. Compulsive polydipsia is also seen in patients with stress/anxiety/obsessive-compulsive disorder (OCD), neurodevelopmental disorders such as autism, bipolar disorder or developmental delay, as well as in patients with psychosis such as schizophrenia.

➤ PP needs to be differentiated from DI (Table 15.2).

TABLE 15.2 Differential diagnoses between PP and DI

	PP	DI
Sudden onset	No	Possible
Otherwise symptomatic	Yes	No
Failure to thrive	No	Yes
Nocturnal PP	No	Yes
Serum Na	<135 mmol/L	Normal or increased
Serum osmolality	<280 mOsm/kg	Normal or >300 mOsm/kg

PRACTICE POINTS

- Children with PP are easily diagnosed by the long history, absence of weight loss or failure to thrive. Low serum osmolality (<280 mOsm/kg) and urine specific gravity <1005 confirm the diagnosis. A specific gravity greater than 1.005 excludes the diagnosis of DI. The water restriction test is the gold standard to distinguish PP from cranial DI.
- The main risk of excessive drinking is the development of dilutional hyponatraemia, as water intake exceeds the water excretion capacity by the kidneys. This can lead to water intoxication with symptoms of cerebral oedema of delirium and vomiting.
- Management includes voluntary restriction of water intake, removing any stress/anxiety and behavioural therapy.

DIABETES INSIPIDUS

➤ The maintenance of water balance is primarily dependent on normal thirst, the hormone arginine vasopressin (AVP, also called ADH) synthesis and renal tubular responsiveness to the AVP.

➤ DI is a heterogenous disorder characterized by a disturbance in water balance that manifests by passing large volumes of diluted urine.

➤ There are two forms of DI: Cranial (caused by deficiency in AVP) and the more common nephrogenic DI (AVP resistance) (Box 15.5, Box 15.6).

BOX 15.5 Summary of both forms of DI

Cranial DI

- Aetiology   A variety of diseases (Box 15.6) that affect the hypothalamic-hypophysial axis.
- Presentation   Polyuria, excessive thirst, hyperthermia, vomiting, convulsion, constipation.
- Diagnosis   Confirming polyuria. Water deprivation test. High serum sodium and osmolality. Urine: Low osmolality. A first morning urine specific gravity more than 1010 makes it unlikely. Urine osmolality >800 mOsm/kg with

serum osmolality <270 mOsm/kg rules out DI. Brain MRI. Measurement of AVP.

- Therapy   Depends on the aetiology. Regular replacement of AVP with desmopressin, which is a synthetic analogue of the hormone AVP.

Nephrogenic DI

- Aetiology   Inability to concentrate urine due to insensitivity of the renal tubules to AVP resulting from mutations in the AVP receptor 2 gene, which has an X-linked recessive inheritance.
- Presentation   As noted earlier.
- Diagnosis   As noted earlier. Genetic testing.
- Therapy   Medications including amiloride and hydrochlorothiazide.

BOX 15.6 Causes of DI

- **Cranial DI (AVP deficient)**
  - ❼ Familial autosomal dominant inheritance
  - ❼ Post-trauma such as motor vehicle accidents
  - ❼ Agenesis of corpus callosum
  - ❼ Sarcoidosis
  - ❼ Pituitary mass adenoma is the most common cause
  - ❼ Autoimmune
  - ❼ Brain tumours such as glioma and craniopharyngioma
  - ❼ Inflammation such as TB meningitis
  - ❼ Drugs (e.g., antiepileptic drugs)
- **Nephrogenic DI (AVP resistant)**
  - ❼ Congenital X-linked
  - ❼ Drugs (lithium, which is used for bipolar disease)

PRACTICE POINTS

- In clinical practice, a child suspected of DI who has daily urine output of <1–1.5 L/day (depending on the age) is very unlikely to have DI (in adults, it is < 2.5 L/day).
- Early morning measurement of simultaneous serum osmolality, urine osmolality and serum electrolytes is essential.
- Although the diagnosis of DI is easy with a classical presentation of polydipsia and polyuria, the diagnosis of mild DI can be delayed leading to high levels of sodium and osmolality, which can cause an encephalopathic picture with brain damage.

GROWTH DISORDERS

The most common endocrine complaints seen at GP surgeries are those related to height (especially cases of short stature), weight (overweight or underweight) and pubertal maturity (premature or delayed onset of puberty).

Short Stature

Core Messages

➤ Normal height is dependent on a complex interaction between genetic factors and hormonal, nutritional and psychosocial components. Children normally have their highest growth rate from birth to 1 year of life (23–28 cm), which decreases by the age 1–3 years (7.5–13 cm/year) and age 3 years to puberty (5–7 cm/year) and increases during puberty (8–9 cm in girls and 10–10.5 cm in boys/year).

➤ Short stature (SS) affects 2.5% of children and is an important reason for consulting primary care physicians, paediatricians and endocrinologists. It comprises about half of referrals to paediatric endocrinology. SS is defined as height <2 standard deviations (SD) below the mean or less than the third centile for age and sex.

➤ Growth monitoring must distinguish normal from pathological SS (Box 15.7). The three most common causes of SS are familial SS, constitutional delay of growth and malnutrition worldwide. In Western countries, small for gestational age (SGA) with no catch-up growth and growth hormone (GH) deficiency are the most common pathological diagnoses of SS.

BOX 15.7 Normal and pathological causes of short stature

- **Normal SS**
  - ❼ Familial short stature
  - ❼ Constitutional delay
- **Abnormal growth disorders**
  - ❼ SGA
  - ❼ GH deficiency
  - ❼ Malnutrition
  - ❼ Skeletal dysplasia
  - ❼ Chronic diseases (inflammatory bowel disease, coeliac disease)
  - ❼ Psychosocial
  - ❼ Chromosomal (Turner's syndrome)
  - ❼ Endocrine (hypothyroidism)
- **Idiopathic short stature, which is a diagnosis of exclusion**

➤ Normal SS includes 'Familial SS' with a final adult height achieved below the third centile. Affected children have short parents and normal growth rate and bone age and enter puberty at the normal time. Their ultimate height is related to their parental height. Children with 'constitutional delay of growth' have normal growth rate but delayed onset of puberty (aged 13 years in females and 14 years in males) and bone age. Because of delayed bone age, they have more time to grow, and they usually achieve a normal adult height appropriate to the family pattern.

➤ Low birthweight (LBW) is defined as a birthweight of <2500 g which includes both preterm neonates (born <37 weeks' gestation with appropriate size for the gestational age) and neonates with LBW for gestational age (SGA). The latter is defined as a birthweight and/or length below the normal <−2 SD.

➤ The GH–insulin-like growth factor-1 (IGF-1) axis is a fundamental component of growth. Genetic defects of this GH–IGF-1 axis include genetic mutations of GH deficiency, GH insensitivity, and low activity of IGF-1.

➤ Girls with Turner's syndrome (TS) present with SS in >90% of cases. Early recognition and treatment with GH can lead to excellent growth.

Recommended Investigations

➤ Full blood count (FBC), C-reactive protein (CRP) or erythrocyte sedimentation rate (ESR).
➤ Function tests for renal, liver and thyroid.
➤ Immunoglobulin A (IgA).
➤ Ca, P, and alkaline phosphatase.
➤ Tissue transglutaminase (TTG).
➤ Karyotyping (or follicle-stimulating hormone [FSH] if karyotyping is not available).
➤ Bone age, skeletal survey (if skeletal disproportion is present).
➤ IGF-1.

PRACTICE POINTS

- Children's growth is like trees; they grow faster in spring and summer; therefore, growth velocity should be measured yearly. Parents of children with SS often seek medical services because of a possible 'endocrine' cause; endocrine diseases are rare – no more than 5% of cases.
- The 9-centile growth charts should be used, which describe growth patterns precisely. They show the 0.4 and 99.6 centiles, and, therefore, only 1 child in 250 lies below or above these lines, which are more significant than the 3-centile growth charts.
- Measuring a baseline length at 6–8 weeks of age is recommended. Measuring the height of both parents is essential in evaluating a child with SS and predicting the ultimate height of the child.
- When evaluating children with SS, it is more important how their growth rate has been rather than where the centile is on the chart.
- The term SS is often confused with growth failure. SS is defined as height less than the third centile with normal annual growth rate, while growth failure is defined as a growth rate <5 cm/year.
- GH is a major counter-regulatory hormone to insulin; therefore, children with GH deficiency may present with hypoglycaemia, particularly during fasting or mild illness.

- Always consider TS when pubertal delay is combined with SS. Signs may be subtle, as children can achieve normal adrenarche, and a few have breast development.
- Although most short children do not have GH deficiency, it should not be missed because it is potentially treatable (Box 15.8).

BOX 15.8 Characteristic features of a child with GH deficiency

- Incidence: 1 in 4000–8000, affecting both sexes equally
- Normal length and weight at birth
- Appears younger than their chronological age (infantile)
- Normal intelligence
- Growth velocity <5–6 cm before the age of 4 years
- Chubby body build with normal proportion between upper and lower segments
- Delayed tooth eruption, high-pitched voice
- Genitalia are underdeveloped for the child's age
- Delayed bone age

When to Refer Children with SS

➤ UK guidance recommends referral of children with a single length or height measurement below the 0.4 centile (<2.67 SD), as this is likely to be associated with an organic cause.
➤ A child whose height is causing serious concern to their parents.
➤ Any growth velocity <4–5 cm/year. This is pathological.
➤ SS with prolonged symptoms such as weight loss, diarrhoea and anorexia.
➤ Any child with SS and evidence of hypoglycaemia.
➤ SS with dysmorphism or suggestive of TS.

Excessive Height (Tall Stature)

➤ Growth is influenced by many factors, such as hereditary, genetic, illness, nutritional, hormonal and psychological factors (Box 15.9). Growth depends on:
  ➢ Nutrition during intrauterine and first few months of life.
  ➢ GH from 6 months onwards.
  ➢ GH, thyroid hormone, adrenal glands and sex steroids.
  ➢ Leptin and insulin contribute to growth through their interaction with the GH–IGF-1 axis.
➤ Excessive height defines children who are above the 99.6th centile for age and sex on the 9-centile chart.
➤ Familial tall stature is the most common cause: Children have a normal growth rate, growth according to the mid-parental height (or with the tall parent in cases of a large discrepancy between parental heights).

BOX 15.9 Main causes of excessive height in childhood

Proportionate

- Hereditary/genetic
- Pituitary gigantism
- Soto's syndrome
- Endocrine causes such as precocious puberty, McCune–Albright syndrome and GH–IGF-1 axis
- Idiopathic tall stature

Disproportionate

- Marfan's syndrome
- Homocystinuria
- Klinefelter's syndrome
- Beckwith–Wiedemann syndrome (BWS)

Recommended Investigations

➤ Urine for homocysteine: Increased, but cystine is low or absent in blood.

➤ IGF-1 and GH in blood.

➤ Plasma levels of FSH, luteinizing hormone (LH) for cases of Klinefelter's syndrome.

➤ Karyotyping for suspected cases of Klinefelter's syndrome (will show 47 chromosomes XX,Y). Molecular genetic testing.

➤ Bone age and skeletal x-ray for a child with precocious puberty (e.g., McCune–Albright syndrome).

➤ Echocardiography for Marfan's syndrome to exclude aortic aneurysm.

➤ Cranial MRI for suspected pituitary tall stature to exclude adenoma.

PRACTICE POINTS

- The child's length or height must be measured accurately. In children younger than 24 months, recumbent length and standing height are not the same; the former is significantly greater. Measurement with tape is inaccurate.
- Obese children are often tall, with a height usually in the 70–99th centile.
- Girls report concern to their GPs about their height at an earlier age than boys. Society perceives tall and slender girls as beautiful, but excessive height as less acceptable than in boys.
- Marfan's syndrome (MS) is the most common cause of disproportionate tall stature (lower body segment > upper segment; arm span > height). Clinical evaluation should include cardiovascular (aortic aneurysm) and ophthalmological evaluation (lenticular dislocation). MS needs to be differentiated from homocystinuria, which is associated with intellectual disability and thrombotic phenomenon.

- Children with MS are at risk of early death because of progressive aortic dilatation. Arachnodactyly and lens dislocation are important clues which need to be differentiated from patients with homocystinuria. *Referral to a paediatrician and an ophthalmologist is important.*
- Children with Klinefelter's syndrome often present with complaints other than height, e.g., gynaecomastia, behaviour problems such a aggressiveness, excessive shyness and antisocial acts such as setting fires and criminal behaviour.
- Tall stature may be caused by precocious puberty. The skin should be examined for café-au-lait maculae to exclude McCune–Albright syndrome, which is also associated with fibrous dysplasia in the bones.
- Children with excessive height are at risk of developing orthopaedic problems such as kyphosis and scoliosis and psychiatric problems such as anxiety, depression and behaviour disorders.

PRECOCIOUS PUBERTY

Core Messages

➤ Normal sexual development begins in girls with breast development, followed by the appearance of pubic hair (sometimes simultaneously with breast development), axillary hair, onset of menstruation, acne and adult body odour. In boys, it begins with testicular enlargement ≥4 mL followed by enlargement of the penis, the appearance of pubic hair, deep voice, acne and adult body odour. These secondary sexual characteristics are accompanied by accelerated growth velocity (8–9 in girls and 10–10.5 cm in boys/year).

➤ Precocious puberty is defined as puberty occurring at an unusual age: <8 years in girls or <9 years in boys. Puberty nowadays starts earlier than in previous generations. The incidence of precocious puberty is 10- to 20-fold higher in females than in males.

➤ The causes of precocious puberty (Box 15.10) are divided into the more common form (80% of cases) of central precocious puberty (idiopathic or with identifiable causes) and peripheral (adrenal and gonadal) causes. In more than 90% of girls and 50% of boys, the cause of precocious puberty is idiopathic, i.e., no identifiable cause.

BOX 15.10 Main causes of precocious puberty

Central Precocious Puberty (GnRH-Dependent)

- Idiopathic (often genetic, including kisspeptin gene)
- Central with identifiable causes (e.g., hamartoma, neurofibromatosis-1, hydrocephalus, meningioma)
- Hypothyroidism

Peripheral (Not GnRH-Dependent)

- Gonads (ovarian cysts, McCune–Albright syndrome)
- Adrenal (e.g., congenital adrenal hyperplasia, tumour)
- Iatrogenic (external sources of sex hormones)
- Teratoma (e.g., in the mediastinum)

Partial or Normal Variant of Puberty

- Premature thelarche
- Premature adrenarche

➤ Central precocious puberty is defined as premature activation of gonadotropin-releasing hormone (GnRH) release, which is triggered and regulated by activators such as kisspeptin protein. The kisspeptin gene (*KISS1*) is a key factor to regulate puberty.

➤ Peripheral causes of precocious puberty are less common compared to central precocious puberty. Typically, there is an absence of testicular enlargement.

➤ Partial precocious puberty includes premature thelarche, which often starts before the age of 2 years as an isolated breast enlargement due to increased ovarian oestrogen FSH. The condition is benign and regresses by time. The children who develop thelarche after the age of 2 years have unpredictable outcomes, and the breast enlargement may persist until puberty. Premature adrenarche (appearance of sexual hair) is due to increased secretion of androgens from the adrenal cortex. Serum dehydroepiandrosterone (DHEA) is increased and diagnostic.

Recommended Investigations

➤ Hormonal assay of GnRH, LH, FSH and sex hormones.

➤ Serum level of I7-hydroxyprogesterone, DHEA, cortisol and aldosterone in cases of suspected congenital adrenal hyperplasia (CAH).

➤ Wrist x-ray to assess bone maturation and puberty: If bone age is within 1 year of chronological age, puberty either has not started or only just started; bone age within 2 years indicates the child is in puberty.

➤ Pelvic ultrasound scan and adrenal visualization for CAH.

➤ CT scan or MRI of the head for all cases suspected of central causes of precocious puberty.

➤ Skeletal survey for bony fibrous dysplasia with precocious puberty and hyperpigmented spots.

➤ Genetic in cases of idiopathic central precocious puberty.

PRACTICE POINTS

- A child with precocious thelarche or adrenarche needs careful evaluation, as these cannot often be easily and definitely differentiated from true precocious puberty. In precocious thelarche, the nipple is characteristically pale, immature, thin and transparent. In contrast, the breasts of genuine precocious puberty are mature with a prominent nipple and dark areola, indicating high circulating oestrogen. In addition, there is no growth acceleration or advanced bone age with partial precocious puberty.
- In any child with precocious puberty, careful search of the skin is essential: Café-au-lait maculae with smooth borders suggest neurofibromatosis type 1 (NF-1), while larger café-au-lait patches with irregular outlines is consistent with McCune–Albright syndrome (polyostotic fibrous dysplasia of bone and ovarian cysts).
- Hypothyroidism can cause precocious puberty; children are short, and the growth velocity is decreased.

DELAYED PUBERTY

Core Messages

➤ Normally, menarche occurs at a median age of 13 years and usually starts 2–3 years after the start of breast enlargement (thelarche). Penile and scrotal enlargement usually occurs 1 year after testicular enlargement.

➤ Puberty can easily be assessed by bone age (wrist x-ray): If bone age is within 1 year of chronological age, puberty either has not or has just started; bone age within 2 years indicates the child is in puberty.

➤ Delayed puberty (DP) is arbitrarily defined as a delay of pubertal changes beyond 14 years in girls and 16 years in boys. The definition includes those children who do not complete their puberty within 5 years from its start.

➤ The cause of DP in the vast majority of boys and in most girls is constitutional. Other causes are listed in Box 15.11.

BOX 15.11 Main causes of DP

Constitutional

Chronic diseases (malnutrition, Crohn's disease, coeliac disease, cystic fibrosis [CF], anorexia nervosa):
- Intensive physical exercise
- Chromosomal (Turner's, Noonan's, Klinefelter's syndromes)
- Polycystic ovarian syndrome (PCOS)
- CNS tumour (craniopharyngioma, meningioma, prolactinoma)

Prader–Willi Syndrome
- Irradiation of the gonads, chemotherapy
- Following bone marrow transplantation
- Androgen insensitivity syndrome (testicular feminization syndrome)

➤ DP is usually assessed with delayed growth and velocity for chronological age. The exceptions to that are boys with Klinefelter's syndrome (47 chromosomes, XXY is the most common pattern), who are tall with long arms and legs, having normal adrenarche but small testes.

Recommended Investigations

➤ FBC: Hb, ferritin, CRP (anaemia with high CRP suggests Crohn's disease)
➤ Screening blood tests for coeliac disease
➤ Hormonal assay: Levels of FSH/LH, GnRH, oestrogen, testosterone, prolactin, GH, 17-hydroxyprogesterone and DHEA assay for CAH
➤ Radiological investigation for suspected case of Crohn's disease
➤ Thyroid function tests (TFTs) for suspected thyroid disorders
➤ Karyotyping for suspected cases of Turner's syndrome (X0) and Klinefelter's syndrome (XX,Y)
➤ Wrist x-ray for bone age
➤ Pelvic ultrasound scan to detect ovarian cysts, tumour or ovarian dysgenesis, testicular ultrasound for tumour

PRACTICE POINTS

- With detailed history and examination, including growth measurement, diagnosis can be established in most cases.
- Remember to use the Tanner chart for pubertal stages, and never forget to obtain the height of the parents and siblings when a child presents with DP.
- While the principal cause of DP in boys is constitutional, girls have more frequent pathological causes, e.g., anorexia nervosa, chronic diseases, intensive exercise or chromosomal abnormalities.
- Once constitutional DP is established, children can be reassured that DP is inherited and physiological and that they will achieve later normal puberty.
- In girls with DP and short stature, TS is the most likely diagnosis. Mean adult height is 143–144 cm. Girls with TS achieve normal adrenarche and axillary hair at the appropriate age; thelarche and menstruation may occur in a small percentage.

Conditions Requiring Referral

➤ If the diagnosis of DP is uncertain or unclear.
➤ If pathological conditions (see the list earlier) have not been excluded. This is the principal aim when evaluating a child with DP.
➤ All girls with an inguinal hernia. They should undergo a pelvic ultrasound scan examination before herniotomy to exclude androgen insensitivity syndrome.
➤ In girls with otherwise normal sexual maturation but delayed menarche and galactorrhoea, prolactinoma is likely. Urgent prolactin level and MRI of the brain should be considered.

➤ For hormonal treatment, which is often indicated if the DP and/or growth are causing distress or school underperformance. Boys with constitutional DP may be treated with oxandrolone at age 11.5 years and testosterone at age >13.5 years and girls with ethinylestradiol or oestrogens.

➤ Girls with TS who may receive GH. Many girls achieve heights greater than 150 cm with early treatment.

EXCESSIVE HAIR

➤ Humans have approximately 5 million hair follicles distributed as lanugo (soft, unpigmented hair that sheds later); vellus hair that is short, fine and light; and terminal hair that is thick, long and pigmented.

➤ Hair growth more than what is expected for age, sex and ethnicity is termed hirsutism or hypertrichosis. It can lead to psychological problems including stress, low self-esteem, depression and social isolation.

➤ While hypertrichosis indicates a non-androgenic excessive vellus hair growth in areas not usually hairy, hirsutism is an androgen-dependent male pattern of hair growth usually in women (present in 5–10%). Androgen stimulates the conversion of vellus into terminal hair.

➤ The most common cause of hypertrichosis is racial or familial, which is frequent in people from the Mediterranean area and Indian subcontinent. The most common cause of hirsutism is PCOS, which accounts for 70–80% of cases. Among the most important endocrine causes are CAH and Cushing's syndrome (CS) (Box 15.12).

BOX 15.12 Main causes of excessive hair growth

- **Hypertrichosis**
  - ❼ Racial and familial hypertrichosis
  - ❼ Congenital hypertrichosis
  - ❼ Drugs (e.g., steroids, phenytoin, cyclosporine, minoxidil)
  - ❼ Syndromic, e.g., Cornelia de Lange's syndrome
  - ❼ Malnutrition, including anorexia nervosa
- **Hirsutism**
  - ❼ PCOS
  - ❼ Precocious puberty
  - ❼ Endocrine causes (e.g., CS, CAH)
  - ❼ Idiopathic hirsutism
  - ❼ Androgen-secreting tumour

Recommended Investigations

➤ Serum testosterone, DHEAS, LH, FSH: Serum 17-hydroxyprogesterone, DHEAS to diagnose CAH; serum prolactin for hyperprolactinaemia.

➤ TFTs.

➤ Pelvic ultrasonography to assess uterus and ovaries.

➤ MRI, particularly if hormonal studies have been inconclusive, and for pituitary adenoma and adrenal and ovarian cysts or tumours.

PRACTICE POINTS

- Any acute and/or severe hirsutism requires investigation to exclude serious underlying causes such as a tumour of the ovary, adrenal cortex or precocious puberty.
- The diagnosis of PCOS is made by at least two of the following three criteria: oligo-ovulation/anovulation, clinical or biochemical signs of hyperandrogenism and the presence of polycystic ovary. Girls are often obese and have hyperinsulinism, insulin resistance and acanthosis nigricans (hyperpigmented area which may also be associated with internal malignancy). They are at high risk of developing T2DM. Androgen excess may cause deepening voice, acne and a masculine body.
- An enlarged and fused clitoris resembling a penis and labial fusion present at birth. A mistaken diagnosis of cryptorchidism and hypospadias is often made. These may be signs of CAH.

GOITRE AND HYPOTHYROIDISM

Midline neck lumps are discussed in Box 15.13.

BOX 15.13 Main causes of goitre and midline lumps

- Goitre
    - ❼ Congenital (e.g., caused by defects in thyroxine synthesis)
    - ❼ Endemic due to deficiency of dietary iodine
    - ❼ Resulting from thyroiditis (e.g., chronic autoimmune thyroiditis)
    - ❼ Drugs causing goitre (e.g., lithium)
    - ❼ Hyperthyroid goitre
- Ectopic thyroid tissue
- Thyroglossal cyst and duct
- Cystic hygroma
- Branchial cyst (usually off centre of the neck)
- Dermoid cyst
- Pharyngeal pouch

PRACTICE POINTS

- Thyroglossal cyst, which develops from a remnant thyroglossal duct, is painless but becomes enlarged and tender if infected. A pathognomonic sign is its upward movement on swallowing and tongue protrusion.
- The usual branchial cyst appears as an insignificant-looking papule on the side of the neck (in contrast to thyroglossal cyst). In terms of surgical removal, it may be quite difficult to trace out its tract.
- Excision of a midline cyst should never be considered before ensuring that it is not a thyroid mass.

HYPOTHYROIDISM

➤ A screening programme for congenital hypothyroidism (CH) has been in place since 1974 in the UK. Early detection and treatment (within the first few weeks of life) of CH through neonatal screening prevent irreversible neurodevelopmental delay and optimize its developmental outcome. Adequately treated children have normal growth, puberty and fertility.

➤ Causes of hypothyroidism are numerous and are summarized in Box 15.14. Hypothyroidism is more common in patients with autoimmune diseases such as T1DM and coeliac disease and in those with Down's syndrome and TS.

BOX 15.14 Classification of the main causes of hypothyroidism

● **Primary Hypothyroidism**
  ❼ Thyroid dysgenesis (absence, hypoplastic, ectopic)
  ❼ Iodine deficiency
  ❼ Dyshormonogenesis
  ❼ Chronic autoimmune thyroiditis (Hashimoto's disease)
  ❼ Drugs (amiodarone, lithium)
● **Secondary Hypothyroidism** (TSH deficiency due to defect of its release):
  ❼ Isolated
  ❼ Association with other pituitary hormone deficiency
● **Tertiary Hypothyroidism** (thyrotropin-releasing hormone deficiency)

➤ Thyroid dysgenesis (athyreosis, hypoplastic or ectopic) comprises 65–70% of CH cases. Dyshormonogenesis usually presents as a goitre that can be detected at 20–22 weeks' gestation. If a fetal goitre is diagnosed, cordocentesis or amniocentesis is performed to assess fetal thyroid function. If hypothyroidism is confirmed, intraamniotic thyroxin injections are performed.

➤ Apart from CH, in iodine-sufficient areas, the most common cause of hypothyroidism is chronic autoimmune thyroiditis (Hashimoto's thyroiditis), which is associated with antithyroid autoantibodies such as thyroid peroxidase and thyroglobulin antibodies.

Recommended Investigations

➤ TFTs.
➤ Autoantibodies, including antithyroid antibodies, and thyroid peroxidase (TPO).
➤ Ultrasound scan may show scattered decreased echogenicity.
➤ Knee x-ray to assess the severity of intrauterine hypothyroidism.
➤ Radioisotope scan.
➤ Genetic testing, as clinically indicated, includes newly available 'comparative genomic hybridization array and whole exome sequencing'.

PRACTICE POINTS

- A newborn with an abnormal neonatal screening result should be referred as soon as possible (within 2 weeks of life) to a specialist centre.
- If the screening result indicates a low thyroxine (T_4) and a high thyroid-stimulating hormone (TSH), treatment should start immediately. If the serum TSH >20 mU/L, treatment should start within the first 2 weeks even if the T_4 is normal. Treatment is less urgent if the TSH is 6–20 mU/L. The recommended dose is currently 15 µg/kg/day, which is higher than the 5–10 µg/kg/day previously recommended, in order to normalize thyroid function rapidly within the first 2 weeks of life.
- TSH normalizes slower than T_4. Therefore, the first goal of treatment is to normalize the T_4 as rapidly as possible. The second goal is to normalise the TSH within 4 weeks. Maintaining a normal TSH below 5 mU/L and T_4 in the upper half of the age-specific reference ranges has been associated with optimal neurodevelopmental outcome. A prolonged period of low T_4 levels (under 10 µg/dL) is associated with a poor neurodevelopmental outcome.
- Foods should not be consumed for at least 30 minutes after taking the T_4 tablet. For young infants, the tablet should be crushed and mixed with breast milk or water. Soy formula interferes with absorption.

TRANSGENDER

Introduction

➤ 'Transgender' or 'trans' refers to a group of individuals whose gender identity differs from the assigned sex at birth. Characteristics of terms related to this subject are shown in Box 15.15. In the UK, approximately 1% of the population aged 16–24 years identify as transgender. In the 2021 census, about 262,000 people aged ≥16 years in England and Wales said that their gender identity was different from that on their birth certificate.

➤ Published literature suggests that transgender people experience significant inequality and discrimination (about 70%). Many also experience loneliness, social isolation, bullying and violence.

➤ Transgender people feel they are medically underserved, as they experience poorer health outcomes and lower quality of life than the general population. They are facing health professionals who lack gender-specific knowledge. They also have a higher incidence of depression and anxiety and increased mortality rates compared to general population.

➤ Primary care professionals and paediatricians can play a key role in supporting children and young people who are transgender or gender non-conforming. They will be seeing a lot more transgender children in the future who may present with totally unrelated medical problems such as gastroenteritis, cough and asthma. Both types of healthcare professionals are encouraged to take on emerging roles as coordinators of care within regional paediatric transgender services. Management of puberty blockers and affirmative hormones for those who may need them are significant issues they may face.

BOX 15.15 Terminology related to transgender patients

• Cisgender	• Any individual whose gender identity matches the sex identity at birth.
• Gender identity	• An internal sense of being a man, a woman or some other gender.
• Non-binary	• A person who does not identify as exclusively a man or a woman.
• Gender dysphoria	• The severe distress and emotional discomfort many transgender people experience because of their status.
• Transsexual	• The desire of some transgenders to seek medical assistance to transition from one sex to another.
• Diagnostic overshadow	• A misdiagnosis attributing a patient's health concerns and problems to their trans status.
• Gender non-conforming	• A person whose behaviour, interests or actions do not conform to the societal expectations based on biological sex.
• Gender role	• Describes how a person presents themself as masculine or feminine in the context of societal expectations.
• GIDS	• Gender Identity and Development Service, to which an increasing number of children have been referred to in England, especially those registered as female at birth.
• WPATH	• The World Professional Association for Transgender Health is an international multidisciplinary organization that was founded in 1979 to provide clinical guidance to healthcare professionals with evidence-based care, education, research and public policy for transgender individuals.

PRACTICE POINTS

- The number of transgender patients presenting for treatment is increasing. It is essential that primary care clinicians and paediatricians attain the adequate knowledge to provide comfort care and improve transgender patients' health outcomes.
- Under the Gender Recognition Act 2004, UK adults can obtain a gender recognition certificate (GRC) if they meet the following criteria:
  - Have gender dysphoria
  - Have lived full time in the acquired gender for at least 2 years
  - Provide a declaration to remain permanently in the acquired gender
  - Are 18 or over
  - Pay a £5 fee

  After obtaining the GRC, the acquired gender can be recorded on the birth, marriage and death certificates.

- Transgender people can request to change their name and gender at any time and do not need to undergo any reassignment treatment. GP practices do not need to wait for any documents, updated birth certificate or GRC to make the changes. The transgender patient will be given a new National Health Services (NHS) number and registered as a new patient. GP practices must inform Primary Care Support England (PCSE) with their name, NHS number and confirmation that a new NHS has been created and the individual is aware of it. PCSE will then send the practice a new patient record using the new details and transfer all medical information from the original record.
- It is good practice in primary care to ask the patient's preferences in terms of the physical examination, especially if they have experienced gender dysphoria related to their body. They may wish to be examined by a doctor of their own gender.

Legal Aspects

➤ The Equalities Act 2010 incudes transgender status among the nine 'protected characteristics that protect them from discrimination, harassment and victimisation'. This indicates that transgender patients must never be refused treatment or care because of their status.

➤ The right of transgender people to privacy and confidentiality was established by the Gender Recognition Act 2004. It states that information about a person's gender recognition process is protected and that disclosing their history without their consent is an offence.

➤ Primary care professionals should ensure that transgender individuals are aware of national screening programmes, including breast, cervical and bowel cancers, and are referred to them if they consent. Screening for transgender and non-binary people is shown in Box 15.16.

BOX 15.16 Guidelines on screening transgender and non-binary patients

Trans-women and non-binary people who are registered with a GP as female:
- Are invited for breast and bowel cancer screening.
- Are not invited for cervical screening and abdominal aortic aneurysm (AAA).

Trans-women and non-binary people who registered with a GP as male:
- Are invited for bowel cancer screening and AAA.
- Are not invited for breast screening but can request it.
- Do not need cervical screening.

Trans-men and non-binary people who are registered with a GP as female:
- Are invited for breast, bowel cancer and cervical screening.
- Are not invited for AAA.

Trans-men and non-binary people who are registered with a GP as male:
- Are invited for bowel cancer and AAA screening.
- Are not invited for cervical screening but can request it.

Medical Management

➤ Several organizations provide clinical practice guidelines for the treatment of transgender youth, including WPATH and the Endocrine Society. Medical intervention is based on pubertal stages (Box 15.17).

➤ The diagnosis of gender dysphoria should be made by a mental health professional with expertise in gender identity prior to considering hormonal therapy.

➤ The aim of medical transgender interventions is to prevent the development of unwanted secondary sex characteristics of the biological sex and to promote the development of desired secondary sex characteristics of the affirmed gender.

➤ Transgender people who are undergoing pubertal suppression should be monitored for height, weight and pubertal staging as well as biochemical assessment of puberty using LH, FSH, oestradiol, testosterone and bone age evaluation.

➤ Medical interventions include pubertal suppression using GnRH agonists, reduction in biological hormone production using progestins and use of androgen receptor antagonists such as spironolactone. Masculinizing hormone regimens consist of testosterone, and feminizing hormone regimens consist of both oestradiol and spironolactone.

➤ Gender surgery procedures may include genital and chest surgeries, breast augmentation surgery, vaginoplasty and orchiectomy.

BOX 15.17 Guidelines for medical intervention based on pubertal stages

● Prepubertal   No medical intervention
● Pubertal   Eligibility for pubertal blockers
● Postpubertal   Eligibility for feminizing and masculinizing hormonal therapy

CHAPTER 16

Musculoskeletal

COMMON MINOR ORTHOPAEDIC ANOMALIES

Toe Walking

➤ This is usually a common finding in healthy children up to 2–3 years of age, affecting around 5% of toddlers without an associated medical cause (known as idiopathic toe walking [ITW]). ITW should be a diagnosis of exclusion with no associated orthopaedical or neurological signs. The condition can lead to a risk of tripping or falling in addition to parental concern.

➤ If toe walking persists beyond 2–3 years, other diagnoses should be considered (Box 16.1). Children with Duchene muscular dystrophy (DMD) and cerebral palsy (CP) may toe walk as the initial presentation of their illness.

➤ Features that suggest a benign nature and a good prognosis of ITW include:

➢ Toddler's age.
➢ Intermittency of toe walking, i.e., sometimes heel–toe walking.
➢ Full ranges of active and passive motion of the ankle joints.
➢ No limitation in ankle dorsiflexion (the upwards flexion of the foot towards the shin).
➢ No associated neuromuscular abnormalities.

BOX 16.1 Causes and therapeutical measures for toe walking

Causes	Therapy
● Idiopathic	● Muscle stretching exercises
● Achilles tendon tightness	● Serial casting
● Neuromuscular dystrophy	● Ankle–foot orthoses
● CP	● Botulinum toxin type A injection
● Congenital talipes equinovarus	● Surgical interventions, e.g., lengthening of
● Autistic spectrum disorder	Achilles tendon

DOI: 10.1201/9781032642888-16

Intoeing (Forefoot Adduction Deformity)

➤ This is a common foot adduction deformity in newborns (almost universal) and young children characterized by the forefoot deviating medially. The condition is usually self-limiting, and about 90% of flexible metatarsus cases resolve spontaneously. Severe forms may persist into later childhood causing stumbling or tripping.

➤ Forefoot adduction deformity may be due to a metatarsal adductus, tibial (internal tibial torsion) or femoral anomaly (femoral anteversion) causing medially facing patellae. Metatarsus adductus is defined as an adduction of the foot at the tarso-metatarsal joint with normal alignment in the mid- and hindfoot (Figure 16.1). About 10% of children with femoral anteversion have acetabular dysplasia predisposing to hip dislocation. Therefore, careful examination of the hip is essential.

➤ In most cases, the deformity can be passively corrected and overcorrected by active manipulation or stroking the lateral border of the foot. This mild degree of deformity usually requires no treatment. Some cases where feet correct to a neutral position but not overcorrect may benefit from orthotics or corrective shoes. Rigid feet which do not correct to a neutral position are usually treated with serial plaster casts.

➤ Radiographic assessment of the condition is utilized in severe cases for measuring the angle between the second metatarsal and longitudinal axis. A high degree of the angle suggests a severe form of the metatarsus.

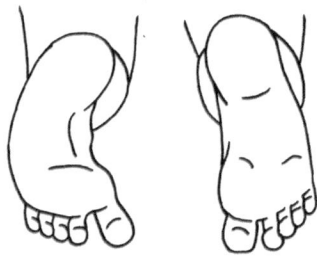

FIGURE 16.1 Intoeing due to metatarsus adductus, more noticeable in the left foot.

Flatfeet (Pes Planus)

➤ This is a common (about 50–60% aged <5 years) and usually considered a normal foot position in the early years of childhood due to ligament laxity, mostly inherited as autosomal dominant. On standing and walking, collapse of the longitudinal arch causes abduction of the forefoot and valgus position of the hindfoot (Figure 16.2). Significant improvement occurs by the age of 6 years. Children with obesity have a higher prevalence of flatfoot than normal-weight children.

➤ Primary care clinicians should distinguish between the two broad types of paediatric flatfoot: Flexible and the rigid flatfoot (Box 16.2). Family history: Associated medical conditions, history of trauma, presence or absence of symptoms (pain, decreased activity endurance) and age of onset help differentiate both types.

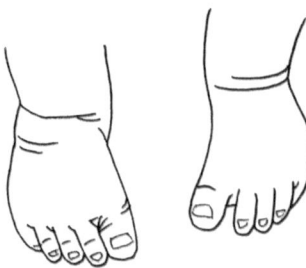

FIGURE 16.2 Bilateral flat feet.

BOX 16.2 Differences between the two types of flatfoot

Type 1 is the common physiological and usually asymptomatic type, defined as an absence or reduction of the medial longitudinal arch on weight bearing and restoring it on not bearing weight, standing on tip toes or with Jack's test (rise of the arch with great toe passively in dorsiflexion). Radiological evaluation is not required. If symptomatic, foot orthoses (specially designed shoe inserts) are beneficial.

Type 2 is the rigid symptomatic type associated with pain and difficulty with walking, often persists into adulthood and may require surgery. It is defined by persistent loss of the medial longitudinal arch in both weight-wearing and non-weight-bearing positions. Radiological evaluation (CT scan is the gold standard) is indicated and mostly shows tarsal coalition (bones grow into one another).

➤ Treatment is not required unless the condition is symptomatic such as pain or abnormal shoe wear. Management includes activity modification, stretching and strengthening exercises, orthoses and reduction of weight in case of obesity.

Clubfoot (Congenital Talipes Equinovarus)

➤ The incidence is around 1–2 per 1000 live births. Most cases are congenital and idiopathic, with a higher male to female proportion of 2:1.

➤ Clubfoot is either unilateral (30–40%) or bilateral (60–70%), positional (most cases) or structural, an isolated deformity or a manifestation of chromosomal abnormalities. Positional clubfoot can be corrected and overcorrected by manipulation. Structural clubfoot is either idiopathic (the most common congenital limb defect) as an isolated abnormality confined to the feet or associated with neuromuscular or chromosomal disorders (Table 16.1). The feet can be discovered by prenatal ultrasonography from 12 weeks' gestation.

➤ The deformity is characterized by metatarsus adductus, cavus foot and equinus position.

➤ Conservative treatment is initiated for most cases with structural clubfoot, including stretching, taping and serial plaster casts. Ponseti plaster casting, weekly or three times a week, has shown to be superior to soft tissue release and has become the

TABLE 16.1 Summary of the three types of clubfoot

Type	Characteristics
Positional	Can be corrected and overcorrected, benign and likely to resolve without treatment. It can be corrected with some overcorrection on passive manipulation.
Isolated	Confined to the lower limbs due to multifactorial causes such as genetic and environmental (e.g., oligohydramnios).
Non-isolated	Syndromic is associated with other congenital diseases such as neuromuscular diseases (e.g., distal arthrogryposis or as congenital myotonic dystrophy) or chromosomal abnormality such as microdeletion or duplication.

gold standard as the first-line treatment. It involves 6–8 weeks of a long leg plaster cast (toe to groin) that requires a change once a week. About 90% require an Achilles tenotomy.

Bowlegs (Genu Varum)

➤ Most cases of bowlegs are physiological and commonly seen in toddlers aged 1–3 years resulting from external rotation of the hip combined with internal tibial torsion (Figure 16.3). It can occur unilaterally or bilaterally. Improvement occurs at the age of 2 years, when it changes to neutral position by 18–24 months and continues to reach genu valgus (knock-knee) by the age of 3 years.

➤ If varus deformity persists or progresses beyond 18–24 months of age, the deformity does not resolve and is pathological. If untreated, it can lead to abnormal joint loading and a subsequent risk of premature osteoarthritis.

➤ Idiopathic tibia vara (Blount's disease, Figure 16.4) is an abnormal progressive angulation below the knee. The condition may occur as infantile (1–3 years), juvenile (4–10 years) and adolescent (>10 years). The infantile form is the most common and is often related to obesity.

➤ Therapy for severe and/or unresolving bowlegs includes braces and unilateral or bilateral high tibial osteotomy.

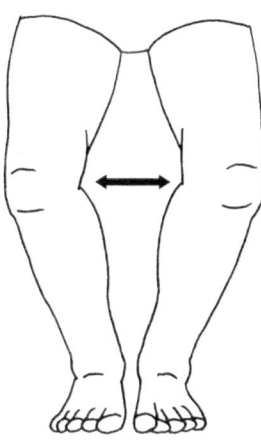

FIGURE 16.3 Bowing of the legs.

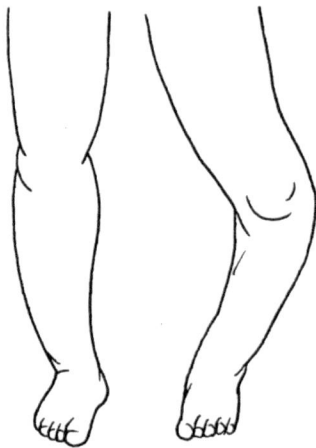

FIGURE 16.4 Tibial bowing (Blount's disease of the left leg).

BOX 16.3 Most common causes of genu varus

● **Physiological** The most common form is physiological and improves by the age of 2 years. X-ray confirms the physiological bowlegs and can exclude pathological causes. Tibial meta-physeal-diaphyseal angle <11 degrees.

● **Pathological**
  ❯ Persistent varus deformity by the age of 2–3 years with an intercondylar distance >5 cm.
  ❯ Blount's disease is uncommon, occurring after the age of 2 years, and is progressive. X-ray of the knee is diagnostic, showing medial tibial metaphyseal 'beaking'. The tibial metaphyseal-diaphyseal angle >16 degrees.
  ❯ Rickets: Other rachitic changes are present, e.g., enlarged wrists. Bone profile and vitamin D level are diagnostic.

Knock-Knees (Genu Valgus)

➤ Genu valgus in children aged 2–6 years is normal and physiological provided that the intermalleolar distance does not exceed 8 cm, as measured by a ruler (Figure 16.5). Within this distance, the deformity can be regarded as minor and should spontaneously undergo a resolution in the next 2–3 years.

➤ In the event of conspicuous and enlarged intermalleolar distance or asymmetrical or unilateral deformities, metabolic, genetic and other causes need to be excluded (Box 16.4). There is a strong association between genu valgus and obesity, which is usually symmetric.

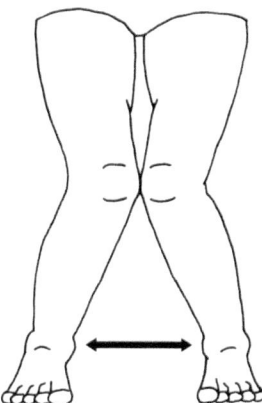

FIGURE 16.5 Knock-knees.

BOX 16.4 Causes of genu valgus deformity

- Idiopathic
- Obesity
- Nutritional, hypophosphataemic rickets
- Post-traumatic
- Renal osteodystrophy
- Osteochondrodystrophy

➤ Investigation includes full blood count (FBC), bone profile and vitamin D level. X-ray of the knees is indicated to confirm the valgus deformity and to exclude secondary causes. Surgery such as hemiepiphysiodesis or osteotomy may be required if the deformity is abnormal and increasing despite conservative therapy.

Syndactyly

➤ Syndactyly, or digit fusion, is found in 1:2000–3000 live births, typically via webbing. It can be isolated (non-syndromic), which is far more common, or syndromic, comprising more than 300 distinct anomalies. Non-isolated syndactyly manifests as nine distinct types with at least eight relevant genes.

➤ Complete or incomplete webbing between the second and third toe is common and normal in children, requiring no intervention.

➤ In syndactyly of the fingers, there may be a shared important neurovascular bundle between the digits. As associated syndromes are numerous, referral is advisable.

Polydactyly

➤ Extra digits or toes occur in approximately 1–2 per 1000 live births and range from a rudimentary extra digit to a fully formed and functioning duplicate digit. About a third of them have a positive family history inherited as an autosomal dominant trait.

➤ In most cases (80%), the polydactyly is an isolated finding (non-syndromic), and in the remaining 20% of cases, the condition (syndromic) is associated with numerous syndromes and chromosomal abnormalities.

➤ At birth it is important to identify any potential syndrome by taking a careful history and performing a physical examination. For example, Carpenter's syndrome is associated with craniosynostosis in addition to polydactyly. Finding polydactyly should lead to examine the skull to diagnose the closure of the sutures.

➤ Treatment of polydactyly is always surgical.

Single Palmar Crease (Figure 16.6)

This is often a normal finding on one hand (about 5% of the population) or both hands. It is sometimes associated with syndromes such as Down's syndrome or foetal alcohol syndrome.

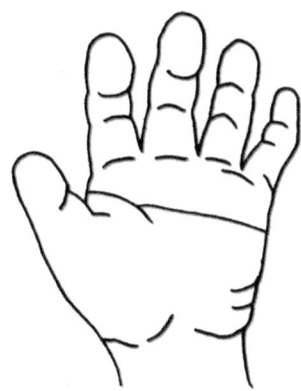

FIGURE 16.6 Single palmar crease.

Musculoskeletal Problems: Pain and Injury

➤ Musculoskeletal (MSK) problems are a common reason for visiting primary care providers and account for 17% of GP consultations each year, including 7–8% of children, with a higher proportion in males than in females. Pain is the most common symptoms of MSK problems, followed by limping, stiffness, muscle weakness and fatigue.

➤ Acute MSK pain is defined as pain lasting <3 months and usually caused by injury, illness or medical procedures. The main caused of MSK trauma are shown in Box 16.5.

> **BOX 16.5** Main causes for consultations due to MSK problems
>
> ### Trauma (Age-Related)
>
> - Head and neck:
> - Upper limb:
> - Lower limb:
>
> - About 15% of all injuries, e.g., head injury
> - About 30%, falls, bicycle injury, sort-related
> - About 50–60%
>
> ### Spinal Diseases
>
> - Trauma
> - Kyphosis, lordosis
>
> ### Joint Disorders
>
> - Arthralgia
> - Arthritis

Investigation (Extent of Tests Is as Clinically Indicated)

➤ In a child with trauma, peripheral pulses and capillary refill time must be checked.
➤ High FBC and C-reactive protein (CRP) will support bacterial infection or arthritis.

➣ Autoantibody screen for autoimmune inflammatory diseases.
➣ Hb electrophoresis and peripheral film for sickle cell anaemia (SCA).
➣ X-ray of the arm excludes fracture or dislocation.
➣ CT scan and/or MRI gives much more detail than conventional x-rays.
➣ Spinal x-ray is indicated if spinal lesions are suspected.
➣ Bone scan in case of suspected osteomyelitis or malignancy.
➣ Urine for proteinuria and to confirm porphyria if clinically indicated.

Management

➤ Guidelines for the management of painful MSK conditions advocate a holistic approach incorporating education, psychological and physical interventions (Box 16.6).

> **BOX 16.6** Management of MSK pain
>
> - Non-pharmacological treatment
>   - ❯ Self-management advice and education
>   - ❯ Exercise therapy, manual therapy/physiotherapy
>   - ❯ Psychosocial intervention
>   - ❯ Complementary therapy (e.g., acupuncture)
> - Pharmacological treatment
>   - ❯ Basic analgesics
>   - ❯ Paracetamol: 10–15 mg/kg 4–6 hourly
>   - ❯ Ibuprofen 10 mg/kg 8 hourly
>   - ❯ Diclofenac 50–100 mg 8 hourly
>   - ❯ Opioids
>   - ❯ Buprenorphine 100–300 micrograms 6–8 hourly
>   - ❯ Co-codamol 30/500 mg 6 hourly as required
>   - ❯ Codeine phosphate: 30 mg 3–4 times/day

Arthralgia (Painful Joints)

➤ Arthralgia indicates joint pain not accompanied by obvious clinical signs of arthritis. Every attempt should be made to localize the arthralgia. Once the painful joint is identified, the differential diagnosis becomes easy (Box 16.7).

➤ Arthralgia may be generalized, involving multiple joints caused mostly by a viral infection, or involve the hip, knee, ankle or temporomandibular joint.

➤ The best approach to a child with arthralgia and normal examination is to perform a careful initial evaluation and inflammatory tests (such as white blood cell [WBC], CRP) followed by periodic monitoring for changes in symptoms or physical findings.

➤ Parents are usually worried that a rapid diagnosis often cannot be made and clinicians are not telling them what is wrong with their child. Informing the parents that there is a plan in place to monitor their child's symptoms should help alleviate parental concern.

BOX 16.7 Main causes of arthralgia

Generalized
- Acute viral infection
- SCA
- Henoch–Schönlein purpura
- Familial Mediterranean fever (FMF)
- Fibromyalgia
- Chronic fatigue syndrome
- Porphyria
- Pre-arthritic stage of juvenile idiopathic arthritis (JIA)

Hip
- Hip pain (e.g., transient synovitis, Perthes disease)

Knee
- Chondromalacia, subluxation, osteochondritis

Ankle
- Sport injury, sprains

PRACTICE POINTS

- Arthralgia in association with acute viral illness should be considered as part of myalgia affecting the tissue surrounding the joints.
- Before diagnosing arthralgia, doctors should ensure that there are no signs of arthritis (red, hot and swollen joint) and no obvious clinical evidence of effusion in the joint.
- The differential diagnosis of arthralgia of the hip includes transient synovitis. Typical history: A child aged 3–7 years wakens with severe groin pain causing refusal to walk or limping. Other causes include Perthes disease or slipped capital femoral epiphysis. The latter affects typically obese short children or those with a rapid growth spurt.
- A painful knee may be caused by traumatic synovitis, haemarthrosis, chondromalacia patella, patellar subluxation or dislocation, synovial plicae or Osgood–Schlatter disease.

- Patellar subluxation is not uncommon and can be detected when the knee is in full extension. Displacing the patella laterally often results in the patient pushing away or grabbing the examiner's hand (apprehension sign).
- A painful ankle is often due to a sport injury (most common cause), referred pain from avascular necrosis of the navicular bone (Köhler's disease) or the metatarsal head (Freiberg's disease).
- Although persistent arthralgia without evidence of arthritis is uncommon in JIA, arthralgia lasting several weeks may occur in the pre-arthritic stage of the disease.
- Knee pain may be a referred pain originating from a diseased hip such as transient synovitis.
- The finding of haemarthrosis (usually in the knee) is indicative of a serious injury to ligaments, meniscus or occult fracture. *Urgent referral is indicated.*

Painful Arm

➤ In children, arm pain usually results from MSK injuries (sprains, strains, contusion, dislocation and fracture). Box 16.8 lists the main causes.

➤ In the absence of dislocation and fracture, a musculoskeletal pain syndrome (MSPS) can be considered. The pain may affect either part of the arm, the whole upper arm or forearm, occurring suddenly or gradually, constantly or intermittently, often associated with burning or numbing sensation.

➤ If there is a history suggestive of injury, e.g., sport activity, the diagnosis is evident. A moderate-severe injury is likely to be followed by an inflammatory response which manifests as pain, spasm, reduced arm movement and redness and swelling.

➤ Less common causes of arm pain include neurovascular, cardiovascular disorders and referred pain from another area such as the neck, chest and abdomen.

BOX 16.8 Main causes of pain in the arm

Trauma-Related

- Sprains, strains, overused muscle
- Viral infection
- Child abuse
- Pulled elbow (nursemaid's elbow)

Non-Specific MSK Pain Syndrome

- Chronic fatigue syndrome (CFS)
- Fibromyalgia
- Reflex sympathetic dystrophy

Inflammatory

- Arthritis (e.g., viral infection)
- Tendonitis and tenosynovitis
- Neuritis (neuropathy)

Spinal

- Cervical nerve root compression
- Brachial plexus

Referred Pain

PRACTICE POINTS

- Muscle pain usually consists of aches, cramps, spasms or twitching. If the pain has a neuropathic component, then there would be a sensation of burning or electrical shock and pins and needles.
- MSPS is a diagnosis of exclusion. The pain is poorly localized, and physical examination is normal except tenderness to light touch over several areas of the arm. Laboratory findings are usually normal. Fibromyalgia and reflex sympathetic dystrophy are variant manifestations of MSPS. Although symptoms often overlap with MSPS, they tend to be prolonged and recurrent.
- Pain in the elbow may be caused by nursemaid's pulled elbow, in which someone pulls hard at child's hand or wrist (commonly when the child falls while the hand is being held by an adult) with the elbow in extension, resulting in subluxation of the radial head.
- Children with fibromyalgia may present with symptoms of inflammatory bowel disease (IBD) (incidence around 50%), migraine or tension headaches (incidence around 50%) or temporomandibular joint dysfunction.
- *Referral of a child with a painful arm should be considered for:*
  - ○ Any ill or feverish child
  - ○ If the arm or hand cannot be used
  - ○ If the pain is severe (crying when the area is touched)
  - ○ In association with numbness or tingling
  - ○ Cause of the pain is not clear
- Children may interpret parasthesias and muscle weakness as pain. Careful history taking and physical examination are essential. The presence of paraesthesia, such as numbness, suggests a neurological condition, e.g., neuritis, or nerve trapping.
- In a young child who presents with unexplained pain, the possibility of child abuse should always be considered. Is this case a safeguarding concern? If worry exists about the wellbeing of a child, this must be reported immediately.

Painful Leg and Limping

The key to an accurate diagnosis is a careful history, thorough physical and neurological examination and appropriate radiological and laboratory investigations.

➤ Pain in the leg is common and caused by many MSK disorders (Box 16.9). Painful limping is the usual presentation.

➤ These disorders may affect the hip (e.g., transient synovitis, avascular necrosis or slipped capital femoral epiphysis [SCFE]), knee (e.g., avascular necrosis, osteochondritis dissecans and idiopathic adolescent knee pain syndrome) or foot (e.g., poor-fitting shoes, trauma and avascular necrosis) or be non-articular pain such as growing pain.

BOX 16.9 Causes of painful leg/limping

Limping with Pain

- Minor muscle strains/sprains/overuse
- Growing pain
- Transient synovitis
- Avascular necrosis (e.g., Perthes disease)
- Arthralgia/arthritis (see 'Arthritis')
- Fracture (e.g., child abuse)
- Malignancy (e.g., leukaemia, lymphoma, bone tumour)
- Sickle cell anaemia
- Spinal disorders (e.g., sciatica)
- Dermatomyositis
- Polyneuropathy

Limping without Pain

- SCFE
- CP (hemiplegia)
- Psychiatric diseases (e.g., conversion disorder)

PRACTICE POINTS

- In a child with leg pain, the shoes should be examined first for poor fit or any foreign body such as toenails.
- The history of growing pains is diagnostic: Non-articular pain occurring at night for at least 6 months and normal physical examination.
- Perthes disease of the hip is not uncommon in children and usually presents aged 5–10 years (mean age: 7 years). Adverse prognosis is related to:
  - Delayed diagnosis.
  - Age at clinical onset: Those who develop the disease aged older than 10 years will certainly develop degenerative arthritis later in life.
- Osgood–Schlatter disease is a common cause of knee pain in adolescents, particularly in those who are active in sports. Typically, the pain worsens with exercise and causes limping. There is often swelling and tenderness just below the knee. Pain lasts weeks or months and usually resolves within 12–24 months.
- Chondromalacia patella (softening of the cartilage on the undersurface of the patella) is also a common cause of chronic knee pain. It mostly occurs in children aged 10–16 years. Pain usually worsens slowly over a year and is typically worse when going upstairs, squatting or kneeling. Full recovery is expected within months or years.
- Long-term use of steroids can cause osteoporosis, fractures and avascular necrosis.
- Many children with hip diseases present with referred knee pain. Examination of both joints is essential.
- In a young child with unexplained pain, child abuse is always a possibility. Careful examination of the skin for relevant bruises and for other signs of possible injury is essential. A skeletal survey may be required.
- SCFE is the most common hip disorder in adolescence; when it occurs prepubertally, an endocrine cause such as hypothyroidism or growth hormone deficiency could well be the underlying pathology.

SPINE

Back Pain

➤ Although back pain in children has generally been less prevalent than in adults, recent reports indicate that around 40% of adolescents suffer from back pain. The prevalence of chronic back pain (CBP) in adolescents over the past two decades has been increasing. Most cases of back pain are nonspecific (i.e., without underlying pathologies). Childhood back pain has a higher incidence of organic causes compared to adults.

➤ Trauma causing muscle strain that settles in a few weeks is the most common cause. More serious causes include infection (e.g., discitis), tumour, spondylosis (injury/fracture of pars interarticularis affecting usually L5), spondylolisthesis (slipping of one vertebra upon another) and spinal deformities (see later). Risk factors for developing back pain are shown in Box 16.10.

➤ CBP is defined as persistent or recurring pain for >3 months. Approximately 1 in 5 children and adolescents experience CBP, with girls experiencing a higher prevalence than boys. Individuals who experience CBP are at increased risk for developing depression, anxiety, social isolation, having more school absences and poor quality of life.

➤ According to a guideline released by WHO in 2020, CBP can be primary, involving one or more anatomical regions that are associated with significant emotional distress and functional disability. Secondary CBP is associated with another condition, e.g., postsurgical or neuropathic.

BOX 16.10 Risk factors for developing back pain

- Family history of back pain
- Overweight and obesity
- Low physical activity and fitness
- Joint hypermobility
- Psychosocial factors (e.g., anxiety, depression)
- Low socioeconomical factors
- Prolonged computer and TV use
- Spinal scoliosis
- Female sex

➤ Back pain in children and adolescents has been shown to predict back pain in adults. The complaint should always be taken seriously. The incidence of back pain in more than one spinal area (cervical, thoracic and lumbar) is higher in children than in adults. Red Flags in children with back pain are shown below.

RED FLAGS WITH BACK PAIN

- Young age (<4 years)
- Corticosteroid use
- Persistent (>4 weeks) or increasing pain, disturbing sleep, pain radiating down to the legs
- Interference with function such as walking, sport or play
- The presence of systemic signs such as fever, loss of appetite or weight, bladder or intestinal dysfunction
- Abnormal signs on physical examination such as tenderness on palpation or pressing the spine

Management

➤ Imaging diagnostics: MRI scan is superior than conventional x-rays in elucidating the cause of the back pain.

➤ Regular physical exercises, which should be monitored.

➤ Children with back pain of short duration, normal physical/neurological examination and no history of trauma are unlikely to need laboratory or imaging evaluation.

➤ Psychological intervention, including psychotherapy or cognitive behavioural therapy (CBT) is important. Screening for psychological and risk factors should be performed using a standardized questionnaire, e.g., Revised Child Anxiety and Depression Scale (RCADS), to assess anxiety and depression.

➤ Assessment for socioeconomic status should be performed, as children living in low-income families are at higher risk of back pain compared to high-income families.

➤ For the pain, NSAIDs are usually prescribed for a few weeks.

SPINAL KYPHOSIS

➤ The normal thoracic kyphosis is composed of 12 vertebrae (T2–T12), with a radiological curvature between 20 and 40 degrees. This type of kyphosis increases with age, and the increase is greater in females than in males. Pathological kyphosis is usually associated with >50 degrees of curve (Box 16.11) and is associated not only with a cosmetic problem but also with a spinal cord stretching, causing pain and neurological deficits.

➤ Congenital kyphosis is caused by congenital malformations of the vertebrae.

➤ Postural kyphosis is a common cause of referral from primary care. Typically, a complete correction of the kyphosis can be achieved clinically and radiologically on hyperextension of the spine. There is a strong association between thoracic kyphosis and obesity. Children usually spend 60–80% of their school day in sitting position, in addition to the sitting at home to do homework and watching TV. This prolonged sitting can cause damage to the intervertebral discs, leading to kyphosis.

➤ Structural kyphosis, of which idiopathic kyphosis (Scheuermann's disease) is the most common form, affects 4–8% of the population. Repeated trauma is the likely underlying cause. It develops in adolescence (typical age 13–16 years) and may become slightly progressive, particularly in boys. Usual presentation is with a mild pain or painless kyphosis with compensatory lumbar lordosis and tight hamstrings. In contrast to postural kyphosis, affected patients cannot actively correct the deformity.

BOX 16.11 Types of kyphosis

Types
- Physiological (20–40 degrees)
- Congenital
- Postural
- Idiopathic Scheuermann's disease

Associated With
- Obesity
- Post-traumatic
- Ankylosing spondylitis
- Achondroplasia
- Neurofibromatosis type 1
- Prader–Willi syndrome
- TB (Pott's disease)

SPINAL SCOLIOSIS

➤ Scoliosis is the most common type of spinal deformity. It is defined as a lateral curvature of the spine of >10 degrees (as measured on the standing frontal radiograph) and vertebral rotation (Box 16.12). It is divided into:

  ➤ Postural scoliosis is a non-structural, functional curvature of the spine due to muscle imbalance or leg length discrepancy. The curve disappears in lying down position.

  ➤ Idiopathic (adolescent) scoliosis (80% of cases). This is the most common condition, affecting 2–3% of children, and occurs as an infantile (birth to 3 years), juvenile (4–10 years) or adolescent form (>10 years). Asymmetry of the posterior chest wall on forward bending is the most valuable abnormality detected on examination.

  ➤ Secondary types of scoliosis (20% of cases) include neuromuscular, CP, joint hypermobility and postradiation scoliosis.

BOX 16.12 Degrees of scoliosis and its severity

- <10 degrees   No scoliosis
- 10–25 degrees   Mild scoliosis

Structural Scoliosis
- >30 degrees   The risk of progression to adults increases
- >45 degrees   Surgery may be indicated with persistent pain
- >50 degrees   Scoliosis will progress in adulthood and cause health problems and reduction of quality of life and may require surgery
- >60 degrees   Scoliosis interferes with lung function

Guidelines on the Management of Spinal Deformity

Kyphosis

➤ Genetic causes have recently identified 53 loci. Genetic testing helps predict the risk of scoliosis progress at genetic counselling.
➤ Children and adolescents are encouraged to participate in specific exercises to prevent scoliosis progression.
➤ All patients with more than mild degrees of kyphoscoliosis should be referred for respiratory function testing.
➤ Prepubertal patients are managed by an exercise programme including hyperextension exercises, observation and repeated examination. Those with >40–50 degrees of kyphosis should be referred for consideration of bracing, which has been established as the most effective non-operative treatment for most mild types of kyphosis, including Scheuermann's disease and kyphoscoliosis.
➤ Post-pubertal patients with kyphotic curves <40–50 degrees who are otherwise asymptomatic and with acceptable cosmetic appearance of their spine require no treatment. Those with kyphosis >60–80 degrees are likely to be symptomatic, and the appearance of the spine is unacceptable; *therefore, referral is required for possible surgery.* Systematic review studies found Pilates exercises to be effective to correct spinal deformities and postures.

Scoliosis

➤ Examination of scoliosis requires full forward bending (Figure 16.7). If the curvature does not disappear on this manoeuvre, x-ray of the spine should be requested. Persistent or more than occasional complaints of aches in the spine are not normal in patients with kyphosis or scoliosis and require urgent evaluation.
➤ Patients with spinal deformities require careful examination for the presence of associated neurological abnormalities. The presence of café-au-lait spots

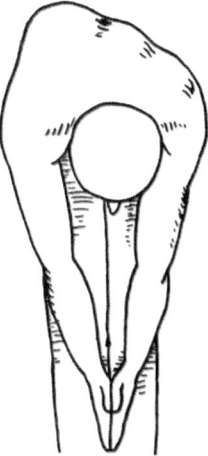

FIGURE 16.7 Scoliosis of the spine may not become apparent unless the patient is asked to bend forward.

(neurofibromatosis type 1), excessive height (Marfan's syndrome), sacral dimple, hairy patches and foot deformity suggests non-idiopathic causes. *Early recognition of such associations and prompt referral are required.*

➤ Scoliosis with curves between 10 and 19 degrees may require observation only with 6-monthly x-rays. Curves between 20 and 29 degrees may require:
  ➣ Referral for possible brace (after 25 degrees).
  ➣ Scoliosis with curves between 20 and 30 degrees usually progresses in prepubertal children but are less likely to do so in postpubertal ages.
  ➣ Scoliosis of >40–45 degrees is likely to continue to progress even after skeletal maturation is complete.

ARTHRITIS

Core Messages

➤ Rheumatic diseases are characterized by an exaggerated autoimmune activity, which can be organ specific (such as reactive arthritis) or systemic (such as JIA) and systemic lupus erythematosus (SLE).

➤ Children with arthritis have a better chance of outgrowing their arthritis and have lower risks of disability compared to adults.

➤ Arthritis may be monoarthritis, oligoarthritis (four or fewer joints) or polyarthritis (five or more joints). The main causes of arthritis are shown in Box 16.13.

➤ Clinical summaries of some types of arthritis are summarized in Box 16.14.

BOX 16.13 The main causes of arthritis*

- Monoarthritis
  - ❯ Septic arthritis (SA)
  - ❯ Transient synovitis of the hip
  - ❯ Monoarthritic JIA
  - ❯ TB arthritis
  - ❯ FMF
- Oligoarthritis
  - ❯ Reactive arthritis (arthritis after GI infection)
  - ❯ Oligoarthritic juvenile rheumatoid arthritis (JRA)
  - ❯ Neoplastic arthritis (leukaemia, lymphoma)
  - ❯ Juvenile ankylosing spondylitis
  - ❯ Lyme disease
- Polyarthritis
  - ❯ Viral arthritis (e.g., parvovirus B10)
  - ❯ Rheumatic fever (RF)
  - ❯ Polyarthritic JRA
  - ❯ Collagen disease (e.g., SLE, dermatomyositis)
  - ❯ Vasculitis (e.g., Kawasaki's disease)

* Some types of arthritis (e.g., FMF) may present as mono-, oligo- or polyarthritis.

Recommended Investigations

➤ Erythrocyte sedimentation rate (ESR), WBC, platelets.
➤ Antinuclear antibodies (ANAs).
➤ IgM-RF usually negative in systemic-onset disease.
➤ Ultrasound scan: Very useful in detecting an effusion or assists in aspiration.
➤ MRI is very sensitive in differentiating SA from osteomyelitis and other causes.
➤ Bone scan: Positive in the majority of cases with SA.
➤ Bone marrow is diagnostic in suspected cases of neoplastic arthritis.

BOX 16.14 Clinical summaries of some types of arthritis

JIA (see next section)

Transient Synovitis

- This is a common cause of limp in childhood aged 3–7 years.
- History of a recent viral upper respiratory tract infection is very common.
- Acute onset of a limp and hip pain in an otherwise healthy child.
- Children typically are afebrile with limited range of hip motion.
- Usually normal laboratory findings.
- It is self-limiting, usually lasting 1–3 weeks.

Viral Arthritis

- Arthralgias are more common than viral-induced arthritis.
- Usually occurs within a week of developing symptoms of a viral infection such as rash; it may precede their onset by a week.
- Arthritis is usually symmetric, self-limiting (may last 2–4 weeks) and bilateral.

Reactive Arthritis (ReA)

- This is an autoimmune arthritis that usually occurs 1–3 weeks after an enteric or genitourinary bacterial infection (*Campylobacter*, *Salmonella*, *Shigella* or *Yersinia*). Arthritis typically affects weight-bearing joints such as the knee.
- Commonly associated with the human leukocyte antigen (HLA)-B27.
- ReA is transient and self-limiting and typically lasts less than 6 weeks. A few patients develop spondylarthritis, uveitis and erythema nodosum.

Septic Arthritis

- SA is almost always monoarthritis. It is defined as positive joint fluid culture for bacteria and/or WBC count in the joint fluid of >50,000 cells/mm (predominately polymorphonuclear cells) with or without positive blood culture (positive in about 50%).
- SA is characterized by an abrupt onset of fever and joint pain, fever is usually high >39.5°C, with severe pain, restricted range of joint movement and refusal to walk.

TB Arthritis

- Typically monoarthritis which follows pulmonary TB.
- Arthritis is painless, persistent in one joint and unresponsive to conventional treatment.

JUVENILE IDIOPATHIC ARTHRITIS

➤ JIA refers to a chronic autoimmune arthritis which lasts at least 6 weeks in children younger than 16 years of age without a known cause. The antigen HLA-B27 is frequently positive. Prevalence is about 1:1000 children, with peak ages of 1 and 4 years, and girls outnumber boys by 3:1.

➤ JIA encompasses seven major types based on clinical characteristics. About 10–20% of all patients with JIA present with systemic onset (Still's disease), characterized by recurrent high fever (quotidian fever) and a fleeting, salmon-pink rash on the trunk and upper extremities. Boys and girls are equally affected with a mean age of 4 years. Other features include generalized lymphadenopathy, hepatosplenomegaly, leukocytosis, anaemia, myocarditis and pericarditis.

➤ The polyarticular onset or adult type accounts for 10–30% of JIA, with an abrupt or insidious arthritis of several joints (more than four joints). This type affects females more than males, with a mean age of 12 years. This group is divided into RF-negative and -positive polyarthritis.

➤ In the remaining cases, the presentation involves monoarthritis or pauciarticular arthritis (accounts for 50–80% of all cases with JIA), affecting predominately females younger than 6 years. Systemic manifestations are usually absent or mild. Autoantibodies such ANA are usually positive, and RF is negative. Children are at high risk of iridocyclitis, which can lead to a vision loss in up to 60%. Iridocyclitis is an important sign. RF is negative.

Principles of Management of Arthritis

➤ Management of children with arthritis is complex and challenging. Early diagnosis and treatment is associated with improved long-term outcomes.

➤ The aim of treatment of arthritis includes monitoring the use of antirheumatic medications, pain and coping, growth, school attendance, psychosocial functioning, physical activity and nutrition.

➤ NSAIDs are used in larger doses and for longer periods for their anti-inflammatory effect than for analgesia alone. Several weeks may elapse before an adequate anti-inflammatory effect has been achieved.

➤ During the past decades, JIA management was mostly dependent on the use of corticosteroids, methotrexate and sulfasalazine. Recently, highly effective biological agents, such as interleukin (IL-1, IL-6) and TNF inhibitors, have dramatically changed the disease outcomes.

SYSTEMIC LUPUS ERYTHEMATOSUS

➤ SLE is a chronic, usually lifelong inflammatory connective tissue disorder of unknown aetiology. Females account for 90% of cases.

➤ Autoantibodies are important for the diagnosis and are responsible for many of its clinical manifestations. The presence of ANA, anti–double-stranded DNA (anti-dsDNA) and antiphospholipid antibodies suggests that SLE is an autoimmune disease.

➤ Clinical features are shown in Box 16.15.

BOX 16.15 Clinical manifestations of SLE

● Skin	● Malar rash, discoid lupus (incidence 60–85%) Photosensitivity of skin rash following sun exposure
● Mouth	● Ulcers
● Joints	● Non-erosive polyarthralgia/arthritis affecting two or more joints
● CNS	● Headache, confusion, seizure, psychosis
● Renal	● Lupus nephritis (nephritic/nephrotic syndrome)
● Serositis	● Pleuritis
● Cardiac	● Pleuro-pericarditis, myocarditis, endocarditis
● Other	● Fatigue, malaise, fever, antiphospholipid syndrome
● Laboratory finding	● High ESR, normal CRP, lymphopenia, thrombocytopenia, haemolytic anaemia, ANA, anti-dsDNA, antiphospholipid antibodies

VASCULITIS (BOX 16.16)

➤ Vasculitis, inflammation of the blood vessel walls of any size, is caused by auto-immune antibodies directed against blood vessels. Immune cell infiltrates involve granulocytes or mononuclear cells.

BOX 16.16

● Small vessel vasculitis	IgA vasculitis (Henoch–Schönlein purpura), granulomatosis polyangiitis (Wegener's granulomatosis)
● Medium vessel vasculitis	Polyarteritis nodosa, Kawasaki's disease
● Large vessel vasculitis	Temporal (giant cell) artery, Takayasu's arteritis

KAWASAKI DISEASE

➤ Kawasaki disease (KD) is an acute multisystem inflammatory disease that principally affects infants and young children: 85% are less than 5 years of age, with a peak incidence at 1–2 years. Initially described by Kawasaki in Japan, the condition has been recognized worldwide. It is the leading cause of acquired heart disease in children. Diagnosis is established by certain clinical criteria (Box 16.17).

➤ The most serious features are those affecting the cardiovascular system:
  ➢ Myocarditis occurs in about 25% with findings that include tachycardia, gallop rhythm and non-specific ST-T wave changes on the ECG. Myocarditis generally resolves completely.
  ➢ Mild self-limiting pericardial effusion may develop toward the second week.
  ➢ Coronary artery aneurysm (CAA) is the major feature affecting an otherwise excellent prognosis. Approximately 20–25% develop coronary artery changes if patients are not treated swiftly. KD may present as sudden death in 1.7%. CAAs

occur in 15–20% of cases. Aneurysms may also occur in other arteries, such as renal, axillary and iliac arteries.

➤ *Because of the cardiac involvement, urgent referral is required for any suspected case of KD.*

BOX 16.17 Diagnostic criteria for KD

Fever persisting for at least 5 days plus at least four of the following:

1. Bilateral, painless conjunctival inflammation without discharge
2. Changes of the oropharynx mucosa, cracking lips, strawberry tongue
3. Acute, unilateral, non-purulent cervical lymphadenopathy >1.5 cm
4. Polymorphous rash, primarily truncal
5. Changes of extremities: Oedema and/or erythema of hands and feet

---

Laboratory findings are not diagnostic but characteristically include leukocytosis with increased neutrophils, mild-to-moderate normocytic normochromic anaemia, almost universally increased ESR and CRP and thrombocytosis, which begins in the second week and peaks at about 3 weeks (mean count 800,000/mm^3). Less characteristic findings include raised aspartate and alanine aminotransferase; increased ASO titre, IgG, IgA and IgM; and pyuria and proteinuria.

Management

➤ Aspirin is recommended at a dose of 30–50 mg/kg/day, divided into four doses. After the resolution of the acute symptoms (usually after 14 days), the aspirin dose is reduced to 3–5 mg/kg/day in a single dose for its antithrombotic effect. Aspirin is continued for 3–4 months if there is no CAA, until CAA resolves (coronary aneurysm <8 mm) or indefinitely if the coronary aneurysm persists (CAA >8 mm). If the patient cannot take aspirin, dipyridamole is recommended.

➤ Intravenous immune gamma globulin (IVIG) plus aspirin reduces the incidence of CAAs. A large single dose of gamma globulin (2 g/kg body weight) infused over 10 hours is more effective than the previously recommended regimen of four smaller daily doses.

CHAPTER 17

Dermatology

INTRODUCTION

➤ About 10–15% of children attending primary care clinics do so because of skin problems.

➤ A specific dermatological diagnosis cannot always be made; classifying conditions into one of several groups, e.g., as maculopapular, vesiculobullous or papulosquamous, is a good start (Table 17.1).

➤ Itching, no matter what the cause, is always worse at night because of fewer external distractions and because the warmth of the bed worsens itching.

TABLE 17.1 Examples of common skin eruptions

Lesion	Lay Term	Examples
• Macule	• Dot	• Freckles
• Papule	• Small bump	• Warts
• Maculopapular rashes		• Viral exanthem, eczema
• Patches	• Patches	• Port-wine nevus
• Nodule	• Big bump	• Epidermoid cyst
• Tumour	• Tumour	• Lipoma
• Plaques	• Raised or thick bump	• Naevi
• Squamous	• Scale covered, scaly	• Squamous cell carcinoma
• Papulo-squamous		• Psoriasis, lichen planus
• Vesicles	• Small blister	• Herpes infections
• Bulla	• Big blister	• Urticaria
• Vesiculobullous rash		• Bullous impetigo
• Pustule	• Pimple	• Infected vesicle, e.g., varicella
• Comedones	• Blackheads	• Acne
• Crusts	• Scabs	• Late stage of varicella
• Excoriation	• Scratch mark	• Eczema

MACULES AND PATCHES

➤ A macula, known in lay language as dot, is a circumscribed, flat area of change in skin colour which is less than 1 cm in diameter. It can be either hyperpigmented (e.g., freckles) or hypopigmented (vitiligo). A patch is a larger area of change in skin colour that is >1 cm in diameter.

DOI: 10.1201/9781032642888-17

➤ Salmon patch is by far the most common vascular lesion in neonates and refers to a midline or symmetrical pink maculae over both eyelids.

➤ Single or a couple of café-au-lait lesions 1–3 cm in diameter occur in about 20% of all healthy children. Café-au-lait spots are the hallmark of neurofibromatosis. Diagnosis is established with six or more lesions over 0.5 cm in diameter in prepubertal and 1.5 cm in diameter in postpubertal individuals.

➤ Although blue patches (known formerly as Mongolian spots) are considered benign, widespread extrasacral lesions may persist in adulthood. They may coexist with some inherited errors of metabolism, e.g., gangliosidosis.

➤ Freckles around the mouth should be differentiated from Peutz–Jeghers syndrome. The latter is autosomal dominant, associated with hyperpigmentation on the lips and mucosae and a risk of intestinal polyps and cancer elsewhere.

➤ Although patches of bruises over the shins are almost universal in toddlers due to frequent falls, bruises on the arm, back, abdomen, thighs and genitalia are highly suggestive of child abuse.

PAPULES AND PLAQUES

➤ A papule, a little bump or pimple in lay language, is a small (<1 cm) solid, circumscribed lesion that is palpable above the skin surface.

➤ A plaque is a solid, circumscribed lesion with its surface area greater than the elevation. Plaques vary in size from 1 cm to a huge size covering part of the body. Plaques can arise directly from the skin or through a coalescence of papules.

➤ Some eruptions have a combination of papules and plaques (papulosquamous eruption), and pityriasis rosea is a typical eruption of this combination. Other examples include erythema toxicum neonatorum, acne, milia, atopic dermatitis, warts, molluscum contagiosum and insect bites.

➤ Acne may appear in newborns as self-limited neonatal acne during 0–6 weeks of life, characterized by papulovesicular eruption on the face, scalp and neck. Acne also appears in preadolescents (7–12 years) and adolescents (12–18 years), affecting about 85% of the last age group.

➤ Psoriasis is a T-lymphocyte autoimmune, chronic inflammatory disease. About a third of patients are children. It may present in infancy as nappy rash. Guttate psoriasis is the most common presentation in older children triggered by streptococcal infection and is characterized by a sudden onset of small red or pink papules 1–10 mm in diameter.

➤ Lichen planus is not that uncommon in children. Lesions are polygonal, flat-topped papules 2–6 mm in diameter. The diagnosis can often be confirmed by looking for white papules on the buccal mucosa.

RED FLAGS

● Erythema toxicum neonatorum is seen in about half of healthy newborns and is often mistaken for staphylococcal pustules. The well-appearing child and asymptomatic rash exclude any infection.

● Scabies is often mistaken for atopic dermatitis or impetigo. Associated streptococcal infection can lead to complications such as glomerulonephritis or rheumatic fever.

VESICLES AND BULLAE

➤ Blister is the lay terminology for both vesicle and bulla. While a vesicle is a fluid-filled raised cavity which is less than 1 cm in diameter, a bulla is greater than 1 cm in diameter. Examples of vesiculobullous eruption include epidermolysis bullosa, herpes simplex virus, herpes zoster, herpetic gingivostomatitis and erythema multiforme.

➤ Important clues for diagnostic purposes: Whether the blisters arise on erythematous skin (e.g., atopic dermatitis) or on normal skin (e.g., epidermolysis bullosa, pemphigus) and whether the blisters are flaccid, meaning arising from superficial layers (e.g., bullous impetigo), or tense, meaning arising from deeper layers of skin (e.g., bullous pemphigus).

➤ Herpes zoster (shingles) is relatively benign except when it affects the ophthalmic division. Protection of the affected eye is essential.

➤ Scabies is a parasitic infestation caused by mites, with typical pruritic burrows found in the webbing spaces of fingers. It is often misdiagnosed as eczema, which can prolong a patient's suffering.

➤ Naproxen, an NSAID used as an inflammatory agent in rheumatic diseases, may cause an eruption characterized by erythema, vesicles and shallow atrophic scars after sun exposure.

RED FLAGS

Serious vesiculobullous conditions include:

- Stevens–Johnson syndrome with lesions involving the lips and mouth, often triggered by drugs.
- Eczema herpeticum is a serious infection caused by herpes simplex virus (HSV), which is invading eczematous lesions. It can lead to death through dissemination of the virus to the brain and other organs or from secondary staphylococcal or streptococcal infection.
- Incising or puncturing bulla should not be performed, for this may trigger infection.
- Herpes simplex and varicella can become disseminated in immunocompromised patients. The child should be admitted and given appropriate treatment of intravenous acyclovir.

HYPER- AND HYPOPIGMENTED LESIONS

➤ Pigmentary disorders are a common presentation at primary care clinics, paediatricians and dermatologists. Melanin (black pigment) plays a key role in determining human skin colour. Other pigmentary determinants include haemoglobin (red), haemosiderin (brown), carotene and bilirubin (yellow).

➤ Most causes of pigmentary disorders are benign, including freckles (ephelides), café-au-lait spots, lentigines and blue patches (formerly known as Mongolian spots). Both post-inflammatory hypopigmentation and post-inflammatory hyperpigmentation commonly occur after an inflammatory process, such as eczema. These will gradually fade.

➤ In some cases, pigmentation can be an external sign of a serious underlying systemic disorder such as melanoma. Multiple café-au-lait spots can be associated with other syndromes (e.g., McCune–Albright syndrome, LEOPARD syndrome, ataxia telangiectasia) which carry a high risk of cancer development

NODULES AND TUMOURS

➤ A nodule (lump or bump) is a solid, usually benign, round <2 cm in diameter that extends deeper into underlying tissues than a papule. Examples are lymph nodes, thyroid or pulmonary nodules. Larger nodules >2 cm are classified as tumours, which can be benign (e.g., haemangioma) or malignant (e.g., lymphoma).

➤ Any congenital midline lesion, e.g., on the nasal bridge may suggest the possibility of dermoid cyst, glioma or encephalocele. The lesion should be imaged because of the high incidence of intracranial connection. If there is a sinus opening with intermittent discharge, this is a pathognomonic sign for intracranial connection.

➤ Although basal cell carcinoma is rare in children, it may result from basal cell naevus, radiotherapy for other malignancies or after excessive sun exposure.

➤ Although paediatric melanoma is rare (1–4% of all melanomas), its incidence is increasing. The traditional criteria ABCDE (asymmetry, border irregularity, colour changes, diameter >6 mm, evolution) is different in paediatrics, which is usually amelanocytic, with tendency for bleeding, with uniform colour and variable sizes.

ECZEMA/DERMATITIS

Clinical Features

➤ Eczema is a chronic relapsing inflammatory skin condition affecting one in five children in the UK. The condition can have a significant impact on quality of life. There is currently no cure for eczema, but it can be managed satisfactorily using the right treatment.

➤ Although the term 'atopic dermatitis' (AD) is often used interchangeably with eczema, AD should be reserved for an eczema with IgE sensitization. Atopy is a genetic predisposition to develop IgE antibodies in response to common allergens such as pollens and house dust mites to produce allergic diseases, including eczema, food allergy, asthma and allergic rhinitis.

➤ Skin care treatments (such as moisturizers) during the first year of life do not prevent the development of eczema and may increase the risk of skin infection and food allergy.

➤ Incidence of eczema is highest in the first year of life and often resolves during childhood. Around 30% of children with eczema develop asthma, and 35% develop allergic rhinitis.

➤ Seborrhoeic dermatitis (SD) is often difficult to differentiate from AD: Pruritus is always present in AD, in contrast to SD.

➤ Secondary infection by staphylococci or *Candida* is common and is the most common cause of treatment failure.

Diagnosis (Box 17.1 and Table 17.2)

The clinical diagnosis of eczema is based on a collection of symptoms such as itch and skin rash. Its pathogenesis involves interactions among the genes environment, immune system and the skin barrier leading to skin inflammation:

➤ In infants aged 2–3 months, the face and extremities are usually affected with erythematous weepy patches.
➤ By the age of around 2 years, eczematous lesions mostly affects the limbs, particularly the flexural areas of elbows and knees, as well as the neck, wrists and ankles.

BOX 17.1 Diagnostic criteria of eczema

● The presence of three or more of the following major criteria:
  ❯ History of itching
  ❯ Visible flexural dermatitis involving the face and limbs, later the popliteal and antecubital creases
  ❯ Chronic or relapsing course
  ❯ Individual and/or family history
● In addition, three or more of the following minor criteria:
  ❯ Dryness of the skin
  ❯ Elevated serum IgE
  ❯ Early age of onset
  ❯ Tendency towards skin infection, especially staphylococci
  ❯ History of food allergy

TABLE 17.2 Clinical features of eczema according to its severity

Mild
● Areas of dry skin
● Lesions affecting a few skin areas
● Infrequent itching
● Undisturbed sleep
● Little impact on daily activity

Moderate
● Areas of dry skin
● Red areas of lesions, with or without some excoriation
● Frequent itching
● Disturbed sleep

Severe
● Widespread areas of skin involvement, with bleeding, oozing or cracking of the skin
● Incessant itching
● Loss of sleep
● Severe impact on daily activities

Treatment (Boxes 17.2 and 17.3)

➤ Primary prevention of eczema is achieved with breastfeeding. Probiotic and/or prebiotic supplements during pregnancy can be beneficial in preventing eczema.

➤ The terms 'moisturiser' and 'emollient' are usually used interchangeably. Emollients are mainly lipid-based creams that smooth the skin, limit water loss and are particularly beneficial for dry skin (xerosis), whereas topical moisturizers provide water to hydrate the skin and are beneficial for all severities of eczema.

BOX 17.2 Treatment of eczema

Mild

- Regular use of emollients (four times/day) and soap substitute.
- Mild topical corticosteroid cream for facial eczema such as 0.5% or 1% hydrocortisone.
- Sedating oral AH for itching and if sleep is disturbed.

Moderate

- Regular use of emollients and soap substitute.
- If bacterial infection is suspected, swabs should be taken from the area and antibiotic therapy considered.
- Corticosteroid therapy, such as betamethasone (Betnovate) or clobetasone (Eumovate).

High

- Referral to a paediatric dermatologist.
- Use of moderate or potent corticosteroids (Box 17.3): Fluocinolone, triamcinolone, mometasone, clobetasol (Dermovate 0.05%).
- Topical calcineurin inhibitors (to block the protein calcineurin that contributes to the skin inflammation), such as protopic 0.03% to treat eczema in children >2 years.

BOX 17.3 Evidence-based treatment

- Numerous emollients are available over the counter, and there is no reliable evidence that one moisturizer is better than another.
- Potent and moderate topical corticosteroids are more effective than mild topical corticosteroids in moderate or severe eczema to achieve treatment success.
- There is insufficient evidence of a benefit of moderate topical corticosteroids compared to potent topical corticosteroids. Effectiveness is similar between once or twice daily use of potent corticosteroids.
- Using topical corticosteroid cream for 2 consecutive days weekly probably prevents eczema flare-ups.
- Topical calcineurin inhibitors, such as tacrolimus, are licenced for children 2 years of age and older as second-line treatment for moderate-to-severe eczema that has not been controlled by topical corticosteroids.
- Systemic immunosuppressive treatments are reserved for the treatment of more severe cases of eczema that have been inadequately controlled with topical corticosteroids and topical calcineurin inhibitors.

Criteria for Referral

➤ Failure to respond to continuing use of moderately potent steroid.
➤ Sleep problem not responding to AH at night.
➤ Recurrent secondary infections.
➤ Associated food allergies.
➤ Growth restriction, psychological problems.
➤ Eczema herpeticum (this is a serious infection caused by HSV, which can cause severe morbidity and sometimes death).

VIRAL WARTS

➤ All warts are caused by various types of human papillomavirus (HPV), which also causes cervical cancer and squamous cell carcinoma. HPV is transmitted by direct contact and autoinoculation.
➤ Warts are estimated to occur in about 10% of children and young people, most frequently affecting the hands and feet.
➤ *Condylomata acuminata* (also referred to as anogenital HPV or genital warts) is a common sexually transmitted disease (STD) worldwide. Lesions are 3–5 mm in diameter, flesh-coloured to erythematous papules with slightly verrucous surfaces. In older children the vulva, the shaft of the penis, urethra and perianal regions are involved. The perianal area is mainly involved in children aged 1–2 years. HPV in the genital area is always a reason to consider the possibility of child abuse.
➤ No single therapy has been proven effective in every patient. Most cases may be best left alone. A decision to treat should be made on case-by-case basis according to experience of the physician, patient preference and the application of evidence-based medicine.
➤ For verruca, a Cochrane review identified topical therapy with salicylic acid as safe and effective. The duct tape method is also very effective. The pooled data from

TABLE 17.3 Treatment guidelines for warts

Clinical Features	Treatment	Comments
• Common warts fingers/ dorsum of hands, face (Verruca vulgaris)	• Leave them alone or topical salicylic acid (daily application of 15–20%) • Cryotherapy (liquid nitrogen) excision	• Salicylic acid and cryotherapy are the most used treatment • Treatment can be painful
• Plantar warts on the soles (Verruca)	• Leave them alone or: Salicylic and lactic acid • In a collodion basis: Duofilm or Salactol paint containing 16.7% salicylic acid and 16.7% lactic acid	• Needs time to get response • May cause allergy; should be avoided in children allergic to elastic adhesive plaster
• On the plane warts (Verruca plana) (flat warts)	• Leave alone or trial with tretinoin 0.025% cream for 4 weeks	• Can cause local irritation on the site of application
• Anogenital warts (*Condylomata acuminata*)	• Topical podophyllotoxin 0.15% cream or 5% imiquimod cream • Surgical removal or cryotherapy	• Twice daily for 3 days, then pause for 4 days, repeat up to 4 cycles

several randomized controlled trials demonstrated a cure rate of 75% compared with 48% in the control group. Cryotherapy is painful and is best avoided in children. In addition, topical treatment is usually as effective as cryotherapy (Table 17.3).

Referral should be considered if warts:

➤ Remain widespread despite treatment for 3–6 months.
➤ Appear atypical or the site is unusual.
➤ Are present in an immunocompromised patient. This condition should be suspected if there is incomplete clearance or resistance to treatment.

RED FLAGS

● *Condylomata acuminata* is a well-recognized sign of child abuse. This is, however, only one mode of HPV transmission. In prepubertal children, anogenital lesions may arise through autoinoculation.
● HPV can cause an infection almost anywhere, including the tongue. Differentiating the lesion from the premalignant leukoplakia is important.

MOLLUSCUM CONTAGIOSUM

Core Messages

➤ *Molluscum contagiosum* (MC) is a common, generally self-limiting skin disease caused by the pox virus, diagnosed by its typical distinct appearance of umbilicated, flesh-coloured, dome-shaped lesions. It affects people of all ages but predominately appears in children 2–5 years of age and rarely in children below the age of 1 year.
➤ A used clinical diagnostic tool is dermoscopy, which enables to diagnose MC easily

---

BOX 17.4 Available treatments for *Molluscum contagiosum*

● No treatment and awaiting natural resolution
● Potassium hydrochloride 5–20% every other day for a week is about 69% effective
● Curettage, which is an effective method with 1–2 sessions
● Cryotherapy, which is an effective treatment with a complete clearance at 3–16 weeks
● Immunomodulatory method using 5% imiquimod cream to stimulate the patient's immune response against the infection

---

RED FLAGS

● Immunocompromised patients, such as those with HIV, are particularly prone to MC. This status should be considered whenever the lesions are multiple, in atypical sites (e.g., perianal, genital, pubic, face and neck) and resistant to therapy.
● Squeezing the lesions is commonly practised. However, this can lead to secondary infection and abscess formation. The practice should be avoided.

➤ Although generally benign, it can be extensive and cause itching and discomfort as well as parental anxiety.

➤ The genital area is commonly affected. Transmission of the MC virus is by direct contact with infected skin, which can be sexual (in sexually active people), non-sexual or by autoinoculation.

➤ When papules are widespread and large, immunosuppression such as HIV infection should be considered.

➤ Treatment is not indicated in most cases because it may be painful and cause scarring. Spontaneous resolution in immunocompetent people occurs within 6–9 months; occasionally, lesions may persist for years. Indication for treatment includes:
  ➢ Social and cosmetic reasons.
  ➢ Extensive disease.
  ➢ Associated with complications such as secondary bacterial infection.

ACNE

Core Messages

➤ Acne is a chronic inflammatory skin disorder of the pilosebaceous unit (hair shaft, hair follicle and sebaceous gland) that is characterized by chronic or recurrent development of comedones, erythematous papules and pustules. Acne usually occurs with the onset of puberty due to an increased production of androgens by the adrenal glands and gonads.

TABLE 17.4 Treatment for acne

Degree	Treatment	Detail
Mild *Uninflamed lesions*	• Gentle skin hygiene with cleansers, avoiding rubbing, picking and squeezing. • Topical retinoids (vitamin A creams, Adapalene, Tretinoin, Tazarotene) • Salicylic acid (Acnisal) solution 2%	• Thin layer of application at night, every other night. It can cause skin irritation and increase effect of sunburn. • Application 2–3 times daily

Moderate
More extensive lesions
	• Topical therapy as noted earlier with retinoids.
	• In addition: a systemic antibiotic for 3 months:
	  ○ Lymecycline
	  ○ Erythromycin
	  ○ Doxycycline
		• Reassess after 3 months.
		• Use alternative antibiotic if there is poor response.
		• Combined treatment with topical and systemic antibiotics is more effective than a single one alone.

Severe *Nodulo-cystic scarring acne, deeper inflammation, failure to respond to therapy*	• Referral to dermatology mainly for isotretinoin therapy.	• Refer urgently if the nodulo-cystic lesions are severe. • Treatment with isotretinoin or co-cyprindiol (Dianette) may be considered (see 'Red Flags').
Maintenance	• Topical retinoid or benzoyl peroxide preparation	

RED FLAGS

- Isotretinoin should be prescribed by secondary care only. It is potentially teratogenic.
- With oral use of isotretinoin, effective contraception must be used in women of childbearing age. Pregnancy must be excluded before treatment. Women on isotretinoin should be advised to discontinue the treatment and to seek prompt medical advice if they become pregnant. Each prescription for isotretinoin should be limited for a supply of up to 30 days treatment. While a combined contraceptive pill is effective, an oral progesterone-only contraceptive is not considered effective.
- Isotretinoin may cause pancreatitis if the triglyceride level is high (above 9 mmol/L) as well as mental health problems.

➤ Factors that increase the risk of developing acne include family history of severe acne, obesity, oily/seborrheic skin, emotional stress, vitamin D deficiency and medications (anabolic steroids, hydantoins, ramipril and cyclosporin). There is evidence that dairy products, chocolates and fatty foods predispose to acne development, while vegetables, fruits and probably probiotics decrease this trend.

➤ About 20% of neonates aged around 2 weeks develop acne, predominately comedones, on the forehead and cheeks, resulting from placental transfer of maternal androgens. It is transient and harmless, and no medical treatment is needed.

➤ Patients should be discouraged from picking or squeezing the lesions.

➤ Mild-to-moderate acne can be treated in primary care. Treatment should be assessed at 2–3 months and should continue for a total of 6 months.

➤ Treatment (Table 17.4) includes oral isotretinoin, which is a very effective treatment for those not responding to topical therapy. Treatment aims:
  ➤ To reduce the psychological trauma on the individual
  ➤ To reduce the severity of the disease
  ➤ To prevent long-term sequalae such as scarring

URICARIA (see also Chapter 5: Allergy)

Core Messages

➤ Urticaria is defined as the daily occurrence of wheals (central itchy white papules or plaques due to dermal oedema), angioedema or both, which last less than 6 weeks (acute urticaria = AU). Angioedema is localized, involving deeper subcutaneous tissues, and presents as pain or burning rather than itching. Lesions characteristically come and go within 2–3 hours and last < 24 hours.

➤ Acute spontaneous urticaria is the most common type of urticaria occurring in 50–75% of cases. It is usually self-limiting, often occurring in association with an upper respiratory tract infection. Antigens, e.g., a virus, binds to a specific antibody on mast cells and basophils to form an antigen–antibody complex, causing the release of mediators, mainly histamine.

➤ Chronic urticaria, defined as daily appearance of wheals for >6 weeks, is frequently associated with increased autoantibody production against IgE receptors, and, therefore, patients are at high risk of developing autoimmune diseases such as Hashimoto's thyroiditis, coeliac disease and rheumatoid arthritis.

Aetiology (Box 17.5)

BOX 17.5 Aetiological classification of urticaria

● Acute spontaneous urticaria triggered by:
  ❯ Infection, such as tonsillitis, Epstein–Barr virus
  ❯ Food (e.g., fish, shellfish, nuts)
  ❯ Respiratory allergens such as pollens, mould spores, mites and animal hair
  ❯ Medications such as penicillin, NSAIDs
  ❯ Genetic (e.g., hereditary angioedema)
  ❯ Collagen-vascular (e.g., systemic lupus erythematosus)
  ❯ Idiopathic
● Chronic spontaneous urticaria is characterized by recurrences of the rash at least twice a week and lasts more than 6 weeks
● Chronic inducible urticaria, i.e., physical (e.g., cold, solar and exercise induced)
● Episodic chronic urticaria

Investigations

The diagnosis of urticaria is clinical, and the vast majority of cases of acute urticaria do not require investigation. Unusual, chronic or episodic urticaria may entail the following testing:

❽ Full blood count (FBC), C-reactive protein (CRP) (abnormalities may suggest autoimmune or collagen-vascular)
❽ Thyroid function tests and antibodies, antinuclear antibody (ANA) for suspected autoimmune disease
❽ Liver function tests
❽ Allergy testing: Skin prick test (SPT) or serum specific IgE test
❽ Physical challenge (reproducibly induced by the same physical stimulus)
❽ C4 (as an initial test for hereditary and acquired C1 esterase inhibitor deficiency)
❽ Skin biopsy for suspected vasculitis

Management

➤ Acute urticaria is a self-limiting disease which usually resolves over days and weeks.
➤ Antihistamines (AHs) are the mainstay of treatment. The use of sedating first-generation AHs (cyclizine, chlorpheniramine) is not preferred due to their significant sedation and short duration of action. A combination of first- and second-generation AHs may be indicated for acute urticaria.

<6 weeks

❽ Avoidance of known triggers.
❽ Trial of second-generation non-sedating AH, including:
  ❼ Loratadine: 5–10 mg, cetirizine: 5–10 mg, fexofenadine: 120–180 mg, desloratadine 1.25–5 mg.
  ❼ For angioedema with life-threating swelling of larynx and tongue, inject adrenaline 1:1000 intramuscularly.
❽ If sleep is disturbed, chlorphenamine (Piriton), 1–4 mg every 4–6 hours depending on the child's age.
❽ Short-term use of prednisolone should be considered in cases with signs of angioedema or if children remain symptomatic while on a maximal dose of AH. Recommended dose: 0.5–1 mg/kg/day.

>6 weeks

❽ Second-generation non-sedating AH. In addition, the following therapeutic measures should be considered for persistent symptoms despite high doses of AH:
  ➤ Omalizumab, which is a monoclonal anti IgE antibody.
  ➤ Cyclosporine 5 mg/kg/day.
  ➤ Antileukotrienes (Singulair) and immunomodulating agents (cyclosporine, tacrolimus).
❽ If there is diagnostic difficulty or failure to respond with 6 weeks of continuous AH:
  ➤ *Referral to allergy specialist.*

RED FLAG

● Cold urticaria is the most common form of physical urticaria. The cooling of skin associated with evaporation emerging from swimming water is hazardous; death may occur in children so exposed.

SCABIES

➤ Scabies is one of the most common skin diseases worldwide, affecting 150–200 million people annually, in particular, those living in poor and overcrowded conditions. In 2017, the World Health Organization (WHO) added scabies to the list of neglected tropical diseases and called for action to achieve eradication.
➤ Scabies is caused by the parasite mite *Sarcoptes scabiei*. The infection can be complicated by group A streptococci and *Staphylococcus aureus*.
➤ Lesions consist of burrows, vesicles, pustules and excoriated papules. Classical sites for scabies lesions include finger webs, hands, wrists and genitalia.

Diagnosis

➤ The gold standard remains visualization of the parasite, or its eggs, or eggshell fragments by light microscope examination following skin scrapings.
➤ Dermoscopy or epiluminescence microscopy are useful tools to confirm the diagnosis of scabies by identifying the typical rash and burrows.

Treatment

➤ Treat patient and all close relatives.
➤ All bed linen and clothes need to be washed in hot water.
➤ Use topical scabicide (treatment may need to be repeated after 1–2 weeks):
  ❼ Permethrin 5% cream is the first line of treatment and is highly effective after a single application. It is applied overnight from scalp to toes. A second application is recommended to eradicate newly hatched mites.
  ❼ Crotamiton cream 10%. Several applications are required to obtain a good response.
  ❼ Malathion lotion 0.5% has a limited efficacy compared to Permethrin.
  ❼ Ivermectin orally, 200 micrograms/kg, 2 doses 2 weeks apart, has a high cure rate close to 100%.

IMPETIGO

➤ This is a contagious bacterial infection of the skin. The infection is classified as primary (direct bacterial invasion of previously normal skin) or secondary, following skin abrasion by insect bites, scabies or eczema.
➤ The most common non-bullous impetigo, caused mostly by group A streptococci (GAS), which manifests as papular, pustular and honey-coloured crusts usually around the mouth and nose. Bullous impetigo, mostly caused by *S. aureus*, consists of a large, fluid-filled bulla, 1–2 cm, usually affecting the intertriginous area such as axilla, groins and the buttocks.
➤ There is a strong association between scabies infestation and impetigo, suggesting that scabies increases the risk of bacterial infection. GAS skin infection is implicated in up to 50% of post-streptococcal glomerulonephritis and rheumatic fever.

Management (Box 17.6)

The healing stage takes up to 30 days without treatment and 7 days following antibiotic therapy.

BOX 17.6 Summary of treatment of impetigo

● For localized, uncomplicated impetigo:
  ❭ Cleansing, removal of crusts: A mild antiseptic such as povidone–iodine may help to soften crusts
  ❭ Topical antibiotic such as fusidic acid
  ❭ Mupirocin (Bactroban) for methicillin-resistant *S. aureus* (MRSA) cases
● For widespread, complicated impetigo, use:
  ❭ Oral flucloxacillin (first choice)
  ❭ Cephalosporin
  ❭ Co-amoxiclav
  ❭ In case of penicillin allergy, use erythromycin

TINEA CAPITIS (RINGWORM)

Core Messages

➤ Of the four types of tinea (*Tinea corporis, unguium, pedis* and *capitis*), *Tinea capitis* is the most common and important type of fungal infection in children.
➤ *Tinea capitis* is a common paediatric infection of the scalp hair caused by fungal infection with dermatophytes which invade the keratin layers. It is a contagious person-to-person fungal infection, frequently associated with poor hygiene, crowded living areas and immunodeficiency status. School-aged children are mostly affected.
➤ The infection is characterized initially by a small papule at the base of the hair follicle, spreading then peripherally to form an erythematous and scaly circular plaque (ringworm) within which the infected hairs become broken just above the scalp causing alopecia of varying degrees.
➤ Until recently, the diagnosis of tinea capitis was established by direct microscopy and culture from scraping or by using a scalp brush. The introduction of molecular techniques using different forms of polymerase chain reaction (PCR) has resulted in identifying dermatophytes faster and more accurately. Wood's lamp is a useful tool to have: Blue-green fluorescence is detectable in a hair shaft infected by fungal infection.

Treatment

➤ Topical antifungals (e.g., topical ketoconazole or antifungal shampoo) are insufficient alone because of the high relapse rate due to the inability to penetrate the root of the hair follicle. However, they can be used with oral antifungals.
➤ Available oral antifungals include:
  ➤ Terbinafine for 4 weeks using the following doses:
    ● 62.5 mg OD for <10 kg body weight
    ● 125 mg OD for 10–20 kg body weight
    ● 250 mg OD for >20 kg body weight
  ➤ Itraconazole 2–4 mg/kg/day for 4–6 weeks
  ➤ Fluconazole
  ➤ Griseofulvin 10–15 mg/kg/day for 6–8 weeks (griseofulvin is still widely used in resource-limited areas)

RED FLAGS

● When a patient presents with diffuse hair loss, *Tinea capitis* is commonly not thought of as a differential diagnosis. This may lead to inappropriate treatment and delay of diagnosis.
● When a patient presents with diffuse scaly erythema, another misdiagnosis of seborrheic dermatitis may be considered.

PITYRIASIS ROSEA

➤ Pityriasis (meaning bran-like) rosea (meaning rose-like) is a common self-limiting skin eruption that usually lasts 2–12 weeks.

➤ The disease commonly begins with a herald patch, followed by the spreading of generalized papulosquamous lesions after a latency period of 10–14 days. The lesions are similar to the herald patch but smaller. Eventually, the rash assumes a 'Christmas tree' appearance.

➤ The cause of this condition is thought to be a viral infection, particularly human herpesvirus (HHV) 6 and 7. The eruption may be preceded by or associated with viral symptoms such as fever, malaise, lymphadenopathy and throat infection.

➤ The disease often requires no treatment, but occasionally oral AH or topical emollients and hydrocortisone may be needed. Low-dose ultraviolet phototherapy was found to be effective.

PITYRIASIS VERSICOLOR

➤ This is a benign skin rash caused by the yeast *Malassezia* species (*M. furfur, M. globose*).

➤ The rash is characterized by multiple scaly hypopigmented or hyperpigmented oval-shaped or rounded, well-demarcated macules/patches, primarily located on the upper trunk, neck and upper arms. Adolescents and young people are predominately affected.

➤ Diagnosis is usually made by characteristic clinical features or, if necessary, can be confirmed by Wood's lamp examination showing typical gold-yellow fluorescence.

➤ Treatment is shown in Box 17.7. The condition tends to persist for years if left untreated. Rapid improvement and cure are usually achieved with topical antifungals. Oral antifungals are used for extensive eruption, frequent recurrence rates or cases refractory to topical treatment.

BOX 17.7 Usual treatment for pityriasis versicolor

- **Topical Antifungals**
  Azoles
  - ❯ Ketoconazole
  - ❯ Clotrimazole
  - ❯ Miconazole
  - ❯ Fluconazole
  Terbinafine
  Butenafine
- **Oral Antifungals**
  - ❯ Itraconazole
  - ❯ Fluconazole

CHAPTER 18

Safeguarding Children

Child maltreatment (abuse or neglect) is common and affects at least 4% of all children in England each year, with some ending in death. In 2016, there were over 50,000 children in the UK identified as needing protection from abuse. Each year, between 1500 and 3000 children in the United States die as a result of child maltreatment. These statistics demonstrate the need for all health professionals to be vigilant in identifying vulnerable children so that effective and preventive measures can be provided for them. Undergraduate education about child protection has been included in the medical school curriculum in recent years.

The purpose of safeguarding children is to:

➤ Promote the welfare of children and protect them from abuse.
➤ Prevent impairment of children's health or development through abuse.
➤ Ensure that all children grow up in a safe and caring environment.

High-profile media coverage of Victoria Climbié and 'Baby P' led to the 2010 government guidance document, 'Working Together to Safeguard Children'. This promotes interagency cooperation and places the onus on health professionals to share concerns and refer or ask for advice if in doubt.

All clinicians working with children should be familiar with:

➤ NICE guideline CG89: When to suspect child abuse.
➤ General Medical Council (GMC) guideline for protecting children and young people. General practitioners are obliged to do safeguarding children training every 3 years to update their knowledge. UK medical graduates must be able to identify the signs that suggest children or other vulnerable people may be suffering from abuse or neglect and know what action to take to safeguard their welfare.
➤ The Royal College of General Practitioners builds on this GMC recommendation, stating that GPs need to be able to act as an advocate for the child in knowing when and how to share concerns about a child who they think might be at risk.

International guidelines on child safeguarding state that doctors, including primary care physicians (PCPs), working with children and young people have a duty to listen and talk directly to the children and to take into consideration children's wishes when making judgment about their best interests. It is good practice to offer to speak to children alone without their parents present if they so wish.

DOI: 10.1201/9781032642888-18

In the UK, all PCPs are entrusted with the responsibility to identify potential child abuse and keep a record of any concerns they may have. They have to obtain level 3 safeguarding competency (RCPCH 2014). PCPs are uniquely placed to respond to any child abuse because they offer services to the same family from birth to death. However, with so many PCPs working part-time and practices containing a large number of patients, this is not always achievable.

The Children Act 1989 and the Children Act 2004 place a duty on the local authority to provide services to children in need in their area. The 2017 Act abolished local safeguarding children's boards and identified three local partners: Local authority, local health authority and the police. Children's services have evolved considerably by shifting from child-focused services to an integrated family-oriented practice with the following advantages:

➤ It concentrates on the care of both underage children and adult family members.
➤ It brings the whole family within an umbrella service rather than offering a single intervention to a single family member.
➤ It improves communication and coordination between the family and the services.
➤ The new service is delivered by small multiagency teams; thus, it is more economical.

The main categories of abuse are:

➤ **Physical abuse** may involve hitting, shaking, throwing, drowning, suffocation, burning or scalding, poisoning or other forms that cause physical harm and injury to a child.
➤ **Sexual abuse** includes penetrative contact (e.g., genital-genital or hand-genital), non-penetrative physical acts (e.g., masturbation, kissing, rubbing or touching outside the clothing) and non-contact activities (e.g., involving children in looking at or in the production of sexual images or watching sexual activities). These activities are usually carried out by an adult or a significantly older child on a child by force and before the age of legal consent.
➤ **Emotional abuse** indicates persistent emotional ill treatment of a child likely to result in persistent and severe effects on the child's emotional development. This form of abuse appears to be the most prevalent. Because of the absence of physical injuries, it tends to be underdiagnosed and underestimated. Emotional abuse can take many forms from failure to provide love, affection, security and emotional support to rejection, intimidation, harassment, verbal assaults and cyber bullying.
➤ **Neglect** is the persistent failure to meet a child's basic physical and/or psychological needs and is likely to result in serious impairment of the child's health or development. It usually involves failure by a parent or carer to provide adequate food, clothing or shelter, to protect the child from physical or emotional harm or danger, or to ensure adequate supervision or access to appropriate medical care or treatment.
➤ **Fabricated or induced illness** (see later).

DIAGNOSTIC FEATURES OF CHILD ABUSE

Diagnostic features of child abuse include the following.

Physical Abuse

➤ An injury that is unexplained.
➤ An injury that is incompatible with the history or with the child's level of development.
➤ Unexplained recurrent injuries.
➤ A delay in seeking medical help.
➤ Certain skin manifestations including:
  ➣ Bruises on the cheeks, buttocks, genitals and back.
  ➣ Bruise marks shaped like hands, fingers or a belt.
  ➣ Black eyes, retinal injuries including retinal haemorrhage.
  ➣ Cigarette burns, producing circular, punched-out lesions of uniform size.
  ➣ Human bite marks.
  ➣ Alopecia in which the hairs are broken at various lengths.
  ➣ Oral injury, frenulum laceration.
➤ Unexplained causes of increased intracranial pressure, with signs of a reduced level of consciousness, bulging fontanelle (head trauma, including subdural haematoma, is the most common cause of death from physical abuse).
➤ Any fracture in an infant too young to walk and fractures that are unusual or unexplained, such as a spiral fracture from twisting rather than transverse from impact.
➤ Unexplained intra-abdominal injuries.

Emotional Abuse

➤ Failure to thrive, particularly in infancy, and developmental delay.
➤ Sudden change in behaviour, e.g., aggressive or withdrawn behaviour.
➤ Poor interaction with parents.

Sexual Abuse

➤ Genitals: Anogenital injury; pain in the vaginal, penile or rectal area; discharge or bleeding; sexually transmitted diseases; pregnancy.
➤ Chronic dysuria, encopresis.
➤ Bruises or bleeding near the genitals.
➤ Sexually transmitted disease.
➤ Sleep disorders, aggression, withdrawal, depression, poor school performance.

Neglect

Maltreated infants suffer from greater developmental disability than older children who were maltreated. Children achieve more motor and developmental milestones during infancy than at any other period in life. In contrast to other causes of developmental delay, neglect-related developmental delay is commonly associated with the following features:

➤ Abnormal behaviour including avoidance, insecure withdrawal and inactivity.
➤ Poor social interaction, including parental interaction, failure to provide adequate supervision.
➤ Signs of neglect are often present, including clothes that do not fit or are inappropriate and poor hygiene in a child who is persistently dirty and smelly.
➤ Delay in seeking appropriate medical attention for illness or injury.
➤ Significant improvement of milestones once the child receives adequate affection and care.

POTENTIAL SITUATIONS FOR CONSIDERING SAFEGUARDING

➤ **Domestic violence and abuse (DVA).**
The connection between domestic violence (DV) and child harm is recognized in UK national guidance (NSPCC 2011). DV is a high-risk factor putting the child at risk of maltreatment (Table 18.1). It is a significant concern in this country, especially following the recent Domestic Abuse Act, which, among many things, defines children as victims of DVA for the first time.
➤ **Asylum-seeking and refugee children.**
Seeking asylum from persecution is a basic human right as outlined in the United Nations Refugee Convention. As also outlined in the Children Act 1989, the UK has a statutory duty to safeguard all children regardless of their country of origin. About 7% of the total asylum applications in 2022 were from unaccompanied minors.
➤ **Child trafficking** is a form of modern slavery with risk of human exploitation, violence against children and child abuse. Modern slavery and human trafficking have become a major global health concern.

TABLE 18.1 Risk factors for child abuse

Parental Risks	Child Risks
Domestic violence	Learning difficulties, physical disability
Drug and alcohol misuse	Behavioural problems
Mental health problems	Chronic illness
Financial difficulty	Prematurity
Single parent	Asylum seeking minors
Young age of parent	
Parent abused as a child	
Families with history of 'induced illness'	

➤ **Fabricated or induced illness** (FII).

FII describes behaviours by a carer that may result in harm (such as poisoning), including:

➤ Deliberately inducing symptoms by administering medication or other substances.

➤ Interfering with treatments by overdosing, not administering medication or interfering with equipment.

➤ Claiming the child has symptoms which are unverifiable.

➤ Exaggerating symptoms resulting in unnecessary investigations or treatments.

➤ Falsifying test results and observation charts.

➤ Obtaining specialist treatments or equipment for children which are not required.

➤ Alleging psychological illness in a child.

FII is associated with significant mortality (around 6%), long-term or permanent injury (7.3%) and long-term impairment of children's psychological and emotional development.

PRACTICE POINTS

One of the strengths of clinicians working in general practice is that they can respond to the needs of multiple family members, including victims and perpetrators of the maltreatment. When the possibility of abuse is being considered, it is important to:

- Take a detailed history from both the child (appropriate to their age and developmental level) and their parent or carer. Look especially for implausible, inadequate or inconsistent accounts of an injury.
- Document the history fully – what was said and by whom. Likewise, for examination and clinical findings – a body map diagram may be useful for multiple injuries and also taking photographs.
- Observe the child's behaviour and interaction with other family members.
- Consider a full examination top to toe, with appropriate chaperoning and consent. All children under the age of 2 years should be fully examined.
- Gather information about the wider family, e.g., from health visitors or colleagues.
- Consider discussing any concerns with the lead colleagues within the practice or organization or with the designated PCP or nurse for the area. There is always a safeguarding lead or team assigned to each practice. Usually there are also regular safeguarding meetings where cases can be discussed.
- Discuss concerns with the parent or carer. In the case of FII, consider how to support the perpetrator. About two-thirds of perpetrators may suffer from chronic somatoform or factitious disorder.

RED FLAGS

- Clinicians tend to be more inclined to engage directly with abusive partners than with their child. Children should not face lack of engagement. Always consider the child's needs and try to offer them a consultation on their own if they so prefer.
- Many clinicians working in general practice seem to have difficulty establishing a link between DV and the potential harm it represents for children. Although most PCPs recognize that DV is a risk factor, some fail to see links between child maltreatment and exposure to DV.
- There seems to be uncertainty about how to solve both confidentiality and safety issues when considering documentation of abuse in records of different family members.

Referral

➤ Everyone has a responsibility for safeguarding children and referring whenever appropriate.

➤ PCPs should consider discussing referrals with a trusted colleague, safeguarding lead or designated health professional before proceeding with the referral. The important key task is to determine whether the child needs immediate protection. If there is an immediate risk of harm to the child, the police should be informed.

➤ PCPs, if certain about child maltreatment, should not wait to confirm the diagnosis before referring to a multiagency safeguarding children, as delay may be detrimental to the child.

➤ It is good practice, if the referral is considered appropriate, to ask parents/carers for consent to refer to children's safeguarding services unless the child's wellbeing will be endangered by doing this. However, the referral should still be made even without consent if there are significant concerns or the police should be informed.

➤ Referral should be made initially by phone, followed by writing.

➤ In cases of serious injury or concern when parental consent is withheld, consider admission to hospital or informing the police.

Index

Note: Page numbers in *italics* indicate a figure and page numbers in **bold** indicate a table on the corresponding page.